THE RESILIENT 9-1-1 PROFESSIONAL

THE RESILIENT 9-1-1 PROFESSIONAL

A Comprehensive Guide to Surviving & Thriving Together in the 9-1-1 Center

Edited by
Jim Marshall and Tracey Laorenza

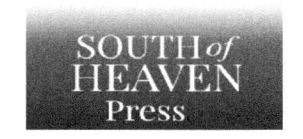

SOUTH *of* HEAVEN Press

The Resilient 9-1-1 Professional
A Comprehensive Guide to Surviving & Thriving Together in the 9-1-1 Center

Publisher's Note:
The Resilient 9-1-1 Professional: A Comprehensive Guide to Surviving & Thriving Together in the 9-1-1 Center brings together an unprecedented group of contributors including 9-1-1 frontliners, their managers, joined by subject matter experts in public-safety, mental health, organizational health, and public administration. Together they deliver powerful stories and fascinating science revealing the health risks faced by "9-1-1Pros" and a full spectrum of solutions to manage these risks and optimize the personal and organizational wellbeing in our 9-1-1 centers. This book is not a substitute for medical care. If you think you, or someone you know, may be experiencing a mental health struggle, please seek the help of qualified healthcare professionals.

If you are considering suicide, please just set down the book and give a call to the National Suicide Prevention Life Line, a fully confidential 24/7/365 help line. Their number is 800-4273-8255. Or text HOME to the Crisis Text Line at 741741 in the United States.

Cover design: Jim Marshall

Copyright © 2018 South of Heaven Press

All rights reserved. No part of this publication may be reproduced, stored in a retrieval system, or transmitted in any form or by any means – electronic, mechanical, recording, or otherwise – without the prior written consent of the publisher.

ISBN 978-1546435273

Published by South of Heaven Press
P.O. Box 280, Petoskey, MI 49770

DEDICATIONS

To my loving sister, Deborah Achtenberg (ENP, Retired), a 9-1-1 pioneer who led me to serve, and become part of the 9-1-1 Family, enriching my life forever; and to my 9-1-1 brother, Michael Stanley (ENP, deceased), whose legacy of support to his 9-1-1 peers will live on. Extraordinary Care Givers both, and champions of the cause to which this book is dedicated.

JIM MARSHALL

To my mom (deceased) and my dad who, intentionally or otherwise, taught me everything I needed to know to become the person I am today. And to Officer Tim Harper (deceased), who made me realize we *must* address mental health issues within our profession. Tim, your life mattered.

TRACEY LAORENZA

Praise for
THE RESILIENT
9-1-1 PROFESSIONAL

"A big thank you to Jim Marshall and team for taking the time to invest in the mental health of our amazing 9-1-1 telecommunicators across the world. I am looking forward to having this book as a resource as we move forward in this ever changing, demanding, stressful yet rewarding career path we have all chosen. Retaining experienced, talented, skilled and healthy telecommunicators is vital to the safety of our communities and its responders. *The Resilient 9-1-1 Professional* is a giant step towards connecting agencies and employees with the tools needed to address the concerns and issues surrounding the extreme stress we encounter."

LISA HALL, ENP
Director
Midland County Central Dispatch Authority (MI)

"2013 was the year that really launched Within the Trenches, true stories from the 9-1-1 dispatchers who live them. The podcast was born out of the need to share dispatcher stories to gain some sort of closure and heal by facing the calls we have buried. It doubles as an educational tool for the general public who has no idea what 9-1-1 dispatchers go through. 2013 also marks a time when I was introduced to Jim Marshall. During our first episode together, he helped me realize that I wanted more out of my dispatch career. I was struggling with a toxic environment that began to leak over into my family life and through talking with him I was able to survive and thrive through the low morale that was, at that time, my dispatch center. *The Resilient 9-1-1 Professional* fills a need in public safety and one that I had the pleasure of receiving face-to-face back in 2013 through his words and guidance."

RICARDO MARTINEZ II, M.A.
Founder
Within the Trenches Podcast and the #IAM911 Movement

"*The Resilient 9-1-1 Professional* is an excellent resource for every emergency services leader. It describes the fundamental stress factors that 9-1-1 dispatchers face. It outlines how to recognize stress, cope and become a more resilient caregiver. Jim Marshall is a gifted therapist who gives energy and hope to us all by shining a bright light in the dark places of our souls and profession. With contributions from many knowledgeable professionals and a pragmatic approach to wellness, this book is a must read."

JAY FITCH, PhD
Founding Partner
Fitch & Associates – Emergency Services Consulting Group

"9-1-1 Professionals, the calm behind the storm. The ones we all rely upon but often forget about. *The Resilient 9-1-1 Professional* is a long overdue book for those who are the first on the front lines to sort out the chaos when it strikes. The emotional toll placed upon our 9-1-1 Professionals has not been addressed until now and these brave men and women who serve deserve to not only survive but also to thrive in life."

SEAN RILEY
President & Founder
Safe Call Now

"For many of us, our response-to-stress skill set was developed in an atmosphere of 'suck it up and deal with it.' As leaders, we must put that part of our past behind us. We need to develop resiliency and recovery skill sets in our people that allow them to 'deal with it' by using tools and resources that are proven effective. I recommend that 9-1-1 professionals purchase this book and use it as a guide for developing those tools necessary to survive and thrive."

JIM LAKE
Director
Charleston County Consolidated 9-1-1 Center (SC)

"Trauma is the business and the bane of emergency service providers. Jim Marshall and Tracey Laorenza's comprehensive book addresses the ways in which trauma affects, and can be managed by, 9-1-1 personnel through personal accounts, professional advice, and clinicians' tales of therapeutic strategies."

ROBIN SHAPIRO, LICSW
Psychotherapist and author of *EMDR Solutions: Pathways to Healing; EMDR Solutions II; The Trauma Treatment Handbook;* and *Easy Ego State Interventions*

"As a paramedic, I believe dispatchers are the TRUE first-responders. They hear terrible things and these sounds create images in their mind that require care. *The Resilient 9-1-1 Professional* will create compassionate leaders who can lend their expertise to dispatchers exposed to traumatic incidents. If you are a dispatcher or a 9-1-1 leader, you want this book!"

NATALIE HARRIS, BHSc, ACP, AEMCA
Keynote Speaker and best-selling author of *Save My Life School: A First-Responder's Mental Health Journey*

"I could not be more excited for this book to be published. It is not only going to fill in cracks in the veteran telecommunicator's foundation but will also give those coming into this stressful but rewarding profession a complete foundation to build on. Every lesson in this book should be taught to every 9-1-1 professional across the nation."

TRACY ELDRIDGE
Public Safety Operations Lead
RapidSOS

"With the intensive, precise nature of the work, its demanding hours and chronic under-staffing, the 9-1-1 dispatcher faces a continuous world of stress. Constantly facing the trauma and tragedy of those we serve, our job requires us to persevere amidst the high standards, ongoing criticism, and frequent lack of recognition. All this can challenge the dispatcher's self-confidence, compassion, and mental health. This book may be a lifesaver for the public safety dispatcher; it's a toolkit well-stocked with resources to maintain one's wellbeing within a vocation that seems to try to erode it – by helping you understand and recognize the elements that breed stress, discovering realistic ways to find equilibrium within that stressful environment, and to ultimately restore a healthy, positive, and rewarding outlook that can support you throughout your career."

RANDALL D. LARSON
Editor, *9-1-1 Magazine*
9-1-1 Supervisor/Trainer, retired

"As 9-1-1 peers, supervisors, managers, and directors, we need to take better care of ourselves and each other. *The Resilient 9-1-1 Professional* is a complete guide for everyone to thrive in this difficult but necessary profession. Every agency is dealing with staffing and retention issues. We have to find ways to be resilient with the difficult calls, overtime, and missed family engagements just to name a few. This guide will show that you are not alone and give you tools to be successful. As a profession, we do a great job of taking care of others. We need to remember to care for ourselves as well. Otherwise, we will have nothing to give."

DON JONES, ENP
Dispatch Manager
Sonoma County Sheriff's Office (CA)

"Extensive research shows Social Worker burnout on account of 'hearing the trauma of others'. And yet, there is little knowledge or credit given to the 9-1-1 dispatchers who may hear the trauma *as it happens*. This book illustrates the gap that needs to be closed as well as how we might close it. This is a fantastic primer that should find its way into all the educational programs for dispatchers."

NICK HALMASY
Founder and Registered Psychotherapist
After the Call

"A must read! Jim Marshall has led the charge in educating the 911 industry in mental health awareness. The mental health of an organization's employees should be top priority; without it, the organization cannot thrive. Jim and his colleagues do an exceptional job addressing this issue and how it affects our psychological, physical, and spiritual lives. This book is one you'll want to own and revisit again and again."

TODD BOROWSKI
Training Coordinator, Peer Support Team Leader
Cobb County 911 (GA)

"Dispatchers are the first first-responder, yet historically they are the last to be remembered in the aftermath of a critical incident or tough call. A book for 9-1-1 dispatchers is long overdue and I'm incredibly happy to see the focus being placed on our emergency dispatchers. *The Resilient 9-1-1 Professional* shines light on how dispatchers experience trauma and that the psychological injury can be healed; it uses stories of traumatic experiences to help dispatchers learn about post-traumatic growth and build resiliency."

HEATHER WILLIAMS, PhD
Regional Peer Support Coordinator
Orange County Sheriff's Department (CA)

TABLE OF CONTENTS

About the Contributors   xv

Foreword: Michelle Lilly   xxi

Preface: Tracey Geary   xxvii

Introduction: Why We Need this Book: Extraordinary Care-Givers Need Extraordinary Resources
Jim Marshall   xxix

SECTION I: WHAT EVERY 9-1-1 PRO & STAKEHOLDER MUST KNOW

1. Golden Glue: A 9-1-1 Dispatcher's Story of Resilience
   Tracey Laorenza   1

2. Days and Nights in the Dispatch Center: What I Saw as a Scientist, Experienced as a Person, and how it Changed Me
   Phoenix Chi Wang   13

3. Understanding 9-1-1 Stress and Nine Unique Risk Factors Faced by Every Dispatcher
   Jim Marshall   25

4. Facing the Impacts of 9-1-1 Stress: The Reality of PTSD and Depression in the Comm Center
   Michelle Lilly, Interviewed by Jim Marshall   40

5. Building the Resilient 9-1-1 Mindset, Part 1: Your Wellbeing Depends on Your Emotional Code
   Jim Marshall   53

6. Building the Resilient 9-1-1 Mindset, Part 2: The ChoicePoints Strategy
   Jim Marshall   65

SECTION II: WHEN 9-1-1 PROFESSIONALS HIT THE WALL: OVERCOMING STRESS-RELATED CONDITIONS

7. The Kevlar Couple's Journey: Courage to Heal & the Power of a New Emotional Code
   Jan Myers — 86

8. Recovering from the Loss of a 9-1-1 Peer's Suicide: My Path Through Trauma into Resilience
   Ryan Dedmon — 100

9. Does Your Console Need a Reboot? EMDR Therapy for Healing Traumatic Stress & Self-Care
   Sara Gilman and Reannon Kerwood — 112

10. When Your Give-A-Damn is Busted: Rebuilding Your Life After Compassion Fatigue
    Jim Marshall — 128

11. 9-1-1 Pros: Sleep for the Health of It! Here's What You Need to Know
    Craig Boss — 140

12. Enough Fat Jokes Already! Seven Steps toward Winning the 9-1-1 Obesity Challenge
    Jim Marshall — 158

13. *"I'm just Sick and Tired of Being Sick and Tired. Help Me."* An EMS Doc's Personal Battle through Self-Medication and Addiction
    Marshal Isaacs — 179

14. "Where was God in All of This?" Recognizing and Traveling Through a 9-1-1 Crisis of Faith to Rebuild Spiritual Resilience
    Jim Marshall — 201

SECTION III: HOW TO SURVIVE & THRIVE TOGETHER: KEY ELEMENTS OF A RESILIENT 9-1-1 CENTER

15. The NENA Stress Standard: The "Shall" Document with Eight Solutions that can Save 9-1-1 Lives
    Jim Marshall — 215

16. The Power of 9-1-1 Peer Support: The First Line of Care and Prevention for the Frontline of Dispatch
    Jim Marshall — 238

17. Choosing and Using Your EAP: How Employee Assistance Programs Can Help 9-1-1Pros
    Randy Kratz and Jim Marshall — 257

SECTION IV: LEADERSHIP THAT GROWS RESILIENT 9-1-1 PROFESSIONALS

18. How to Inspire Employees to Stay and Excel: The Power of Servant Leadership
    Lora Reed, Interviewed by Jim Marshall — 272

19. The 9-1-1 Leader as Stress-Risk Manager: Recognizing Your Role as the Center's SRM
    Jim Lanier, Interviewed by Jim Marshall — 285

20. How a 9-1-1 Director Engaged His Employees to Boost Morale and His PSAPs Major Metrics of Success
    Ivan Whitaker, Interviewed by Jim Marshall — 297

21. Eight Reflections for 9-1-1 Leaders Pursuing Resilience, from Forty Years at the Helm
    John Dejung — 310

22. Leading the Next Generation 9-1-1 PSAP: Managing the Risks of Real-Time Video Interactions
    Jim Marshall — 324

23. "No One Left Behind": Safeguarding the Mental
    Health of 9-1-1Pros in the Aftermath of Mass
    Casualties and other High Impact Events
    Jim Marshall   337

Afterword: Jim Marshall   356

Acknowledgements   358

Appendices
Chapter 17 Appendix   362
Chapter 19 Appendix   366

About the Contributors to
The Resilient 9-1-1 Professional

Craig Boss, MD, D, ABSM, D, AAFP, is the medical director of the Munson Healthcare Charlevoix Hospital Sleep Center in Charlevoix, MI. He completed medical school at the College of Human Medicine at Michigan State University and subsequently completed his residency in Family Medicine at Ft. Bragg, NC. Following his residency, he served as a faculty member and ultimately as assistant residency director at the Eisenhower Army Medical Center Family Medicine Residency program in Ft. Gordon, GA. After leaving the Army in 1997, he practiced full spectrum Family Medicine including outpatient, inpatient, and emergency medicine. In 2006, he completed his Sleep Medicine fellowship at the University of Michigan and has devoted his practice to Sleep Medicine. Dr. Boss is excited to help 9-1-1Pros "Sleep for the Health of It!" He is a passionate teacher and has earned several teaching and clinical awards. He speaks nationally on topics of Family and Sleep Medicine.

Ryan Dedmon, MA, is the Outreach Director for the 911 Training Institute. He coordinates a Crisis Intervention program for advanced officer training at the Regional Criminal Justice Training Center at Golden West College in Southern California. Ryan worked in law enforcement for nearly 12 years, a majority of which were spent in a police dispatch emergency communications center. In 2012, the Southern California chapter of APCO International named him "Telecommunicator of the Year", the highest honor for public-safety dispatchers in Southern California. Ryan is a California POST-certified Academy Instructor and has a Masters of Arts in forensic psychology. He is a contributor to *9-1-1 Magazine* and the *Journal of Emergency Dispatch*. Ryan blends his education and experience behind the console to help dispatchers and police officers battle acute and post-traumatic stress.

John Dejung, MBA, ENP, is currently the director of emergency communications for Dane County (WI), having been so since 2009. From 1997 into 2009 he was the Minneapolis 9-1-1 director. Both Centers are approximately 20 seats, and serve a population of about 500,000, with a crew of 75 Telecommunicators. For the 20 years prior to working in 9-1-1, he was a Coast Guard officer, commanding 3 ships and serving in a variety of other assignments, both ashore and afloat. He has been active at the local and national levels with both NENA and APCO. John graduated with a Bachelor of Science degree in Civil Engineering from the U.S. Coast Guard Academy and from the University of Wisconsin – Madison, with a Master's in Business Administration.

Sara G. Gilman, PsyD, LMFT, has been a licensed Marriage and Family Therapist since 1986, and is EMDR Therapy certified and past-president of the EMDR International Association. Her 2017 doctoral dissertation focused on the effects of cumulative traumatic stress exposure in first responders and the use of EMDR as an early intervention. She is a former San Diego rural firefighter/EMT and served on the San Diego CISM Team. As co-founder and president of Coherence Associates, Inc., she consults with agencies to build strong peer support teams, and trains personnel in "Peak Performance and Mental Toughness." She was awarded Fellowship status with the American Academy of Experts in Traumatic Stress for her extensive work in utilizing EMDR with first responders following critical incidents; and co-authored *Reaching the Unseen First Responder With EMDR,* a chapter in a textbook for clinicians, *Eye Movement Desensitization and Reprocessing (EMDR) Scripted Protocols and Summary Sheets: Treating trauma, anxiety and medical related conditions* (Springer, 2015).

S. Marshal Isaacs, MD, FACEP, FAEMS "Marshal" is the medical director, UTSW/Parkland BioTel EMS System, Dallas Fire-Rescue Department, Prehospital Emergency Medical Services, Parkland Health & Hospital System for the City of Dallas (TX).

Reannon Kerwood, MA, LMFT, is an EMDR therapist and first responder program coordinator for Coherence Associates, Inc. (CAI), a group mental health practice in Encinitas, CA. She specializes in treating first responders, military and trauma survivors. In 2014, as an intern under the supervision of Dr. Sara Gilman, Reannon experienced significant positive outcomes with utilizing EMDR Therapy with first responders following critical incidents. She is a regular speaker to first responder groups throughout San Diego County. Additionally, she is trained and certified in Domestic Violence and Sexual Assault Crisis Intervention, Anger Management, Advanced Cognitive Behavioral Therapy (CBT), EMDR Recent Traumatic Episode Protocol (R-TEP), and Critical Incident Stress Management (CISM).

Randall Kratz, MS, LCSW, PC is a licensed clinical social worker and professional counselor in the state of Wisconsin with FEI Behavioral Health. He has worked as both a counselor and a supervisor in outpatient and hospital settings for over 15 years. He has been a workplace consultant for over 20 years providing employers and employees with assistance for traumatic stress, conflict management, organizational change, substance abuse, work/life balance and other challenges affecting the resiliency of people and organizations.

In the past five years, Randy has worked more exclusively with first responder workplaces including 9-1-1 dispatch, law enforcement and fire/rescue providing critical incident stress management services, EAP consultations and counseling interventions. Randy is an experienced adult educator. He has presented at many conferences and workshops both regionally and nationally.

Jim Lanier, ENP, MPA, is the technical services division manager for the Alachua County Sheriff's Office in north central Florida. Jim has been involved in public safety for over 30 years with experience in firefighting, EMS Paramedic, and 9-1-1. Jim holds a Bachelor of Science degree in Emergency Management and has a Master's degree in Public Administration. In addition to being a NENA Emergency Number Professional (ENP) Jim is a Fire, Medical and QA Instructor with the International Academies of Emergency Dispatch and a member of the IAED College of Fellows. Jim greatly values his experiences as a field first responder, but the 9-1-1 world and the people within it are where his path and passion have led him. Jim was a co-founder of the 911 Wellness Foundation.

Tracey Laorenza, BS, is currently the communications coordinator of a public safety department at a college in Massachusetts. She is editor for South of Heaven Press, and co-editor of The Resilient 9-1-1 Professional. For eighteen years, Tracey was a 9-1-1 police and fire dispatcher; sixteen of which she served as a dispatch shift leader for a suburban police department in Michigan. She was also an instructor within the 9-1-1 Dispatch Academy at Oakland Community College (MI), as well as with Macnlow Associates (MI). Tracey holds a Bachelor of Science degree in Criminal Justice from the University of Massachusetts at Lowell. She will complete her Master of Arts in English and Creative Writing in May 2018. Tracey is also an assistant coach for a women's college softball team.

Michelle M. Lilly, PhD, is an associate professor of Clinical Psychology at Northern Illinois University (NIU). She completed her doctorate at the University of Michigan (UM), followed by a post-doctoral fellowship at the Psychological Clinic at UM where she treated clients presenting with a range of anxiety- and stress-related disorders. In 2009, Dr. Lilly joined the faculty at NIU where she started the Trauma, Mental Health, and Recovery research lab. Her research focuses on cognitive and emotional factors implicated in the development of post-trauma psychopathology, including PTSD, depression, and somatic symptoms. Shortly into her academic career, Dr. Lilly became interested in the psychological and physical effects associated with the unique challenges inherent in the work of 9-1-1 professionals, resulting in numerous completed and ongoing projects with this population.

James Marshall, MA, LLP, is a psychotherapist and Director of the 911 Training Institute. He now educates telecommunicators in personal resilience and 9-1-1 call mastery, and advocates in the 9-1-1 industry to support these causes. "Jim" has been a licensed clinician for over thirty years and was the founding chair of the 9-1-1 Wellness Foundation. He co-chaired the workgroup that authored the industry's first *Standard on Acute/Traumatic and Chronic Stress Management*, and co-authored *Reaching the Unseen First Responder With EMDR*, a chapter in a textbook for clinicians, *Eye Movement Desensitization and Reprocessing (EMDR) Scripted Protocols and Summary Sheets: Treating trauma, anxiety and medical related conditions* (Springer, 2015). Jim earned his Masters of Arts in clinical psychology from Wheaton College (IL).

Jan Myers, MA. As a career 9-1-1 professional, and now a practicing mental health clinician, Jan has been involved in quite a few projects to support 9-1-1 resilience and prevent PTSD: developing and delivering courses for the California (CA) Peace Officer Standards and Training (POST)—including production of a DVD entitled, "Dispatchers: Career Resiliency," a course for Trauma Exposure and Management for CA Dispatchers, helping write the National Emergency Number Association (NENA) Standard on 9-1-1 Acute/Traumatic and Chronic Stress Management, and facilitated the development of the first guide on Line of Duty Deaths and Catastrophic Illness/Injury for Oregon Law Enforcement agencies. Jan also served as a co-founder of the First Responder Support Network providing peer and clinical support for First Responders suffering from work related stress injuries and was a co-founder and board member of the 911 Wellness Foundation.

Lora Reed, PhD, has served as a consultant with 9-1-1 since the 1990's. Her focus is about workplace improvement through employee recruitment, selection, retention, organizational culture, personality/job-fit, and Servant Leadership. Her 2005 dissertation focused on personality & Servant Leadership relationships to employee retention. In 2009, Lora became one of first three Greenleaf Scholars, for her Servant Leadership research with 9-1-1 folks. Her 2015 landmark study on leaders, followers, and organizational citizenship included voices of over 850 U.S. communications center employees. Original scales, modified specifically for 9-1-1 employees in the study, were created by Lora and two research collaborators, presented at *Academy of Management* and published in *Journal of Business Ethics*. Lora was research director for 911 Wellness Foundation (2013-2016) and has published numerous articles and presentations. She serves on her local CISM team in Southwest Florida.

Phoenix Chi Wang, PhD, is a sociologist specializing in culture, work and the state and bureaucracy. Based on her three-year fieldwork at a PSAP in New England, her doctoral dissertation examines the experience, process and consequence of the work of 9-1-1 dispatchers. She has published in peer-viewed journals such as Politics and Society, and American Journal of Cultural Sociology. She earned her Ph.D. in Sociology from Harvard University in 2017 and currently works as a staffer on Capitol Hill. Her legislative portfolio includes: telecommunication, science, space and technology, agriculture, energy, environment, natural resources and women's issues. She acknowledges support from National Science Foundation for her dissertation (Award No. 1539822).

Ivan Whitaker, MBA, has more than 20 years of experience in the field of public safety. He has an MBA in Leadership with a concentration in Organizational Development. Ivan has served in several leadership roles including EMS Management and Director of a Public Safety Answering Point (PSAP). In his most recent role prior to transitioning to Priority Dispatch Corp., Ivan managed more than 145 employees who answered 1.2 million calls per year. His experience in the field, emergency room, and 9-1-1 communications center provides a well-rounded view of the pre-hospital setting. His specialties are PSAP consolidations and organizational development, data-driven response deployment plans, emergency dispatch (ED) protocol implementations, the development of quality improvement programs, and PSAP accreditations. Ivan is a paramedic, EMT, and Emergency Medical Dispatch (EMD) Instructor and has trained many paramedics, EMTs, and EMDs

FOREWORD

I must honestly admit that, like most people, I had never considered the duties of a 9-1-1 professional until about a decade ago. My emphasis as a clinical psychologist and researcher trained in the field of psychological trauma had always been on the impacts on those directly involved in the event. This is called *direct exposure*. I focused on understanding and assisting survivors of assault committed at the hands of another person. I didn't work with "vicarious traumatization" (VT). VT, also called Secondary Traumatization, refers to the psychological impacts experienced by those, like therapists, who come alongside the traumatized person. I say this sheepishly given the audience of this book, but to be fully transparent, I had always thought of vicarious trauma exposure as "Trauma Lite."

Then one day, Heather Pierce, my student at the time, described to me the seven years that she had worked as a 9-1-1 professional before returning to school. I was instantly astounded by my own ignorance of the profound challenges inherent in the profession. This may have been the point at which I looked up a stock photo of a 9-1-1 call center console. I knew that I had to do something. I was driven by the question of how anyone could perform the duties of a 9-1-1 professional without being affected. Heather was driven to bring a voice to the concerns that had grown within her during those years in the profession.

Reflecting on the 9-1-1 Professional's intense engagement with callers and field responders made me question how psychologists have defined direct exposure. These dispatchers answer a call and hear the voice of a person at the height of distress, begging for help as they face life-or-death consequences. In my professional (and personal) opinion, that is pretty darn direct exposure to trauma! So, Heather and I teamed up to conduct a pilot project looking at the prevalence of PTSD in 9-1-1 telecommunicators. Our results received attention in the national news (Chapter 4).

It was a surprise to me that this initial study made national headlines. Apparently, members of the media were just as struck as I had been to realize that the 9-1-1 telecommunicator is also a first responder, exposed to and impacted by traumatic stress. The public also needed to learn what our study made clear: there was a profound need for more research, intervention, and public discourse on the psychological toll created by 9-1-1 work. I truly believe that most people could not survive, let alone thrive in doing the emergency dispatcher's job.

With pleasure, I became more involved in supporting the 9-1-1 family. Over the past eight years, I have continued to study the psychological and physical consequences of work in the 9-1-1 industry (see Chapter 4). 9-1-1 professionals are gifted individuals with abilities and a commitment to service that most people rely on during some of the worst moments of their lives. This is not an overstatement. Work in the 9-1-1 field requires exceptional cognitive skill and resources. The telecommunicator's work is complicated by their repetitive exposure to potentially distressing events. It is high time for the development of better prevention and intervention efforts aimed at bolstering resilience and good health in this vital population. This book can lead us in these efforts.

One of the greatest gifts given to me in this work has been the people. Since the first study came out in 2012, I have had the opportunity to meet more and more frontline 9-1-1 professionals, managers, directors and administrators. My travels to state and national conferences have not only afforded me the chance to hear stories of difficult calls and painful endings, but also to witness considerable strength and resilience. In the process, I have been able to meet extraordinary and tireless individuals who have committed their careers and lives to the betterment of 9-1-1 professionals. Among these individuals, Jim Marshall comes immediately to mind.

When I first met Jim, he had long been spearheading health and stress reduction initiatives through the 9-1-1 Wellness Foundation; a non-profit organization that he and others built in response to the needs he saw within the industry. I can only imagine some of the resistance he received as he tried to champion for better services and resources for 9-1-1 professionals. My own experience has taught me that discussion of mental health needs among 9-1-1 professionals is not always a welcome topic. I think few would deny that Jim Marshall was ahead of his time in recognizing and responding to these needs. Since then, his passion and commitment has only grown. Currently, Jim's 9-1-1 training institute provides trainings and resources that tackle 9-1-1 stress and wellness from multiple angles and modalities. He is working to develop innovative resources such as a nationwide registry of therapists who provide evidence-based intervention for telecommunicators struggling with PTSD. I am consistently inspired by his passion for, and commitment to, the wellness of 9-1-1 professionals.

This book represents a labor of love. Jim has brought together a unique collection of 9-1-1 professionals, mental health practitioners and other subject matter experts to help achieve three major objectives:

- Discuss the short and long-term psychological impacts of work within 9-1-1

Foreword

- Help 9-1-1Pros learn to build resilience in the midst of a job where exposure to distressing events is repetitive and relentless
- Provide encouragement and concrete assistance in preventing and treating conditions such as PTSD, compassion fatigue, addiction, and sleep problems.

In the Introduction, Jim tells his own story, as the brother of a dispatcher and a trauma therapist who was "adopted" by the 9-1-1 family. He describes how the dispatcher's role as the Very First Responder, and the risks they face, made the writing of this book an absolute necessity. The volume begins officially in Chapter 1 with dispatcher Tracey Laorenza's remarkable account of a life-changing call and her battle to reclaim resilience. In Chapter 2, Phoenix Chi Wang describes how living with 9-1-1Pros in the comm center for three years changed her life. Jim builds on these accounts in Chapter 3 by describing nine stressors unique to 9-1-1 that may increase the dispatcher's risk of PTSD and other stress-related conditions. Next, in Chapter 4, I describe key findings of my research on the prevalence of PTSD and depression in 9-1-1. Jim then leads us into hopeful terrain with two chapters focused on how to prevent PTSD and build a resilient mindset upon a healthy Emotional Code and use of a strategy he calls ChoicePoints™.

Jan Myers, a 9-1-1 professional (now mental health professional) leads us into Section Two. She tells her compelling personal story of how she and her husband (a police detective) shed the stigma tied to PTSD in the quest for healing (Chapter 7). In Chapter 8, Ryan Dedmon describes his journey of recovery in the aftermath of his mentor's suicide. This is a timely topic given the startling and concerning rate of suicide among first responders currently occurring in our country.

In Chapter 9, clinicians Sara Gilman and Reannon Kerwood will help you discover an effective, evidence-based intervention for PTSD called eye movement desensitization and reprocessing (EMDR). In chapter 10, Jim Marshall weaves together his personal story with the story of a dispatcher, both striving to heal and regain their professional commitment and passion in the face of compassion fatigue.

In my travels to 9-1-1 conferences, I have rarely left an event without at least a few 9-1-1 professionals asking me about sleep concerns (predominantly insomnia) and/or physical health concerns (predominantly overeating and obesity).

In Chapter 11, sleep doctor Craig Boss provides information on how to enhance sleep among 9-1-1 professionals. Then in Chapter 12, Jim tackles the under-addressed topic of food and obesity in the 9-1-1 culture, offering 9-1-1 professionals seven steps to understanding and dealing with the challenge. Whereas conditions such as PTSD and depression may be seen as natural outcomes of 9-1-1 work, conditions such as addiction are often and unfortunately seen as moral issues over which individuals have control. In Chapter 13, physician Marshal Isaacs sheds light on the struggle by revealing his own personal battle with, and recovery from, addiction. Jim finishes Section 2 with a chapter (14) on how 9-1-1 work can challenge or alter one's faith and beliefs, and how to regain faith in the face of repetitive exposure to events that may often seem unfair or ungodly.

Sections 3 and 4 of this book rightfully focus on 9-1-1 center-level factors that must be addressed to achieve wellness in the workplace for all 9-1-1 professionals. Jim begins in Chapter 15 by introducing the NENA stress standard published in 2013. The stress standard was the first of its kind to focus exclusively on the importance of stress reduction in the 9-1-1 environment. He describes several of the solutions provided for in the Standard so that leaders and their teams understand how to put them into action.

To transform the health and wellness of 9-1-1 professionals, our comm centers must become a culture in which self-care and an emotionally supportive peer environment are actively encouraged. To help achieve these objectives, Jim presents two training models that empower 9-1-1Pros for resilience through peer support (Chapters 16). In Chapter 17, EAP expert Randy Kratz joins Jim to describe a best-practice model for employee assistance programs. He clarifies what 9-1-1Pros and their leaders should expect from EAPs and how to use them wisely.

Leadership takes the center stage in the final section of this book. Without strong and thoughtful leadership, the culture changes required to protect the health and wellness of employees in the 9-1-1 industry cannot occur. In Chapter 18, Lora Reed introduces the concept of servant leadership and its power to inspire highly-stressed employees to remain motivated and committed. In the next two chapters, two seasoned and forward-thinking 9-1-1 directors discuss the pivotal role of leadership in identifying and managing stress in their centers. Jim Lanier describes the mindset of the leader as "Stress-Risk Manager" (Chapter 19) and in Chapter 20, Ivan Whitaker tells how his 9-1-1 team helped him boost morale and key metrics of success under huge time and fiscal restraints.

Foreword

In Chapter 21, John Dejung provides eight insightful reflections on key aspects of leadership applied specifically to the role of the 9-1-1 manager.

The final chapters focus on two timely issues with the profound potential impact on 9-1-1 professionals. In Chapter 22, Jim explores the potential implications of NG9-1-1 on employee health, particularly real-time video call-taking and dispatching. He describes the evaluation and planning needed to protect the health and wellness of 9-1-1 professionals from increased exposure to traumatic stress anticipated with the roll out of these technologies. In the final chapter (23), Jim offers a preliminary "open source" model for strategic planning to assure short and long-term care for all dispatch personnel after "High Impact Events". Mass casualties resulting from gun violence and terrorism may be the most pressing social and public health issue of our time. As Jim urges, call centers need systematic care plans in place before 9-1-1 professionals handle these atrocities. Failure to do such advance planning greatly enhances risk for adverse impacts on the dispatcher and the 9-1-1 center.

I recommend this book to those brave 9-1-1 professionals who are strong enough to perform a stressful and often thankless job. I also recommend it to spouses and loved ones of 9-1-1 professionals, to field responders and their families, government officials, the news media, and the general public. This comprehensive resource can help us each do our parts to support the strong souls who carry us through some of the worst moments of our lives.

Michelle Lilly, Ph.D.
Associate Professor of Psychology
Director, Trauma, Mental Health and Recovery Laboratory
Department of Psychology
Northern Illinois University

PREFACE

Let me start off first with a couple questions to my fellow dispatchers. Have you ever looked at your console and said, "That's it, I'm done?" Or turned to your partner and noticed they were struggling and you didn't know what to do or say to help them? You're not alone. And that's one of the driving forces behind this book. To let all dispatchers and call-takers know you're not alone. There *is* help—in many forms.

As you journey through these pages, you will meet several people who have been touched by the 9-1-1 dispatch profession. Some of these people are, or have been, dispatchers themselves. Some are therapists, scientists, and even medical doctors. There are directors, and those who have served in the military. We are your authors. Our chapters will cover many facets of a world that deals with trauma on a daily basis. We have pooled our knowledge, our experiences, and our genuine concern for the health and wellbeing for *all* 9-1-1 Professionals to create this guide to help you survive and thrive in the 9-1-1 world.

As you walk through these pages, our hope is for you to become physically, mentally and emotionally healthier than when you turned the first page. We hope for a more *resilient* you.

But, this book is not just for dispatchers!

To the rest of our readers, I would like to welcome you to the unknown. Each moment of a dispatcher's shift is just that: unknown. With each ring of the telephone there could be a child screaming for help; a mother who has lost her child; an elderly male who woke to find his wife has passed away in her sleep; an irate driver stuck in a traffic jam because a mile ahead someone has been killed in an accident the driver can't see; or it could quite simply be a lonely, elderly woman calling for the time, because she has no one else to call. Let's not forget the calls about the weather, road conditions, inquiries about when the electricity will come back on, the raccoons out in the daylight, and a myriad of other calls that are answered daily.

You are about to experience some of the most heart-wrenching experiences dispatchers are required to handle. You will witness their steps from the depths of darkness into the bright light of resilience as they become stronger, healthier, Extraordinary Care Givers.

You will walk along-side therapists who have fought to bring to light the trauma suffered by dispatchers. Hopefully you will begin to wonder compassionately about the dispatch profession. And I assure you, it *is* a profession.

Dispatchers are a proud, yet humble group. But we are suffering. We have always been the nameless, faceless voice on the other side of the receiver, answering your calls and cries for help. Now it is your chance to help us.

Tracey Laorenza
Co-editor
The Resilient 9-1-1 Professional

INTRODUCTION
The Heart of this Book

Jim Marshall

Why the Life of the 9-1-1 Dispatcher Matters So Much

I'm eager to tell you a personal story about this certain very demanding "dispatcher"[1] I know. But before we get there, bear with me for a few moments.

If you're an emergency telecommunicator or a 9-1-1 leader, I want to thank you on behalf of all our contributors to this book! We offer *The Resilient 9-1-1 Professional* to you as individuals who deserve great support, and to you as members of your 9-1-1 center team facing incredible stressors increasing each year. We invested in this project to honor and equip you to excel and *be well* in the extraordinary work you do as our Very First Responders. Within these pages you'll find remarkable stories defining the stress challenges facing your 9-1-1 centers (also known as Public Safety Answering Points, PSAP). But, as these stories unfold, you'll also discover an encouraging, comprehensive vision of how you can master those challenges. *The Resilient 9-1-1 Professional* represents a vital resource that needs to be in the hands of every telecommunicator to boost their resilience and their performance. Ultimately our hope is for you to "survive and thrive together", enjoying a great quality of life at work and at home.

Yet, this book is also a must-read for every citizen who depends on 9-1-1 to excel in response to your call. You are the first members of the greater group we call 9-1-1 stakeholders—the many folks who serve, work with, or benefit personally or organizationally from the 24/7/365 work of our 9-1-1 professionals. Their welfare and performance depend on all 9-1-1 stakeholders being educated about, and invested in, doing their parts to support the resilience of the Very First Responder. 9-1-1 stakeholders also include:
- The family members of our 9-1-1 professionals

- Our field responders (law enforcement, emergency medical, and fire service)
- Our 9-1-1 center governing bodies (leaders of field response and 9-1-1 agencies)
- The local, state and federal government officials who decide how the 9-1-1 system will be designed, operated, and funded
- The private-sector partners who provide products and services to run our 9-1-1 centers.
- Leaders and members of our 9-1-1 associations who set industry standards, educate and advocate for our PSAPs
- Health care professionals who research, deliver care and guide advocacy efforts

Finally, this book is also offered to educate our local, state and national TV, radio, print, and social media organizations whose journalism must be informed to accurately report about 9-1-1's work to the public and all stakeholders. This is a challenging task since, as journalists, you need to understand the nature of the 9-1-1Pro's vital role in helping save lives.

Telecommunicators face a unique set of psychological stressors. They are among a group I refer to as ECGs: "Extraordinary Care-Givers". They provide services to people who are in life and death circumstances, the outcomes of which are unpredictable. So, ECGs face a high likelihood of being exposed to traumatic events. Emergency dispatchers function as the heart of emergency response systems of all developed nations. Few people can do their complex job, a job they typically perform under enormously stressful conditions. Which often includes chronic understaffing and overtime, constant 360° scrutiny from all stakeholders, and a lack of respect long afforded our other first responders. They are the Very First Responders. They are the very first to hear the screams of children and parents without warning. It is the dispatcher who gathers the vital information to inform and equip the field responders they'll then send to the scene. 911Pros shoulder an enormous sense of responsibility for the safety of their field responders and every citizen in danger they assist.

Introduction

Yet, as I write these words, our emergency telecommunicators are still categorized by the federal government in the United States as "clerical" workers. (Many good folks are working hard to achieve this reclassification and I'm convinced it will happen, as the reality of the work 9-1-1Pros do becomes clear to those who must know. Hopefully, this book will help in the effort.)

Here's my point. If we wish to assure the personal wellbeing and the viability of our telecommunicators and our 9-1-1 centers for the future, all of us as stakeholders must ascend together to prioritize and systematically support them. New research, journal articles and conference presentations on 9-1-1 stress are essential to this effort. But they are grossly insufficient. To assure that every 9-1-1 Professional can excel *and* be well, their 9-1-1 centers, state governments and our nation(s) must each have defined 9-1-1 resilience plans. This book is a tool to help achieve such plans at each level.

So, this book is for all of you, 9-1-1 professionals and stakeholders. The health, and future, of our 9-1-1 workforce, and our 9-1-1 system, may depend on the commitment you make to read and apply what you find between these pages. We're in this together! So, thank you for reading.

Now for the story I promised!

The Sit-Along that Opened My Eyes

In 1986, I was mired deep in the swamp called *grad school*. I was training in clinical psychology at Wheaton College in Illinois, where I learned all kinds of stuff about "psychopathology"—the mental illnesses, what factors drive them, and how you diagnose and treat them. Then one day, on a visit back to my home state of Michigan, my sister, Debbie said, "you know, you've never seen where I work. Why don't you come with me tonight?" I didn't know that was a possibility—hanging out with a dispatcher at a police station. Sounded cool to me. We went through a back door of the police station, wandered down a dark hall and entered a dimly lit, windowless little room. There was one desk, a phone, a radio, a little card box, and a cast-aluminum IBM Selectric. Do you know what that is? A 50-pound electric typewriter.

She introduced me to the dispatcher who was just wrapping up her shift and within a few minutes it was just us sibs together. Across the room there was a folding table with a bunch of snacks on it. So, this was my sister's "9-1-1 Center." "So, what's this gig about? What do you actually do?" I asked her.

Debbie said, "Well, the phone rings, I answer it and figure out if the caller needs emergency medical, fire, or police help, and I just send The First Responder."

Okay, that sounded easy enough. It was kind of like a customer who enters a grocery store, and they bring a loaf of bread and a half-gallon of milk to the cashier. The cashier checks the price, rings it up, bags it and that's it. In a few minutes a call came through. I wheeled my chair a little closer so I could hear but couldn't make out what the person wanted.

Debbie spoke in a soft, calm tone as she looked toward me with a smirk and rolled her eyes, repeating, "So, your neighbor's dog pooped in your yard, and you want us to arrest the owner?" I quickly covered my mouth to contain my laughter. Debbie held her finger to her lips, and, coupled with a fierce look, sent me a clear non-verbal message, *Shut up. You're gonna get me in big trouble!* The agency policy was to send an officer for a "wellness check," so my sister assured the lady that an officer would be by soon. She dispatched an officer, and, within the next half hour, handled a few more equally momentous calls. Now I knew what my sister's job was.

"Wow," I said. "Piece of cake! You are a smart girl, Sis. This is a government position, right? That means you probably get good benefits, with great retirement. And here I am racking up huge debt for grad school. I'm gonna end up a poor therapist still huffing away at age 70, but you'll be retired by 52!" I was jealous and also impressed by the apparent savvy of her job choice.

She just smiled and said "Yeah, well."

Debbie was never one to waste her words. In retrospect, that smile and her two word reply to me meant, *You clearly don't get it. Wait a while longer, and maybe you will.* It didn't take long for that mental shift to happen.

Introduction

Within minutes, a call came in. I don't recall the details, and couldn't hear the full exchange, but my sister shifted in her chair instantly. She went from the relaxed slouch she'd been enjoying, to what appeared as if she were leaning toward the caller. It was a domestic violence call. I could hear the female caller screaming. My sister quickly engaged her with that same calm tone, but with faster speech, asking a stream of questions that were clearly designed to identify the most critical factors needed to assess safety. She would tone the radio, relay that information to her officer, re-engage the caller, helping her to calm down, and attempt to separate people from other people on scene.

My gut was churning as I sat a few feet away listening and wondering with my psychology brain: *how did she know to ask all those questions; how did she calm that lady down so fast; what kind of intelligence does it take to do this?* It didn't occur to me at the time to ask the most important question that would, years later, become the question leading to my own work in the 9-1-1 industry, *what kind of emotional drain and toll does work like this have on my sister and other dispatchers over a year, a decade, a career?* In the moment, I felt like a presumptuous fool, thinking about my initial impression of her job, based on only a few minutes of observation.

Within minutes after this call had begun, an officer arrived to a scene that was far more stable, and safer for everyone, than when this lady first called. I was absolutely flummoxed. Then Debbie said, "Okay, ma'am, you did a good job; now I'm gonna go. You just talk with my officers and they will help you from here, okay?" Then she spun around in her chair, and, without a breath, resumed our chat about my psych class, "So you were telling me something about the difference between schizophrenia and--what? Bipolar Disorder?"

I was proud of her and embarrassed at the same time. She had just schooled the puffed-up psychologist-in-training. "Wait a minute! Debbie, when I asked you what this gig was, you told me you just figure out what type of emergency it is and then you send what you called The First Responder. I'm a little confused. YOU just responded first—and you did intervention. So why do you call the officer the First Responder?" If you're a telecommunicator and you've done this job for more than a few years you can guess her reply.

Oh, well," she said, "I'm just the dispatcher."

My sister stopped minimizing the real complexity and significance of her role within a couple years (except when she used that phrase strategically with irate callers, as in: "don't shoot the messenger—I'm just the dispatcher!"). I was absolutely blown away by what I witnessed my sister do that day; especially since, in those early days of 9-1-1 work, there weren't any Standard Operating Procedures (SOPs), protocols, or training manuals, to educate and guide the telecommunicator in how they should manage calls such as that domestic violence call. Debbie had to learn the hard way how to handle every call type that came to her desk. It wasn't until years later that she talked about how it impacted her emotionally when, without training, she had to handle calls from mothers screaming into her phone, "My baby's not breathing! Please help me, send somebody, tell me what to do right now!"

Debbie was a pioneer. So were all the 9-1-1Pros who started in that era. She will bristle at this claim when she reads it, but it is true. She simply began writing call-taking SOPs, hiring procedures, a training manual, and even a telecommunicator competency test. She began researching and found a new approach to managing medical calls developed out in Utah using protocols. As her respect for her new-found profession grew, Debbie began leading, as her union's president, to improve the working conditions and employment terms that telecommunicators deserved; terms that might help them choose to stay on board doing such hard work.

In the meantime, I completed my Master's degree in clinical psychology and took my first job as the staff psychologist at a regional referral psychiatric facility in Northern Michigan. My task was to help the psychiatrists diagnose new or returning patients and make treatment recommendations. The doctors became frustrated that so many folks they'd already diagnosed and treated kept failing out in the real world and needed to return for hospitalization. Sure, some folks improved and moved on with their lives, but many did not. I began to wonder, *what are we missing? Are we mis-diagnosing them, are the medications just not effective?* But as a clinician, still green around the gills, how was *I* supposed to answer these questions?

I was way over my head in this first assignment, sucking air through a straw in the deep end of the pool.

Introduction

But as the saying goes, you either learn to swim or you're going to drown. My sister had learned to swim in the 9-1-1 pool. Now it was my turn to survive my own high water as a clinician. So, I poured over patient charts, studied clinical textbooks, got extra supervision, and sought the insights of senior colleagues. I was learning to swim, but the greatest help came one day from a sad little lady sitting across from me in an evaluation room.

As I sat trying to figure out the underlying factors driving this woman's recurrent, seemingly untreatable, life-threatening depression, I had my light bulb moment. Per standard clinical protocol, I'd been doing all the "right things." I conducted a structured clinical interview, administered personality tests, and now I was running her through an "intellectual assessment"—you know, an I.Q. test. "Okay, Betty, if you put these puzzle pieces together the right way, they'll make something. Do your best and work as quickly as you can…Okay, now say these numbers forward…now say them backward…Now put these blocks together so that the pattern on the top matches the pattern in this diagram. Ready? Go."

With stopwatch in hand, I felt a bit guilty dragging this tired, despairing patient through what must have felt like a torture test. Then it struck me: *Gee, Mr. Wizard, you want to understand this person, right? Really understand what's driving her depression? Well then back up, forget the structured clinical interview, and be yourself! Get human with this human!* So, when I finished the I.Q. test, I shoved it aside and said something like, "You know what? I need to apologize. You're trying so hard to cooperate with all this psycho-testing stuff, but I'm not sure I've really invited you just to teach me what your struggle is all about; to tell your story however you want. We're done with the testing. If I just shut up and promise to just listen, would you please teach me?"

Miracle of miracles! When given a genuine chance, and convinced I was actually listening, this woman (and hundreds of others over the next couple years) spoke words that may have never been said out loud before. And her story—many of their stories—revealed a history of severe traumatic stress that had never been recognized. So it had never been treated. It's no wonder that she kept coming through the hospital doors! For sure, many folks have chronic illnesses, like Schizophrenia, that will likely require repeat hospitalizations, but many of our patients' illnesses, though perhaps genetically based, may have been turned on and complicated by trauma.

Medications alone could only do so much to prevent suicide, self-injurious behavior and recurrent hospitalizations. Unless we could help *heal* the underlying traumatic stress, many of these "revolving door patients" were being set up for repeated failures. Of course, many of these admissions began with a call to 9-1-1. Year after year they (or their loved-ones) called, earning these struggling souls yet another nickname: Frequent Flyers. No bonus points were awarded. Just shame.

I faced a similar challenge as a new therapist in my outpatient work. My first few dozen clients saw me as a sincere, young guy eager to help. With the lessons learned from my patients in the hospital, I worked hard to listen to my clients' stories. Even though I didn't feel that I was doing enough to help them, these new clients were grateful and began telling others, who struggled with trauma, to seek my help. Let me offer my apologies in advance to readers who might find this offensive, but there is only one way to explain what happened in terms that 9-1-1 professionals will relate to; I became known as the clinical "shit-magnet." Some of you know from personal experience exactly what I'm talking about!

By no means does this term degrade my clients. It refers to the inordinately huge mass of collective suffering carried into my practice by a caseload full of good folks struggling with Post Traumatic Stress Disorder (PTSD), other trauma-driven issues, and struggles with suicide. Therapies back then could not heal PTSD and I knew my clients deserved better. I became well-acquainted with a sinking feeling each time our hard work in treatment failed to bring them relief. By the end of my third year in practice, it felt like I was *going under*. I nearly bailed out of the profession; but I got support, more training and gained traction in helping those on my growing caseload. But still, treatments for PTSD could not promise healing. It just helped in "managing the symptoms," and that wasn't good enough! Then, fortunately, in my fourth year as a therapist, the Calvary came!

A pioneer, named Francine Shapiro, developed a treatment called EMDR— Eye Movement Desensitization Reprocessing-- which I still call The Whacky Eye-Movement Therapy (see chapter 9). I was extremely skeptical when I read a claim from her doctoral dissertation.

Introduction

She claimed that nineteen out of twenty-two people with PTSD in her initial study who had failed to find relief despite years of treatment, were completely (or nearly) symptom free after only one ninety-minute session of EMDR (199). This was a seemingly crazy claim, but my desperation to find more effective ways to help people eclipsed my skepticism. So, I flew to California and got the training. Within a week of my return to Michigan, I was using this EMDR (which was then experimental) with my clients most severely impacted by PTSD. The results were profoundly positive and encouraging; not only for my clients but for me.

Later in this book, you will learn much more about EMDR and its great value for 9-1-1 professionals. Yet I bring it up here because it is key to this story: I would have never lasted as a therapist if I had continued to helplessly watch as my clients suffered with flashbacks, self-injury, and suicide risk. Nor would I have become an educator in the 9-1-1 industry; I would have little to offer. Over the years, as my sister Debbie and I continued our visits, trading stories about her calls and my clients, she realized that telecommunicators needed the same help I'd learned to provide my clients. Then, after twenty years as a telecommunicator, she retired and was asked to establish the 9-1-1 Dispatch Academy at Oakland Community College (OCC, in Michigan).

When she rolled out her academy curriculum, she recognized that the stress management training available at that time was geared more toward field responder stress; so, she asked me to create a curriculum designed especially for telecommunicators. I initially refused, "Debbie, I'm not goin' into the training room with 9-1-1Pros as a teacher when I've never even sat at that console. That's disrespectful!"

In her soft, commanding, veteran dispatcher voice she responded, simply and to the point, "I'll tell *you* what is disrespectful. When I ask you to train my people and you refuse! Either you do it, brother, or I'll break your arms." Well okay then.

Debbie still denies that she threatened me with bodily harm, and she's probably correct, but, trust me, she was very persuasive!

She was also right. Several months later, after a lot of research, collaboration with Debbie, and sit-alongs at 9-1-1 centers, I arrived in the class room for the first day to launch the course *Survive &Thrive Together in the 9-1-1 Center*™. That was the end of my ambivalence about teaching 9-1-1 professionals, and the beginning of my immersion in the 9-1-1 community that has deepened ever since. In that first class, telecommunicators jumped into intense conversation with me about their stressors. We identified approaches and skills that they could use to manage that stress, and they deeply affirmed the need for training to prevent PTSD and boost their resilience.

Many of my early 9-1-1 students entrusted me privately with their stories about the collision between their personal struggles at home and the stored-up trauma from their worst 9-1-1 calls. They needed help hearing the good news: that PTSD and trauma-driven struggles could be healed with EMDR. And they needed help bridging to that help. I began referring telecommunicators to my clinical colleagues wherever I went, eventually throughout the country. I held these conversations as sacred. These talks began happening, too, with 9-1-1 leaders who had grown up in the emergency response field following the old-school "Suck it Up" Emotional Code (See chapter 5). They weren't sure what to do with their own piled up stressors or how to help their personnel prevent the impacts of stress, but they were willing to learn. At that point I realized I was in 9-1-1 for good.

My clinical knowledge combined with these many conversations with 9-1-1Pros, and growing knowledge of the work demands in comm centers soon convinced me of one thing: telecommunicators in the United States likely experienced PTSD at a rate much higher than the national incident rate. The National Emergency Number Association (NENA) had also grown concerned about this risk and began offering sessions on 9-1-1 stress at their annual conferences. In 2006, they asked me to write articles in their journal to promote awareness, prevention, and to help 9-1-1 professionals realize that there's healing for PTSD.

Others had also grown increasingly concerned about the stress-related risks of working in 9-1-1. For years, before this upsurge of awareness, and my involvement in the 9-1-1 industry, Jim Lanier (currently of Alachua County Sheriff's Office, FL) and his wife Sharon, a nurse, had spoken at 9-1-1 conferences about stress risks facing telecommunicators.

Introduction

Then in 2008, Roberta Troxell conducted a study on Compassion Fatigue among 9-1-1Pros. Her study confirmed our convictions, indicating that 16.9% of four hundred and ninety-seven 9-1-1Pros acknowledged symptoms fitting Compassion Fatigue —a mix of *"burnout"* from cumulative stress and *post-traumatic stress* from exposure to others' trauma. (We'll explore Compassion Fatigue more fully in chapter 10.)

In 2011, Jim Lanier and I, joined by Rick Galway and many of this book's contributors, co-founded the 911 Wellness Foundation (911WF). The goal of the Foundation was to advance research, education, policy and intervention to protect and boost the wellbeing of 9-1-1 professionals. We were fortunate to join with many other mental health and 9-1-1 professionals to launch a NENA effort addressing the stress challenge. Eventually this workgroup produced the *NENA Standard on Acute, Traumatic and Chronic Stress Management*. This standard, approved in August, 2013, states that "all 9-1-1 Public Safety Answering Points (PSAPs) shall establish Comprehensive Stress Management Programs" (NENA 23).

The 911 Wellness Foundation closed its doors in February of 2017. After some good success in raising the profile of the wellness issue in the 9-1-1 industry, we concluded that our best work in the future would be achieved by supporting new initiatives of NENA and APCO International, our 9-1-1 membership and standard-setting organizations. Hopefully this book will help in these association efforts.

Now you know the history that energized the pursuit of *The Resilient 9-1-1 Professional*. Many lives have joined together to make this resource a reality, with the hope that you can join us in making the future of life in the 9-1-1 center the very best it can be, to uphold and to support the Very First Responder.

Enjoy!

Jim Marshall

A Final Important Word about PTSD & PTSI: When it Comes to Trauma, Labels Matter!

Throughout *The Resilient 9-1-1 Professional*, we refer to and describe PTSD, Post Traumatic Stress Disorder. This is the term officially used by the American Psychiatric Association referring to specific and serious impacts a person may experience from exposure to traumatic stress. Yet, the contributors to this volume also want you to think about PTSD as PTSI: Post Traumatic Stress *Injury*. Our military personnel and first responders are often less apt to get help for a "disorder;" unfortunately, there is a stigma attached to that label. And here's the fact: struggles with post-traumatic stress incurred in the line of duty *are* an injury. So, for the person experiencing the struggle, PTSI is the most accurate and helpful label to remove the stigma associated with traumatic stress impacts. Yet, the label PTSD is also accurate and has important value in advocating for these injuries to be taken seriously and supported adequately.

Just for a moment, let's put set aside concern for the stigma attached to the word *disorder*. This word literally simply means that something is out of its regular order in a way that is creating difficulty and risk for the person. (Hypertension, or high blood pressure, is also a disorder.) Traumatic stress impacts can certainly throw a 9-1-1Pro's life and wellbeing out of order. When stress injuries incurred in the line of duty result in "disorder," the 9-1-1Pro deserves treatment to heal. Policy makers and insurance companies must take responsibility for assuring this care, and they are more apt to do so when they recognize that PTSI is also PTSD. There is value in recognizing both PTSD and PTSI. I hope you find this recognition valuable as you read about PTSD and its healing throughout the rest of the book.

Works Cited

"NENA Standard on 9-1-1 Acute/Traumatic and Chronic Stress Management." *National Emergency Number Association (NENA)*, 2013, p 23, c.ymcdn.com/sites/www.nena.org/resource/resmgr/Standards/NNA-STA-002.1-2013_9-1-1_Ac.pdf.

Shapiro, Francine. "Efficacy of the Eye Movement Desensitization Procedure in the Treatment of Traumatic Memories." *Journal of Traumatic Stress*, vol. 2 no. 2, 1989, pp. 199-223, onlinelibrary.wiley.com/doi/abs/10.1002/jts.2490020207.

End Notes

[1] Throughout this book we use the terms dispatcher and telecommunicator interchangeably referring to all those who take 9-1-1 calls from the public and or dispatch field responders. I also use the term 9-1-1 Professional, or 9-1-1Pro, referring first to the frontline dispatcher but also to all 9-1-1 team members, including supervisors and directors.

SECTION I

WHAT EVERY 9-1-1 PRO & STAKEHOLDER MUST KNOW

CHAPTER 1
Golden Glue:
A 9-1-1 Dispatcher's Story of Resilience

Tracey Laorenza

It was 2003, and I was five and a half years into my dispatch career. Like most dispatchers, by that point I had handled calls about births, deaths, broken bones, and I even had someone call to report their husband's wedding ring getting stuck on his penis (she did repeatedly assure me he had unusually large fingers). But on July 9, just after the start of my shift, the worst call of my career came in.

Dense fog rolled through the area, and a misty rain spit down. My partners and I sat at our positions with our breakfast and first cups of caffeine. Around 7:30 a.m. the shrill trill of the 911 line pierced the quiet room. Before she could even be asked, "What is the location of your emergency." a heavily accented female screamed, "My house is on fire." Through broken English and jagged sobs, she pleaded for someone to save her children, followed by a harrowing scream. We couldn't get any more information from her. But, as with most major incidents, several more phone lines began to ring: both emergency and non-emergency. The callers provided all the information we needed: it was a mobile home situated in the middle of a trailer park, occupied by two adults and four children, and flames were visible from the front. Within one minute of the first call, my partners and I toned the fire department, requested mutual aid from neighboring fire departments, notified the ambulance company and had the sheriff's department on the way.

The mother had not hung up the phone, so we listened to the open line. She tried to regain access to the home; each effort was thwarted. What made her hold onto that phone, we will never know, but it was our life line as much as it was hers. Time seemed to stand still. There was nothing more we could do. I felt helpless.

Suddenly, she spoke rapidly in Spanish and another voice was audible in the background; her teenage son had made it out. Despite her obvious pleas, he made several attempts to go back in, but the flames beat him back just as they had her. As she yelled for him to stop, glass broke in the background. She screamed and dropped the phone.

After what seemed an eternity, the boy picked up the phone and told us his father had broken through a window carrying his youngest sister. He said his father was only able to hand his sister to his mother before collapsing to the ground, where he now lay unconscious. He and the little girl were both badly burned.

The fire department was updated right away, and they requested a medical helicopter for transport. The call was made, but the request was denied. The dense fog, a remnant from the previous day's intense summer storms, grounded the helicopter. It would be up to the fire fighters and ambulances to transport the victims. However, they arrived only to discover a home fully engulfed in flames and announced it would be a defensive assault only.

The two remaining children were found hours later in their shared bedroom, pronounced dead at the scene. The father would die at the hospital the next day, succumbing to his wounds. The infant would remain in the hospital for an extensive period due to the severity of her burns. The teenage son and mother would recover from their minor injuries and be released from the hospital within a couple of days.

Despite the array of calls I had handled in the previous five years, I had not lost a child; now, in one call, I had lost two. The fire department had not lost anyone to a fire in over six years; in one call they lost three. I was heartbroken. I went home to my apartment that night and cried. I screamed into my pillow. Then quiet sobs wracked my chest. The world turned into a blur. I heard nothing. I felt nothing.

When the tears stopped, and I could take a full breath again, I rolled over and stared out the window as if the darkness could soothe me. I searched through the helplessness and pain for answers. Nothing came.

After a sleepless night, I returned to work, game face on. Word came that there was going to be a debriefing, and the dispatchers were invited. Understand, in 2003 it was not a popular thing to invite dispatchers to a debriefing session. Dispatchers "just answered the call," they are not affected like a fire fighter or police officer who actually sees the scene. It was a *big damn deal* to get invited to this. But my partners said they didn't need it, they weren't going. So, reluctantly, I said the same. I was horrified my partners were fine and I wasn't. I thought something was wrong with me. So, I showed nothing, I said nothing. I put my head down and I grinded through the day working police radio, then I was off for three days.

Golden Glue: A 9-1-1 Dispatcher's Story

On my days off, I did something I had never done before, nor since—I went to the scene. I was drawn to it. As I drove there, I played the incident out in my head as it had been relayed days before. But this was not the first time I had been to their house. I'd been transported there the minute the details started coming in. As the incident unfolded over the phone, I pictured the house, the view from the front, from the side, and the neighbors' houses. I did a quick sketch of the scene in my head to better help my responders; this is a dispatcher's curse, and blessing.

The house was just a burnt remnant now. Teddy bears, cards and signs inundated the front walk, spilling over into the street. The broken window was now boarded up. The spot where the father fell was marked with a cross and candle. As I knelt beside it, a tidal wave of pain washed over me. My eyes flooded with tears which spilled down my cheeks and soaked my tee shirt. I mourned the loss of a father who gave his life to save his children. I cried for the children who couldn't be saved.

I went to the house five times that weekend. I don't know what I expected to find. I was searching for something, but I never found it. Some of you may think I was just weak, that I should have sucked it up and moved on. Believe me, so did I. After five years of training classes with other dispatchers, I had heard many stories about that "one call" other dispatchers couldn't quite get over. But I never thought *I* would come across something I couldn't handle. Not me. Well, guess who was wrong. And dealing with it didn't get any easier from there, either…

In the days that followed the fire, I learned the father was an immigrant who spent his life working to earn money to buy a house and bring his wife and children to the United States. When he bought this home and moved his family in, they became fixtures of the community; everyone knew them. The community held fund raisers and gatherings for the family. Like me, the community was suffering.

I went back to work at 7 a.m. the following Monday. Even though tears still came at the first thought of the fire, and I couldn't sleep very well, I thought I was doing okay. However, when I entered the dispatch room, I realized it was my turn to work the 9-1-1 lines and the fire radio; I ran to the bathroom and threw up. Staring at the remains of my breakfast, a bead of sweat dripped into the toilet. I couldn't move. Fear glued me to the locker room floor. My eyes stung from what felt like an endless flow of sweat. I let the fear wash over me, fighting it would only make the process last longer.

When I could pull myself off the floor, I looked in the mirror. My eyes were puffy and red, and tracks of tears and sweat crisscrossed my cheeks. Sweat had even bled through my undershirt and left dark stains on my heather gray uniform shirt. I looked just like I felt. With a heavy sigh, I threw water on my face to erase the evidence, and rinsed the bitter bile taste from my mouth. I put on a clean work shirt, and with a quick run of my fingers through my hair I was presentable. I walked back to dispatch.

No one noticed the different shirt, no one made mention of how long I had been gone. I sat at my position, slid my headset on and plugged in. It was 7:21a.m.; my boss would walk through the door in thirty-nine minutes. The 9-1-1 line lit up. I hesitated. A second ring. I blinked. A third ring. I reached to answer, and my hand shook. Self-doubt was winning. Swallowing a lump of bile, I pushed the button, "9-1-1, what is the location of your emergency?"

"This isn't an emergency, I just wanted to let you know there is a car broke down in the middle of the road." My shoulders dropped from my ears. My chest loosened. And a ragged breath escaped my mouth. After getting the necessary information I disconnected the call.

I looked at my partners, they were busy and didn't realize what had just happened. Alone with my thoughts, my hands trembled. Silently I begged for the 9-1-1 lines to stay quiet. I looked at the clock again: 7:26 a.m. I could feel my nose and eyes swell as the emotions gripped again. Tears welled, but I held them at bay. I had to do something, but what? I couldn't excuse myself; I had just gotten back from the bathroom. I was trapped. My breathing was short and rapid. Why was time moving so slowly?

Finally, it was 8 o'clock, and my boss walked through the dispatch door. Before he could even get his key in his office door I said I needed to talk to him. Unplugging my headset, I excused myself and nearly ran into his office. Tossing the headset on his desk I blurted, "I'm done...I can't do this job anymore." It was 8:01, he hadn't even gotten his coat off.

"What? Why? Tracey, sit down."

I sat and told him everything I could remember about the past five days. Not one tear fell as I told him. No sweat dripped down my back. My hands were steady as could be. I had learned, when I was just a child, never show anyone when you're scared. I thought the best thing to do was to just stop dispatching. I thought everything would be fine if I just stopped doing what reminded me of the pain.

Golden Glue: A 9-1-1 Dispatcher's Story

But he wouldn't accept my resignation. He said to go home and take a few days off; to allow the healing process to happen. If I felt that I really wanted to quit in a week, he would think about accepting it. Reluctantly, I took his advice.

I wasn't told to see a therapist. I wasn't even asked if I needed one. There wasn't anyone to call. Not that I would have. I had to do the therapy thing when I was a kid, I knew it wasn't for me. So, I went home to my empty apartment. I got on the internet and looked at flights to go home (my family lived 850 miles away). The prices were ridiculous. I turned the computer off, packed a bag, made sure I had someone to check on my cat, got in my car and drove home. I arrived at my sister's door at 10:30 p.m., "Surprise!"

I spent five days surrounded by family and friends. Not once did I tell them what happened. *They wouldn't understand. They're civilians,* I told myself. I don't know many dispatchers who talk about what we deal with outside of work. So, I wasn't about to go down the dark road with them. Why would I want to bring these horrific deaths into their world? It was my job to protect them from this type of stuff. I simply told them I came without calling because I wanted to surprise everyone. We all had a wonderful time being with each other. It would be years before I would tell any of them what had happened that July day—twelve years and 206 days, to be exact. And even then, I would diminish the severity of the trauma.

After my week away, I went back to work and told my boss I was fine; I could do it. And I did—by avoiding 9-1-1 calls and working the fire radio, at all costs. I stopped talking on the telephone to anyone, other than my mother and my sister, unless I absolutely had to. The crying stopped, but the dreams didn't; not for months. I heard the mother's scream over and over, but never saw her face. Whenever we got a house fire, I would sweat, and my hands would shake. It wouldn't stop until the situation was over.

No one ever knew. My boss never asked again how I was handling everything. Life went on. I grew hard, gruff. Brick by brick a wall went up. I didn't do any of it consciously. I didn't even know I did it at all, until 2007, when I attended my first Jim Marshall training class, *Survive and Thrive*. It was a Saturday morning (I know, I know, who goes to training on a Saturday…) and I was sitting in the back row, as I always did. As an introvert I did not like to draw attention, and, as I learned when I was very young, if I don't make eye contact I don't get called on. The actual content of the material from that day escapes me. But I do remember, as the day wore on, I began to realize I was neither surviving nor thriving in my work life.

I hung on Jim's every word. I wanted to ask questions but was too shy to raise my hand. The class didn't solve my problems, but I did go home a little stronger than I had been before the class.

While I did not meet Jim on that day, I was friends with his sister, Debbie. She had retired from dispatch and created a dispatch academy which she asked me to join as an instructor. We worked closely together, and one day, while creating a customer service class, we ended up talking about how shitty I was at customer service. For whatever reason the conversation followed a crooked path to me divulging, for the first time in five years what had happened, from start to finish, during the call and what life was like since then. In the kindest possible way, she blurted, "My God, you have PTSD (Post Traumatic Stress Disorder)."

I have been through a lot in my life: sexually abused as a child, physically abused in a domestic violence situation as a young adult and lost two pregnancies and a marriage as an adult. After all of that, it seemed incomprehensible that a "simple" call at work would be what finally brought me to my knees, let alone result in PTSD. I told her, "Only soldiers get PTSD, or police officers and fire fighters, but certainly not dispatchers." She shook her head and told me I had a lot to learn.

We discussed PTSD and dispatching at length that day. Everything she mentioned rang true with me. I certainly showed symptoms, such as reliving the event, avoiding things that reminded me of the event, and a negative change in feelings and beliefs. Yet, I never sought to have Debbie's impression confirmed, thus PTSD was never officially diagnosed…And she and I never discussed it again.

As time wore on, the wounds scarred over. The nightmares stopped. The trill of the 9-1-1 line no longer triggered fear. I even handled the murder of two small children, and the loss of an elderly couple to a fire, amongst several other distressing calls. But nothing ever again affected me like that fire call. I wouldn't let it. I came into work, I did my job, and I went home. I didn't open up to anyone. I stayed behind my brick wall. (Pretty helpful, don't you think?)

Understand, I had gutted things out my entire life. The after effects of the fire would be no different. I accepted I was "broken," and pushed on. I threw myself into training. I went to every type of training I could get my hands on, especially stress management classes. I found ways to relieve stress in and out of work. I found Nature to be a healer.

Golden Glue: A 9-1-1 Dispatcher's Story

Walking through the woods or around water, armed with my camera always at the ready to capture shots of animals and birds, became my passion. I focused on taking care of everyone else. But I never discussed the call again, not once. It would still be years before I had someone bring me face to face with myself.

In March 2011, my mother had a massive stroke. The doctors said she wouldn't survive. I rushed home to be with her and my family as she clung to life. She defied the odds and clawed her way back, but not without some difficulties. She suffered significant mental, and some physical, damage. Then, within a couple of months, my favorite aunt had a massive heart attack and died. Living 850 miles away had become unbearable. My work suffered significantly.

One afternoon a command officer, I'll call him Adam, called dispatch looking for information. I didn't know the answer to his question. And I was so preoccupied with thinking about my mom, it didn't even dawn on me to find the answer to his question. I simply said, "I don't know." Within ten seconds of hanging up on me, he burst through the dispatch door, and told me exactly what he thought of my awful performance. He found what he was looking for in less than thirty seconds then walked out in obvious disgust.

Five minutes later, my boss called me into his office and the conversation went something like this:

"What the hell happened between you and Adam? He's demanding to see the two of us."

"I fucked up. I knew it when it happened. I tried to talk to him when he came in here, but he wouldn't let me speak. It was bad."

"I've noticed you've been off your game lately. How're things going with your mom?" We spoke for nearly twenty minutes about my mom and my struggle with being away from her and the family. Then he dropped the hammer. "Tracey, Adam wants your title."

You see, all this time I was not only a dispatcher, I was a shift leader. I was responsible for what happened in dispatch during my shift. I was supposed to be leading by example…I was failing miserably.

But then he threw me a life line, "Are you willing to let me handle the conversation with Adam? If so, will you be willing to work on fixing your performance?"

When I reassured him I was willing, he said, "I want you to sit in his office and keep your mouth shut. Let him say whatever he has to say. Got it?" I agreed, and we walked to Adam's office.

I learned two very valuable lessons the day I was called up to that office. The first was my boss had my back. He knew what had been going on at home and extended a helping hand. He was the kind of leader I wanted to be. The second thing I learned was exactly what type of leader I never wanted to be. Adam had no interest in me as a person. He didn't ask how things were going with me. He didn't ask why I had behaved the way I had. He didn't ask anything; he just pointed out how disappointed he was in my performance. I sat tight lipped and stoic. I didn't say a word, just as I had promised. Please understand, I'm not excusing my mediocre performance; I accepted and owned my mistakes then as I do now. But, imagine the difference it would have made, had Adam treated me with *compassion* and *empathy*.

True to his word, my boss handled the conversation with Adam. He assured him he would work with me. I had my work cut out for me, but I was ready. Following my boss' lead, I threw myself headlong into reading every book I could find on leadership. I started with *QBQ: The Question Behind the Question* by John Miller. (I highly recommend this book to every leader, regardless of your position.) I read George W. Bush's *Decision Points*, Collin Powell's *It Worked for Me*, Captain D. Michael Abrashoff's *It's Your Ship* and the list goes on. I learned how to change my approach with being a Shift Leader. I started asking myself, "What can I do to make things better for my shift? How can I be better?" (But I wouldn't learn the answer to that until January 31, 2016.)

I mentioned earlier that there was someone who brought me face to face with myself. In February 2015, my mother passed away suddenly. Hers was the eighth and most traumatic death I had to face between 2011 and 2015. Just a month later, I was involved in divorce number two. My life was spiraling, and there wasn't a damn thing I could do about it. Life is a funny thing, though. It tends to bring people into your life when you need them most.

When this person walked into my life, it was quite literally the lowest point I had ever reached, and still no one knew it. Like everything else, I gutted it out. Yet, for the first time in my life, someone said, "enough with the bullshit, I'm not going anywhere until you talk to me." And he didn't. He patiently spent hours talking to me over many, many months daily. He asked questions no one had ever asked before, and I answered them all, candidly and honestly. He listened as I sobbed—never saying a word.

Golden Glue: A 9-1-1 Dispatcher's Story

He would refute me every time I said I was broken. He helped unravel visceral fears, pains, and horrors from my childhood right up until the present. I unpacked all the baggage I had been carrying since I was seven years old. Brick by brick he helped me destroy the bunker I had constructed around myself to hide who I really was. I had never been more vulnerable, nor freer in my entire life.

One day, during those many months, he gave me a gift: a ceramic bowl that had been broken and glued back together with gold. Gold ran through the bowl like blood through a body. It is a Japanese art called Kintsugi, which teaches us that broken objects are not something to hide nor throw away. Instead, they are to be displayed with pride. The art uses a precious metal, liquid gold, liquid silver, or lacquer dusted with powdered gold to bring together the pieces of a broken pottery item, and at the same time enhance the breaks (Carnazzi). It was a reminder that I wasn't broken anymore, I was healed. (Coincidence that it was a *thin gold line* that held the pieces together? For those readers who don't know, police officers are referred to as the Thin Blue Line, fire fighters as the Thin Red Line, EMS as the Thin White Line, and dispatchers are referred to as the Thin Gold Line. We are the nameless voices that bring calm to the chaos. The glue that holds things together.) Truth be told, I would not come to know just how healed I was until tested…

It was an unseasonable warm Sunday in January, 2016. There was low hanging fog, and a misty rain spitting out of the sky. The window in dispatch was open, to get some fresh air; my partners and I hoped to shake the cobwebs that had settled in our brains. It was the start of our third twelve-hour shift in a row, and we were already anxious to go home. There wasn't a whisper on either the police or fire radio, and the phones hadn't rung since we took our seats over an hour ago. It was a slow start to our Sunday. One of my partners announced her son was coming to visit. Soon after, the little eighteen-month-old dynamo barged through the door with his grandmother in tow. He gave us high fives and squealed in delight seeing his mom. He giggled and toddled around showing off his light-up shoes.

We were having a grand old time, until the shrill trill of the 9-1-1 line broke up the fun. My partner answered with, "what is the exact location of your emergency?" quickly followed by, "do you see flames?" The initial angst I always felt with house fires was settled as soon as she asked, "Are you able to get everyone out of the house?" She confirmed the caller's response was yes when she responded, "good, the fire department is on the way," she disconnected the call. *Good, just a house fire.* We let out a collective breath and sat back in our chairs.

Little did we know then, but our caller, the homeowner, had lied to my partner. He did not get everyone out of the house. There were five young men living in a secret labyrinth in his basement, and none of them would be found until it was too late. There was only one ingress/egress, and no functioning smoke detectors. They never had a chance. The caller was more afraid of getting in trouble than helping save their lives.

It was a somber, brutal day. But I couldn't be prouder of my team. They did everything right. All the right questions were asked, and all the right steps had been taken. There was nothing we could have done differently to change the outcome. But that didn't stop the guilt, pain, or sadness...

Everything I learned in the thirteen years between fires came into play. I immediately let a member of the command staff know my partners and I were struggling. When I found out we were offered the chance to be part of a debriefing with the police officers and fire fighters who responded that day, I immediately said I would be attending, in hopes my partners would, too. I also requested someone who specifically worked with and understood dispatchers and trauma: Jim Marshall, the Saturday morning instructor who I now considered a friend. There wasn't anyone else I trusted with our wellbeing, and he readily answered the call. I asked my boss to check in with my team to make sure they were doing okay. I too checked in with them, even after the dust settled, and the debriefing was over, when everyone else went back to their normal routines. I knew in that moment I had come full circle. I had no lasting effects from this tragedy. Once I allowed myself to go through the emotional healing process, my life continued as it had prior to the incident.

Later that year, I made the decision to leave my department and return home after a nearly twenty-year absence. But I didn't leave the field. I now dispatch for a campus police department at a small college. Life is fabulous, and even on the darkest days there is the hope for a brighter tomorrow.

As the Kintsugi technique suggests, we shouldn't just discard broken objects. When something of importance breaks, it doesn't necessarily mean it is no longer useful. Instead, we should try to repair broken things, because sometimes in doing so the object becomes more valuable. This holds true for dispatchers. With a little help from our peers, perhaps a therapist, or a boss who extends a hand, dispatchers can recover from traumatic events, and become even stronger in their abilities to serve as a *First* First Responder. This is the essence of resilience. Each of us should look to deal with traumatic events by discerning the positives from negative experiences, take the best from the worst and teach ourselves that these experiences make each person extraordinary (Carnazzi).

My hope for all of the dispatchers reading this is that none of you suffer as I did, for as long as I did. Dispatchers are fixers. It's what we do; what we are born to do…and we are good at it. But we must remember to take the time to fix ourselves. There are many options available now, and you will read about many of them in the pages that follow. So, please, don't hesitate to reach out. If you feel broken, there *is* glue to put you back together again. None of the effects of our job need be permanent. Learn from my mistakes, failures and successes. Let the Thin Gold Line glue your "broken you" back together again. Continue the journey through these pages and learn what steps you can make to produce a stronger, more resilient you.

Questions for Reflection

To get the most from this chapter, you are encouraged to write your reflections here (in both the Kindle and paperback versions of this book).

- What was your main take-away from reading this chapter?

- What specifically made it valuable to you?

- How can you apply this take-away concretely to improve some aspect of your personal life and or efforts to support the wellbeing of 9-1-1Pros?

Additional Resources

Abrashoff, D. Michael Captain - *It's Your Ship*

Bush, George W. - *Decision Points*

Covey, Stephen R. - *The 7 Habits of Highly Effective People*

Maxwell, John
- *21 Irrefutable Laws of Leadership*
- *21 Indispensable Qualities of a Leader*
- *The Difference Maker*
- *Developing the Leader Within You*
- *The Power of Attitude*

Miller, John G.
- *QBQ (Question Behind the Question)*
- *Flipping the Switch*
- *Outstanding!*

Pausch, Randy with Jeffery Zaslow - *The Last Lecture*

Powell, Colin General - *It Worked For Me*

Sullenberger, Chesley "Sully" Captain - *Highest Duty*

Works Cited

Carnazzi, Stefano. "Kintsugi the Precious Art of Scars." *Lifegate*. June 2017. **www.lifegate.com/people/lifestyle/kintsugi**.

CHAPTER 2
Days and Nights in the Dispatch Center: What I Saw as a Scientist, Experienced as a Person, and how it Changed Me

Phoenix Chi Wang

Editor's Introduction

If you work in the 9-1-1 industry as a dispatcher or a center manager you might ask, "Why do I need to read an outsider's account of what life in the 9-1-1 center is like? I live it every day!" Fair enough. But that's just the point: sometimes we need an outside perspective when we're immersed in our work. As a sociologist, Phoenix Chi Wang came to the comm center looking for answers to good research questions. Yet, she is no typical scientist, or outsider. Phoenix entered the center with humility, and eyes trained to see new dimensions of a reality that's been sitting in front of us all along. Over the next three years, something happened that was far more than Phoenix bargained for. When she left, she carried not just data and a doctorate in her hands, but people in her heart, and a remarkably deep understanding of life in the PSAP.

I asked Phoenix to share this unique experience, because it is full of fresh insights that must be considered in the face of a future that will demand even more of the human beings sitting those consoles. So, it's a must-read for all 9-1-1 stakeholders who care about assuring the vitality of our dispatchers, and the industry that depends on them. This chapter is not an academic recital of statistics. It is Phoenix's account of how she came to understand the true nature of 9-1-1 work, how a group of 911Pros became her "9-1-1 family," and how they changed her life *personally*. Her powerful perspective can help us to reflect more deeply on the work-life stories told by telecommunicators within the pages of this book.

Phoenix's gratitude for these 9-1-1Pros, and what she discovered about their work lives, has inspired her to continue advocating for their wellbeing beyond her graduate studies into her professional work. Her story is one which resonates deeply with me as clinician-trainer, another outsider who was adopted into this unique family of our Very First Responders. Enjoy!

JM

Scientist in the 9-1-1 Center

I spent nearly three years living among forty dispatchers at a Public Safety Answering Point (PSAP) observing their work life. From September 2013 to July 2016 I listened to them manage thousands of 9-1-1 calls, which was the focus of my doctorate project.[1] And here's my confession: I don't think I would have made it to the end of graduate school if I'd studied any topic *other than* 9-1-1 dispatchers. I wouldn't have been passionate enough to spend those years of my young life, day-and-night at a single research site. But what I witnessed among these 9-1-1 professionals was extraordinary. It fueled my passion and drove me to push through the challenges and frustrations that bring down many graduate students at a high-pressure Ivy League institution. And in the end, these dispatchers became my "9-1-1 Family."

Since the dust settled on my doctorate work, I have returned to the 9-1-1 center for visits. These 9-1-1Pros have invited me to their parties, sent thoughtful gifts to my apartment and even posted unconditional likes and thankful comments on a Facebook page I created just to hang out with them. That's the weird thing; they did so much to help *me*. They helped me become a more thoughtful and compassionate social scientist and a Harvard Ph.D. But most importantly, these dispatchers helped me become a stronger and more resilient human. I feel so indebted for their support, yet they treat me as if I did a lot for *them*. So, if I can tell their stories through my research in a way that's even half as meaningful as their influence on me, I'll consider it a success.

Some of the stories I've taken with me from the 9-1-1 center may seem familiar to the general public because they're about handling loss, pain or whatever life throws at us on a whim. Yet, here's what is unique about such stories as experienced in the 9-1-1 center: dispatchers face all this human toiling on a daily basis… not just in their own lives, but in the lives of their colleagues in the center and on the road, as well as with callers on the phone—*all at the same time.*

I also carry PSAP stories within me that outsiders to 9-1-1 would not likely imagine. After all, how many people in this country know what the 9-1-1 dispatcher's job actually is, what a 9-1-1 center looks like, and what it feels like to work in one? How many times do dispatchers have to explain to their therapists—if they ever go to one—what they do before they can even start talking about what the problem is? How many citizens, policy makers or journalists have ever toured a PSAP? Even dispatchers can be unaware of what their colleague sitting next to them experiences, as they are often isolated by their headsets and forced to move on to the next call.

The Unknown 9-1-1 World

A PSAP is a world unknown to the outside world it serves. Yet, these dispatchers embraced my presence so openly. I believe they want and need to be understood by all 9-1-1 stakeholders and the public they serve. So, I hope this chapter will help provide a fresh perspective of the dispatcher's work life. Let me start with one of the main arguments from my 9-1-1 research.

I see the 9-1-1 dispatcher's daily work as far more than relaying messages to field responders and communicating with callers. They are the key link that organizes and shares essential information between two distinct worlds: the "messy reality" of the every-day world in which real folks struggle, and the "official world" of the well-structured, clean-cut institutions—law enforcement agencies, fire departments and emergency medical organizations. The common misconception is that 9-1-1 dispatchers are "just answering the phone." But this notion doesn't do justice to their crucial work serving the public and communicating with field responders. Using Computer Aided Dispatch (CAD) systems, they perform the most important work in the PSAP—what I call "coding" the calls. This is where the vital connection between the two worlds takes place. The 9-1-1 dispatcher listens to calls often full of ambiguous, confusing and perhaps misleading information. They then translate it into *one single* CAD code—*robbery, electric odor, man down,* and so forth.

I believe that once we fully realize how critical the dispatcher's work is in bridging these two worlds, it can change the way they see themselves, and how they are perceived by their colleagues and the public. Nobody else straddles and brings these two worlds together like they do.

Imagine This: A Bigger View of The Dispatcher's Role

Imagine you and I are standing on the observation deck of the Empire State Building. To the official world of institutions gathering important data, this is just a building with an address: 71 Broadway Manhattan, New York City (NYC). But from our perspective, the Empire State Building is everything beneath us, full of sounds, smells, and sights. We can see countless details of life unfolding in real time. And if NYC is your home town, looking below may trigger memories of your childhood in a certain neighborhood, driving your first car on a certain street, or hanging out with your college friends. You may even hear live music that reminds you of a heart break. Amidst that moving mass of real life below, are also nitty gritty crises in many forms—complex, confusing and personal. This is the flesh and blood, messy reality that floods into the 9-1-1 professional's headset with each caller in distress.

If you're a dispatcher reading this right now, you're hopefully thinking, *Yep, that's my life at work!* You are expected to make sense of the caller's message, however confusing or ambiguous, then quickly translate it into something short and straightforward, then identify it with an incident type—a CAD code that field responders can use to deliver the right help. You are bridging the caller in the messy reality to the responders in the official world.

So, as strange as it may sound, 9-1-1Pros are the government-appointed producers of knowledge that often carries life-and-death consequences. There are numerous occupations that do similar work: foresters report on the number and variation of vegetation, surveyors knock on your door asking census questions, and cartographers turn three-dimensional land masses into two-dimensional maps. However, unlike many other professional "connectors" of the two worlds, the 9-1-1 professional has to build that bridge urgently, at extremely high stakes.

What makes it even more difficult, is that most 9-1-1 calls are charged with emotions—people panic, babble, scream, pant, bawl, curse, contradict themselves or abandon the conversation half-way, and often lie. You, the 9-1-1Pro, are talking to them during the most vulnerable and helpless moments in their lives. So, your success at bridging "the messy reality to the official world" depends on your ability to be a patient, empathetic, skilled and decisive conversationalist who controls the phone communication. What a huge task! You try to jump into the minds and hearts of the callers, instantly capturing the nature of the incident, and assigning a code in the CAD system so that you can quickly assure them, "help is on the way." And you may be doing all this while you're hungry, sleep-deprived and alone, separated from the rest of the world by the headset you are wearing. Oh, and your PSAP is probably short-staffed, struggling with high rates of burn-out and turn-over.

Maybe you have never thought about your job the way I do, or perhaps you have. Either way, hopefully you are convinced that what you do is important and meaningful, especially given all the stress and other costs of doing your work.

What Your 9-1-1 Peers Taught me About the Dispatcher

During my three years in the comm center, my 9-1-1 folks taught and told me a lot about their work experience that I believe is common among dispatchers. One important thing I learned is that your relationship with your colleagues on the street is deep, and often complicated. You may feel love and respect for these responders. You may have grown up with, or attended the same school as some of them. You may even be related, or married, to them. The last thing you want is to see something terrible happen to any one of them. So, just receiving or sending those two code words--*Officer Down*--can be life changing.

But sometimes you also feel invisible. That your job, which you do proudly and skillfully, is regarded by certain people you work with as easy, safe, and even dispensable. You may have chosen 9-1-1 work versus road work because you like to be behind the scenes. Or, you may have been an officer, firefighter, or medic, or perhaps aspire to become one. In any case, you've probably noticed that there are some subtle, or not so subtle, differences between the way you and your sworn colleagues in the field are treated, discussed and paid. Your relationship with some of them may be laced with tension. If you haven't come to terms with all this, you may end up stuck feeling resentment about these differences.

Yes, there is an obvious difference between your work and your field response colleagues'—you aren't on the road. There may be times when you wish you were, so you could see everything with your own eyes instead of just picturing it over and over again in your head. You never *see* the incidents, but in another way, you *always* see them. With only your audio connection to the caller, you strive to make that leap from the call to the code by visualizing all the details of an event in your mind that you can't see or reach physically. There may be some bad calls that you want to get over, but they linger in your mind for days, months, years, and even decades.

Many of you say you're glad you're not on scene. Yet, many of you wish you were, to get the rest of story about some of the toughest calls—to have *closure*. You wonder what happened to the mom looking for her son, to the 90-year-old woman living alone who broke her hip, to the homeless guy who was beaten up again, or to the college kid who called in a panic after wiring all his money to a scammer. But you don't have time for closure. You have to pick up and move on to the next call, leaving you without time to answer the painful hypothetical questions, like: *What else could I have done? What if I had done or said something different? Was it my fault?* So those questions may follow you home. These are all aspects unique to the 9-1-1 work experience that fuel stress on the job. Layers of visceral memories can pile up over time until they seem like just a blur without any articulation.

But 9-1-1 professionals are tough.

The Mental Toughness of 9-1-1 Pros

My 9-1-1 folks are the bravest and most enduring people I know. For example, I remember Jimmy striding into the room, laughing through his lungs, taking 9-1-1 calls, then bantering and exchanging *Seinfeld* lines with Stevie next to him. Then after his shift was over, he drove to the hospital to take care of his 6-year-old son who just had brain surgery. Or Sheila who told me about her long painful divorce and her mom with Alzheimer's, then took a call from a crying woman divorcing her husband, "I understand. Believe me; I'm going through a divorce myself." Nothing ever stopped my 9-1-1 family from being humorous, bad-ass and fearless: abdominal surgery, aching knees, infidelity, dying pets, spouse on disability…nothing. It pained and warmed my heart at the same time to see their bright and brave smiles every day, knowing clearly what they were going through and struggling with.

I believe there are countless 9-1-1 professionals out there who are fighting their own wars, just like the 9-1-1 folks I know. Maybe you are one of them and you take tremendous pride in it. It's likely you plan to continue approaching your 9-1-1 work with the same "bring it on…it is what it is" attitude. To be honest, that's a gift I took with me from hanging out in the PSAP, and from which I still benefit greatly today. I learned to joke and laugh about the problems I had. I learned to block negative thoughts out of my mind. I learned to normalize all the weird, shitty and terrible things in life while still living it whole-heartedly. And I learned to do it all while multi-tasking. As I mentioned earlier, I probably wouldn't have survived graduate school without spending the majority of my waking hours during my dissertation years with my 9-1-1 family.

A Second Look at How We're Handling our Stress

As important as your mental toughness is, you didn't create the stress and traumatic events you're exposed to while working as a 9-1-1 dispatcher. As my research shows, 9-1-1 stress is created by the demands and expectations of our society, the larger public safety system, and from the 9-1-1 communication system. So why should you handle it (combined with all your personal life stress) alone? Maybe you've thought about, even sought out, a more organized way of dealing with stress, but you can't find the help, or don't know where to start. Helping you succeed in managing your 9-1-1 stress should be a responsibility shared by all of us who benefit from your service: the public, our government, industry vendors, and researchers like me. We should all work together to help the 9-1-1 profession gain the recognition and status as a profession that it deserves. All the contributors to this book share that belief, and that's why we've written these chapters. So, I'm glad you're curious and concerned enough to read on and learn more about how to do great self-care and support the 9-1-1 family in this effort.

My Own Struggles with Stress and Self-Care

In January 2014, when I was 5 months into my 9-1-1 fieldwork, I had to deal with a relationship breakup and some harsh criticism on my dissertation in the same week. Let me be clear: if you fail your dissertation you fail graduate school. At that point I had already spent more than 5 years in graduate school. Both my personal and academic life fell apart within days. As a result, I developed what is clinically known as *Acute Stress Disorder* (ASD). I didn't feel safe and had trouble falling asleep. I went to the theatre with my friends and found myself unable to sit through scenes with minimal violence. I kept going to my PSAP every day, listening to 9-1-1 calls and taking field notes. I was struggling, but there was no way I was going to give up. Not after 5 months of learning the ropes— how my listen-only phone operated, how CAD worked, what the response plans were, what the police, fire and medical units did and needed, what all eleven fire channels were for, what PRO-QA did, what Shot-Spotter was, and everything else. I was finally beginning to get it. I had access to the most exciting research site I could dream of, and I was not going to take a break or quit just because my new year started badly. I also needed the brisk, sarcastic "we've seen it all" energy in the PSAP. It made me feel alive and my problems seem trivial.

Through that period, I coped with my own problems and setbacks as my 9-1-1 friends did: by distancing myself from my negative feelings, making light of them and throwing myself quickly back into the game, so I could regain my groove. But, in retrospect, there were a few other things that were also important to do. I'm sharing my stressors, and what I did to cope with them, hoping it will help you face yours.

First, I needed support and perspective from my 9-1-1 family. Fortunately, they were able to give it to me, along with more wisdom than I had asked for. I had to force myself out of my room and seek out friends to stay with, so I had a basic dose of human interactions. I also actively, and purposefully, sought to articulate my thought processes and private feelings—confusion, shame, frustration, guilt, fear, hopelessness and anger—battling in my mind at the time. I did this by talking to my family and friends, and by writing down the feelings. I found that articulating problems and emotions gave them a concrete shape and size, as if I could see them in front of me. That's how I realized they are much smaller, weaker and easier to defeat than when still stuck inside in my head. These methods of self-care come from my mother, a doctor, as well as from a therapist I visited at Harvard University Health Services. I also learned that there is an infirmary at school which would open its doors to me if I had urgent needs.

March 17, 2014 marked the 8th anniversary of my father's passing. That afternoon, after waiting eagerly for months, I finally received a letter of response from an academic journal. They rejected the paper I had spent four years working on for publication. By nightfall I felt as if I was going to collapse. I left my apartment and walked into the infirmary. Three days later I was discharged, able to resume my research in the PSAP again. By the end of the spring semester I had produced exactly 100 pages of double-sided handwritten notes. I was back on track.

If you search Acute Stress Disorder online, you will see that it shares many symptoms with Post-Traumatic Stress Disorder (PTSD). But if those symptoms last longer than a month the diagnosis is likely to be PTSD. I was fortunate that my ASD resolved before it progressed to PTSD. I believe my illness was so short-lived because I was blessed with several types of important support:

- My whole 9-1-1 family who had my back
- Friends who offered space and company
- Timely advice from trained and experienced professionals
- Well-organized and funded care organizations with sufficient resources to address the specific challenges faced by their client population (Harvard students)
- A rather flexible daily schedule
- The option of not going to the PSAP or listening to 9-1-1 calls if I wasn't up to it.

I was able to resolve my stress issues easier than a 9-1-1 dispatcher, because what I was going through was quite different. Although my stressors were a huge deal to me at that moment, they weren't uncommon. Breakups and academic failures are issues that most family, friends and therapists are apt to relate to, far easier than the trauma 9-1-1Pros are exposed to in a PSAP. Without all those supports, I couldn't have bounced back so quickly. So, I'm left wondering, how much access do our dispatchers have to the full range of support they need? Not to mention that a great number of them have been suffering from PTSD already (See Chapter 4).

This book is a project that attempts to bring together as many of those factors that contributed to my resilience as possible, but on an organizational level. Here is what I hope this chapter, and the others in this book, will help to do:

- Build a more supportive 9-1-1 family across the country
- Call for more responsive peer-support and counseling programs that grow in number,
- Offer professional suggestions on resilience and self-care
- Provide some much-needed public education on the 9-1-1 profession
- Plead for well-funded facilities and agencies with trained personnel specializing in 9-1-1-incurred stress and PTSD
- Support 9-1-1 leaders in pursuit of fully staffed 9-1-1 centers, which would enable more flexible hours and give 9-1-1 dispatchers room to seek the help they most need.

I urge these PSAP improvements not just as a sociologist, but as a survivor, who is attuned to the struggles our 911Pros face, and who knows what it took to overcome her own.

My late father, whom I mentioned earlier, used to be a Simultaneous Interpreter in the United Nations. With headset on, he was tasked to instantly translate between Mandarin (Chinese) and English during high-stake UN conferences. After each of his 30-minute shifts, he left with his shirt soaked in sweat. It wasn't until I started writing up my dissertation, and using the word *translate*, that I was struck by the huge similarities between his job and my 9-1-1 folks.' At that moment, I realized that he had led me from heaven to this work in the 9-1-1 center— I was meant to study 9-1-1 dispatchers. And that conviction grows stronger every day. My 9-1-1 research, and the insights I've shared here, matter to me professionally *and* personally. I hope they will matter to you, too. Not just moving you to pause and ponder, but also to help shape the policies and practices impacting 911Pros' wellbeing in your PSAP, and in our country. Supporting you through this work is the least I can do for my *9-1-1 family*.

※

Questions for Reflection

To get the most from this chapter, you are encouraged to write your reflections here (in both the Kindle and paperback versions of this book).

- What was your main take-away from reading this chapter?

- What specifically made it valuable to you?

- How can you apply this take-away concretely to improve some aspect of your personal life and or efforts to support the wellbeing of 9-1-1Pros?

Additional Resources

On the work of connecting messy reality to the official world, you can read a classical book on this topic: James Scott's *Seeing Like a State*.

On the dilemmas and struggles of government employees to serve citizens, you can check out Michael Lipsky's *Street Level Bureaucracy*

End Notes

[1] Dr. Phoenix Wang Chi succeeded in completing her project resulting in her approved dissertation: Wang Chi. 2017. *Discretion, Cognition and Embodiment in Process: Days and Nights with 911 Dispatchers*. Harvard Library. Cambridge. But her 9-1-1 family still just calls her Phoenix.

CHAPTER 3
Understanding Stress and the Nine Unique 9-1-1 Risk Factors Faced by Every Dispatcher

Jim Marshall

Understanding Stress

Humans can handle enormous physical and psychological demands. We can come out the other side of disasters even stronger than we were before, like surfers reappearing from a monster wave we never thought they'd survive. It all depends on two things: what's thrown at us, and what we're prepared to do with it. World-class surfers are always hunting for the biggest waves to get the best rides. But they also know that the bigger the wave, the greater the risk they'll end up in harm's way. So, they must carefully assess what they'll be up against; and their skills must match the challenge.

The National Institute of Occupational Safety and Health (NIOSH) defines job stress as "… the harmful physical and emotional responses that occur when the requirements of the job do not match the capabilities, resources, or needs of the worker." (Sauter). With that definition in mind, as we recall the 9-1-1 stories of Tracey and Phoenix (Chapters 1 and 2, respectively) it's obvious that the dispatcher's work life is apt to be super stressful.

So, to decrease dispatcher stress, and make it manageable without setting them up for trouble, 9-1-1 stakeholders must work to assure that, as a general rule, the demands placed on them don't exceed their "capabilities, resources or needs." And dispatchers must adopt the Resilient 9-1-1 Mindset and Skillset, using the resources and supports we provide them.

In this chapter, we will first unpack some fun science to explain "the stress experience;" then we'll explore *The Nine Unique 9-1-1 Risk Factors*. In essence, we're going to do good stress-risk assessment, just like those surfers do, by studying the waters in which dispatchers are expected to survive and thrive. Then in the coming chapters we'll explore solutions related to these stressors. So, let's get some good upfront knowledge of stress to prepare us for this exploration of 9-1-1 risk factors.

A day in the Life of Momma Z, Zig and Zag[1]

Let's take a quick trip south of the equator so I can lay out some key stress facts for you in black and white. Imagine a Momma Zebra in all her striped glory, lazing in the tall grass of the West African savannah. She's flanked by her two baby zebras, Zig and Zag, names she gave them as life-saving instructions, "When the lion stalks, you *Zig*, and you *Zag*!" Her tail is swatting flies from their little hides as she tells them the tale of how she and Daddy Z met. In these cozy, relaxed moments when she senses they are safe, her brain's "brake" is turned on; she's operating from her parasympathetic nervous system (PNS).

The PNS doesn't demand much of her energy supplies. It helps her do the mundane every-day duties of life on the savannah, like forage for food, take care of the kids, and play. It only uses the resources (blood, sugar, hormones) demanded for these basic tasks. Right now, she has no cause to stomp on the "gas pedal," which is her sympathetic nervous system (SNS). There's no physical threat, no need for her brain or her feet to run in high gear.

Lions, on the other hand, are constantly on the prowl and they burn so many calories in these supper hunts they must eat something the size of one Momma Z (or two smaller versions) every three days just to survive. After crouching and spying from bushes just yards from the Zebra family, Leo erupts from his hiding place, springs into action and races toward them at full tilt. Momma Z bolts into flight as the decoy, keeping her kids on the down-low. The chase is on! In the moment when she sees the lion, she accurately perceives him as a *Stressor*—a threat demanding immediate action. She must activate her *Stress Response*. This is a series of internal changes enabling her to run quickly, zig, zag, and thwart Leo's advances. She has to step on the gas pedal. Instantly her hypothalamus and pituitary order up a hormone power fuel that morphs into adrenalin and cortisol, with a little help from her adrenal cortex.

These stress hormones fuel her Stress Response, the mojo she needs to escape Leo the Lion and regain safety. Her blood pressure spikes as sugar supplies dump into her blood which then rushes through her brain to enhance quick thinking and vigilance; it rushes through her body enabling agility and speed. And, in case Leo's claws rip her belly open in the hunt, it also fires up her immune system to fend off infection, so she can heal and remain alive to raise her kids. After a few minutes of chase, Momma Z successfully zigged and zagged her way beyond Leo's teeth. Dizzy and defeated, he dragged his sorry tail back to his big bush where he collapsed into a sleeping heap. Zig and Zag were still hiding, huddled safely together in the tall grass.

Within 90 seconds after sensing that she and the kids were safe again, Momma Z stepped on the brake and stopped producing that hormone super fuel. Now she can "rest and digest" (Harvard Health 1). All her systems (neuro, endocrine, cardio, circulatory, etc.) could return to the normal mode of functioning, preventing her from depleting energy reserves that she may need for the next chase. This balanced state within and between all her systems is called *"homeostasis."* To be healthy, that's the state all mammals, us included, need to spend most of our time in.

So, as we travel from Africa to the 9-1-1 center, you'll now know exactly what I and our other writers mean when we use the terms, *stressor, stress response, and balance*. And, keep this in mind: humans tend to activate the same full-blown stress response as Momma Z—even when our lives are not at risk. So, each time a 9-1-1Pro experiences one of our Nine Unique 9-1-1 Risk Factors they may activate the same life-or-death stress response as Momma Z did. Also, like Leo, stressors don't always exceed our reserves in a single event. Sometimes the greater risk is that they will occur too often over time, *gradually* depleting our resources. For these reasons, we need to identify those nine unique 9-1-1 risk factors, and then read the rest of the book to learn how to reduce and manage them to enjoy high resilience and performance.

Our list of 9-1-1 risk factors (stressors) here will be far from complete—there are many other stressors that telecommunicators experience, many they often consider more upsetting (on a daily basis) than those on our list. Veteran dispatchers in my classrooms have often chimed in together about such stressors that, in combination, over the years really get to them: "It's not the big, bad calls that bother me the most, it's the annoying calls…working short-staffed…it's mandatory overtime for months on end…it's my coworkers…our administrators…new CAD!" (CAD stands for Computer-Aided Dispatch, software used to gather and send data from callers to field responders.)

These are all examples of what I call common 9-1-1 stressors. Let me be clear: common does not mean *minor*! The cumulative impact of these common stressors is very serious and must be addressed (as we will in the last section on 9-1-1 Leadership). Our list is limited to those nine stressors that are *unique to 9-1-1* and represent special risk factors. They are related directly to the telecommunicator's duty at the console dispatching and call-taking. Here's the list, which we'll entitle…

9-1-1's Nine Big Risk Factors

#1: No warning Before Potentially Traumatic Calls
#2: The big "C" of 9-1-1—Lack of Closure
#3: Telecommunicators are Psychologically On-scene but Physically Unable to Reach It
#4: 9-1-1Pros "Send their Own" into Harm's Way
#5: Limited Sensory Engagement with Those on Scene
#6: High Call Volume and Frequency
#7: The Crazy-Tasking Demand
#8: Little to No Downtime to De-stress
#9: Lack of Appreciation and Professional Respect

If you're a frontline 9-1-1Pro, as you read the description of these nine risk factors, I invite you to reflect on how *you* and your co-workers have experienced them in your 9-1-1 center. This will be a helpful exercise preparing you to apply the knowledge we'll offer you in the rest of the book.

If you're not a 9-1-1Pro, your first glance at this list may prompt the same reaction I witnessed when I have presented it to my clinical colleagues at conferences, for example: "I never thought of their job this way before! What incredibly stressful work!" The explanations below should help shed a lot of light on a profession that has been "out of mind" for most of our citizens, because telecommunicators are "out of sight". They are not on scene. As you read the description of each risk factor, try an exercise: first imagine you are the dispatcher at the console. Wonder what it would be like to experience that specific risk factor; then think about your role (supervisor, 9-1-1 director, governing board member, etc.) and ask, *how could I use my role, my influence and our resources to best support our 9-1-1Pros in the face of this work stressor?*

9-1-1 Risk Factor #1:
No warning Before Potentially Traumatic Calls

9-1-1 professionals provide their field responders with the *who, what, when, where* information about the scene they will face. The 9-1-1Pro assesses and reports what's happening on scene, including tragic events that are either in progress or have just occurred such as suicide, homicide, domestic violence, etc. which pose potential danger to the responder. This upfront information allows field responders to begin visualizing and thinking about how they will approach the scene, their objectives, and their strategy. It also empowers them to prepare tactically and psychologically before being exposed to potentially traumatic events.

By contrast, due to the very nature of the 9-1-1Pro's role as the Very First Responder, they receive no warning before the calls they handle. The sounds of human suffering that explode into their headsets come in hot and unfiltered: the responder in a panic shouting, "officer down"; the mother screaming that her baby isn't breathing; the father whose speech is indecipherable between groans after discovering his son's suicide. The list goes on and on. The 9-1-1Pro is repeatedly exposed to potentially traumatic events without any chance to prepare or buffer mentally.

Telecommunicators are the first to receive highly charged, emotionally loaded information from callers in distress with no warning. Humanity, raw and uncensored, floods directly into the headset and mind of the telecommunicator: all the cruel, violent, ugly, rude, obnoxious, and heart-breaking bits of so many human lives. And since it comes without warning, there are more important questions we must ask and must be answered to assure their wellbeing:

- How does this lack of warning affect the way in which the brain stores and sorts through this potentially traumatic information?
- Does exposure to all this stimuli without warning increase the risk that the telecommunicator will be psychologically affected compared to the field responder sent to the same call?
- What is the best way to prepare our 9-1-1Pros to manage this kind of unbuffered input that is part and parcel to their jobs?

9-1-1 Risk Factor #2:
The big "C" of 9-1-1—Lack of Closure [2]

Throughout the country, when I have asked telecommunicators what one of the most stressful parts of their job is, they almost always say it is the lack of closure after dispatching responders to high-risk scenes, or after calls with folks for whom they feel the most empathy; usually children and the elderly. Seldom does a telecommunicator know the outcome of the call after they disconnect from the caller.

As we know from the story of Momma Zebra, production of cortisol for zebras and humans stops about a minute and a half after we perceive a threat to be over (Mate' 31). But it's difficult for a 9-1-1Pro to experience closure to a life-threatening call when they must disconnect from the caller before any life-or-death outcome is known. If you're a 9-1-1Pro, you're apt to still be jacked up emotionally until you experience some type of closure. Unlike Momma Z, your brain still believes the lion is prowling, so it keeps producing stress hormones to help you survive—you're still in fight-or-flight mode. So, telecommunicators make attempts to create their own sense of closure by affirming they did a good job, then, hopefully, processing it with their peers (when time permits).

These self-soothing strategies are good and often necessary but are not always *sufficient* to resolve the internal distress or prevent it from stockpiling in your mind and body. Ideally, you will achieve more emotional release by gaining certainty about the result of your intervention with the caller. Even then, after tragic outcomes, knowing the reality doesn't guarantee that you've fully processed the event. But here's the point: the greater your sense of closure, the greater the chance you'll stop producing cortisol. That is a good thing because manufacturing too much cortisol too often can deplete your resources and set you up for health problems. Cortisol has a long half-life, meaning that it flows through your blood stream for minutes to hours after you stop its production. That's why striving for closure is important. So 9-1-1Pros and their leaders need to ask:

- How could we improve the dispatcher's experience of emotional release after tough calls and dispatch experiences?
- Respecting legal restrictions, what can we do to maximize and expedite the scene information dispatchers need to fully let go of the experience?
- What kind of support does a 9-1-1Pro need when tragic calls occur? (Certainly, the definition of "tragic" and the type of support needed vary by person, but it's important for dispatchers to brainstorm this question about themselves and as teams.)

9-1-1 Risk Factor #3:
Telecommunicators are Psychologically On-scene but Physically Unable to Reach It

As telecommunicator Lisa Rouse of the Royal Canadian Mounted Police said to me (referring to tough calls such as those involving children in danger), "you want to jump in your car… to go help them, but you can't. So, my job, really, was my voice." If you've never sat at a 9-1-1 console in real-time, it can be hard to realize how stressful it is for 9-1-1Pros to *not* be able to physically reach those in peril that they're striving to help save. But our finest 9-1-1 leaders do "get it" and this realization is a must if they're going to take care of their personnel.

In 2011 I moderated a workshop exploring how 9-1-1 stressors can impact the personal health and relationships of 9-1-1Pros. After the session, a police chief and his buddy, a fire chief, came to me with urgent looks on their faces.

They asked me to step into the hall. I had no clue what they wanted, but I sure was curious. The police chief was energized and adamant, "Jim, we want you to pass on a message to 9-1-1 folks as you continue your travels and presentations. As officers, we've got our Kevlar, we've got our weapons; we've got strategies and tactics that we can implement right there on scene, in person. We can often get the bad guy and save the people who are at risk. But the telecommunicator can't reach the scene *physically*. That must feel awful. A lot of *helplessness*. So, tell them we said they have the harder job—tell them we get it." Well, that certainly got my attention.

Then his buddy the Fire Chief jumped in, "Exactly my point. Not only can we usually reach the scene, we put on our turnout gear and other equipment which allows us to get into the fire and reach the people. We can help save people with our own hands. But the telecommunicator can't reach that scene--they have a harder job." I never forgot their message.

If you're a 9-1-1Pro you're all too familiar with Unique 9-1-1 Stressor #3. If you're a 9-1-1 stakeholder, hopefully you, too, can see the point: carrying responsibility to help save the lives of callers and field responders without being able to reach the scene, can produce helplessness that is unique to telecommunicators. This helplessness, coupled with their strong sense of responsibility, is quite an emotional load to bear. What those two leaders at the conference shared with me helped accentuate a message critical to all 9-1-1 stakeholders. We must equip telecommunicators with the ability to tolerate such extraordinary stress and optimize their resilience. This is not an option. But our directors can't achieve this mandate if the funding isn't provided.

9-1-1 Risk Factor #4:
9-1-1Pros "Send their Own" into Harm's Way

Our veterans of war know that going into the front line of battle is a horrible thing. And when they return home seriously injured or dead, their commanding officers experience a psychological devastation we as civilians cannot fathom. But I believe dispatchers can. Every day dispatchers send their colleagues into harm's way: scenes fraught with the danger of death. And when the dispatcher loses a responder with whom they often have some kind of personal attachment, they can suffer *survivor's guilt*.

This guilt, coupled with self-blame and a sense of failure, is captured in a phrase I've heard telecommunicators strain to say aloud, "if I hadn't sent her, she wouldn't have died." Whenever a telecommunicator makes a statement like this in my class, their colleagues react at once with an empathy so strong and uniform that you know they too dread or have experienced this themselves. They will almost always come to the telecommunicator's rescue, seeking to ease the guilt by offering statements of comfort: "If you hadn't sent them, somebody else would have…You can't stop what happens to them in the field…It's your job to send them; you did the right thing even though the result was bad." Each of the statements is true and important for a 9-1-1Pro to hear. Yet, as essential as they may be, such attempts to comfort are often not *enough* to release the telecommunicator's survivor's guilt.

Certainly, grief is a normal response for anyone who loses someone they care about. But what makes *survivor's guilt* so predictable among dispatchers when field responders die? It's the unique nature of their relationship. At the end of the day, what matters most in the heart of every dispatcher? This is a question I've asked over 1,000 dispatchers in group settings, and invariably their answer, almost in unison is: "Everyone goes home." 9-1-1Pros feel an enormous sense of responsibility for protecting their field responders. Yet, ironically, they ultimately have no control over what happens out there. Dispatchers strive to gather and deliver every bit of information they can for their responders' safety. But once those responders arrive on scene, what unfolds is a result of many variables beyond the telecommunicator's influence. Coupled with the fact that they are physically safe from the danger into which they're sending their friends, the guilt can become exponential.

We must recognize that 9-1-1Pros don't just experience stress after "Officer down" incidents. They may also experience big *anticipatory anxiety* about these incidents in two ways: as highly intense anticipation in the heat of the moment *during* a high-risk incident not knowing how it will turn out, and, as an ongoing worry about the future: *when will Officer Down happen on my watch?* Both types of anticipation can fuel ongoing hypervigilance and over-activation of stress hormones, a factor in developing Compassion Fatigue and Chronic Stress Response. So, we can see that if dispatchers and their leaders do nothing in the face of Risk Factor #4, the impacts can be serious for our 9-1-1Pros both personally and for their performance. The good news is that it is possible to heal the traumatic impacts of a line-of-duty death with help from Evidence-Based Treatment—specifically, *trauma therapy* proven effective in resolving PTSD symptoms (see Chapters 8 and 9). Yet we should also explore the answers to these questions:

- Should basic 9-1-1 training always include frank discussion about the possibility of experiencing such Survivor's Guilt?
- Are 9-1-1 personnel prepared to provide support when field responders perish or survive injuries inflicted on-scene?
- What protocols for care of the dispatcher, as a survivor, should be put in place after such an event?

9-1-1 Risk Factor #5:
Limited Sensory Engagement with Those on Scene

As of this writing, with very few exceptions in the U.S., dispatchers can only share an auditory data connection with callers and their field responders through phones and radios. They can hear them and speak to them but cannot actually see them. Consider this: visually impaired people learn to compensate for their sensory deprivation. As a result, they develop auditory attunement and spatial awareness superior to sighted individuals. Likewise, experienced 9-1-1Pros develop a heightened ability to listen, often hearing things through the phone or radio that others would not notice. Then, combining skillful inquiry and strategic use of their own voices, 9-1-1Pros can offer a powerful emergency response. At the same time, such superb auditory attunement to the caller or responder's voice may lead to greater emotional distress when the sounds of tragedy ring in their ears.

When there are perceived risks of death or significant injury on scene, the inability of 9-1-1Pros to actually *see* what is occurring, likely increases their Emotional Labor. In nearly every session of Survive & Thrive, I've asked my students three questions, which many will answer almost in unison. The first is, "Do you visualize the scene you're dispatching?" Their answer: "Yes."

So, although dispatchers can't literally see the scene, nearly all of them still use their *imagination* to connect with the people and events on scene through their visual channel, not just their auditory channel. Then I ask, "When you visualize, do you imagine the best or the worst possible scenario?" Their answer: "The worst."

After warning them that I'm about to appear very naïve, I ask the third question: "Why in the world would you do that to yourself—imagine the worst instead of the best?" If you're a responder, you know the answer to this question: "To be as prepared as possible."

This is a universally employed strategy among telecommunicators: using visual imagination as an aide to consider all possible factors; it stimulates great interrogatory questioning. And it can also buffer the 9-1-1Pro's mental health if doing so boosts their sense of ability and confidence in call management. Yet, there's a downside. Dispatchers who struggle with bad calls often report that it isn't just the sounds that haunt them. It is also the images they recall in their minds. And remember, those imagined scenes may be worse than the actual scene. Even if a dispatcher later gains more accurate information about the scene from field responders, the original traumatic sounds and images can remain locked in the nervous system. Such unresolved information can cause repeated distress when retriggered. Fortunately, it can be reprocessed and drained of its potency with Evidence-Based Treatment (EBT, see Chapter 9).

If a 9-1-1Pro you know suffers in a big way with past 9-1-1 images as we've discussed here, consider offering this support:

- Welcome them to "talk it out" with you, to tell their story about the call or radio experience(s). Just listen and acknowledge their distress without interrupting or trying to "fix" it.
- Affirm to your peer that this distress is very common among telecommunicators. They aren't weak or weird for experiencing it.
- Encourage them to read Chapter 9 in this book to learn about healing that is now possible.
- If they are willing, offer to help your peer find and make an appointment with a qualified therapist (using the guidance offered in Chapter 9).

"The Big H" of 9-1-1

Before exploring the last few 9-1-1 Risk Factors, it's important for us to define one major reason why the first five factors are so potent in increasing risk for the telecommunicator. You may have already identified it: helplessness. Each factor may decrease the sense of empowerment to change difficult circumstances. We know from the science of traumatology that when one feels helpless to change traumatic events to which they're exposed, the risk of psychological fall-out is greater. That is why I call helplessness *The Big H of 9-1-1*. Let me be clear, I am not saying dispatchers are actually helpless to influence those struggling on scenes. Countless times, our 9-1-1Pros have played a major, if not the greatest role in helping save lives. We are speaking here about their subjective experience of helplessness. "I just feel like I could have, should have, done more!"

9-1-1 Risk Factor #6:
High Call Volume and Frequency

How many calls does a 9-1-1Pro take (whether call-taking, radio dispatching, or in a combined position) during an eight-hour period? Surely that number varies greatly depending on which hours and shift you're working, current staffing, your service area's demographics, and many other factors. Yet, for most telecommunicators the answer is simply, *a lot!* To gain an objective perspective of how much raw, emotionally-loaded human contact a 9-1-1Pro experiences, we need to ask another question. How many calls do field responders handle during that same eight-hour time span: six, eight, or maybe ten? The telecommunicator handles many times more calls or radio dispatches in that time period.

The frequency of calls is a significant stressor due to the sheer number of informational bits that the 9-1-1Pro's brain must process related to each call. These bits are often highly charged by the energy of the caller's emotional distress. If these super-charged data bits stay active as unprocessed memories tied to the residual over flow of stress hormones, we can expect the 9-1-1Pro's quality of sleep to suffer. Yet, among the multitude of calls, those that are non-emergent can be *especially* exasperating for the dispatcher. Abuse of the 9-1-1-line drives frustration and resentment, further draining their energy reserves.

So, as we reflect on Risk Factor #6, High Call Volume, we need to consider another key question:

- How can our telecommunicators successfully clear these emotionally-charged data bits from their nervous systems during, and at the end of the shifts, so they are more able to "leave everything at the comm center" when they go home? (See Chapter 5.)

9-1-1 Risk Factor #7:
The Crazy-Tasking Demand

Scientists tell us that humans don't actually multi-task; rather, those who appear to be great multi-taskers, like 9-1-1Pros aren't actually doing many things *simultaneously*; they're shifting speedily from one task to the next. Consistent with findings from a landmark Stanford Study (Ophir), I define multi-tasking as work activity involving rapid cognitive movement (requiring shifts in concentration) between two or more tasks. And when this multi-tasking involves big time emotional labor as it does for 9-1-1Pros, I call it *Crazy-Tasking*.

For sure, whether taking calls, dispatching, or doing both at one console, 9-1-1Pros are mentally processing a huge volume of emotionally-infused data bits as they work with callers. We identified high call volume as Risk Factor #6. The term Crazy-tasking recognizes that in addition to high call volume, there are many other duties in the 9-1-1Pro's job description they are expected to perform. These tasks may be compounded by additional responsibilities assigned to the 9-1-1TC [telecommunicator] on location at the law enforcement agency such as handling warrants, clerical duties, and processing inmates....9-1-1TCs [also] routinely monitor numerous phone lines, access multiple computer applications, and monitor video and alarm information systems (Marshall 186).

Certainly, workers in other fields also are assigned many tasks. The difference is that few occupations combine a multitude of demands in addition to the responsibility for helping save lives. Dispatchers do a great deal of *emotional labor* (EL). EL measures the degree to which certain tasks can drain our energy reserves. In the first major study of 9-1-1 stress, Roberta Troxell discovered that 9-1-1Pros experience an unusually high level of EL, which contributed to Compassion Fatigue (Troxell, see Chapter 10).

9-1-1 Risk Factor #8:
Little to No Downtime to De-stress

First, let me define what I mean by "downtime." It is the time available for the responder to practice self-care: use resilience skills, seek peer support, participate in a group debriefing, read an engaging book, simply use the bathroom, or even just eat a meal without gulping. The amount of actual time available to a 9-1-1Pro for downtime between calls and radio work certainly varies, depending on many factors (shift, hour of day, staffing levels, and more).

Law enforcement officers, medics and firefighters generally have more downtime than dispatchers to practice such self-care. They also have more time free from the expectation to interact with the public. (Surely, available downtime varies for field responders too. I am referring here generally to the relative amount of time they have available.) Because of the telecommunicator's frequency of calls, it's not only more difficult to find downtime, it's harder to wind down psychologically during the brief gaps between calls when they occur. As said previously, they are also less apt to shut off the production of stress hormones from prior calls. Therefore, 9-1-1Pros are more at-risk of accumulating acute stress experiences leading to chronic stress. This produces a stress cascade. The more stress is accumulated, the more intense the response to the next stressor, further using up energy reserves. Can you see how this cascade could play out in the attitudes and exchanges among telecommunicators on the floor? To avoid a strict disciplinary approach when support should be provided first, 9-1-1 leaders must respect the correlation between under-managed, cumulative stress *and* 'negativity'.

9-1-1 Risk-Factor #9:

Lack of Appreciation and Professional Respect

9-1-1Pros, like most field responders, don't want to be patronized or glorified for their professional work. They are uncomfortable with praise and generally get more reward from the intrinsic value of doing emergency response than accolades from others. Most are proud of the service they perform, and many have told me how much they love the work itself. Yet, telecommunicators are also humans doing a job that most folks could not perform technically or endure psychologically. The stressors we've already identified, combined with often excessive work hours, and chronic understaffing (common at most U.S. 9-1-1 centers) can make it very difficult for even the most dedicated 9-1-1Pro to maintain their motivation, positive attitude, and desire to stay in the profession. In APCO's Project RETAINS, dispatchers reported that feeling unappreciated at work was a significant factor contributing to the poor retention rate within the profession (The Compiled Reports…).

Feeling under-appreciated is closely tied to feeling under-respected. Let's face it: unless you've done 9-1-1 work yourself, or have closely observed it being done, you may have the same idea of dispatchers as I did in 1986—they just answer the phone, and send the *real* responders, right? Whether we're citizens, members of the media and press, psychologists, or even 9-1-1 industry leaders, we are all capable of ignorance; a lack of insight about the extraordinary demands placed on 9-1-1Pros, and the risks to which they are exposed. This doesn't mean we don't care. It just means we'll probably fail to do our part to support 9-1-1 professionals getting the help they need to survive and thrive—unless we truly recognize their unique stressors described in this chapter. Providing essential support and resources is the nitty gritty form of respect that they need most of all. That's why I hope you'll keep reading this book.

Conclusion

Dispatchers, their leaders, and all 9-1-1 stakeholders can ask the following questions to help address the nine unique 9-1-1 risk factors:

- To what extent do these risk factors affect the psychological wellbeing and thus the physical health of our telecommunicators?
- Are we equipping 9-1-1Pros and their leaders to optimally manage these risk factors?
- What are the costs if we fail to equip them this way, in terms of performance, retention, morale and quality of life for the telecommunicator both at work and at home?

Every one of these 9-1-1 risk factors can be managed, if we face them head on, together.

⋘⋙

Questions for Reflection

To get the most from this chapter, you are encouraged to write your reflections here (in both the Kindle and paperback versions of this book).

- What was your main take-away from reading this chapter?

- What specifically made it valuable to you?

- How can you apply this take-away concretely to improve some aspect of your personal life and or efforts to support the wellbeing of 9-1-1Pros?

Additional Resources

You'll find value reading all the sources cited below. But for enjoyable, less-technical, reading about the fundamentals about human stress experience consider Sapolsky's *Why Zebras Don't Get Ulcers* (see End Note 1 below). But also read the very encouraging and immediately helpful *Upside of Stress* by Kelly McGonigal (2015).

Works Cited

APCO Institute. *The Compiled Report Synthesizing Information from the Effective Practices Guide and Retains Next Generation.* 2009. www.apcointl.org/doc/conference-documents/personnel-human factor/282-project-retains-compiled-report-2009/file.html.

Marshall, James and S. Gilman. "Reaching the Unseen First Responder: Treating 9-1-1 Trauma in Emergency Telecommunicators." *EMDR Scripted Protocols: Treating Trauma and Stressor-related Conditions,* edited by M. Luber, Springer Publications, 2015, pp 186-7.

Mate', Gabor. *When the Body Says No: Understanding the Stress—Disease Connection.* John Wiley & Sons, 2003, pp 31-33.

Ophir, Eyal et al. "Cognitive Control in Media Multitaskers*." Proceedings of the National Academy of Sciences,* 15 September 2009.www.pnas.org/content/106/37/15583.

Sauter, S et al. "Stress…At Work." *The National Institute for Occupational Safety and Health (NIOSH),* 1999. www.cdc.gov/niosh/docs/99-101/.

Troxell, Roberta. "Indirect Exposure to the Trauma of Others: The Experience of 9-1-1 Telecommunicators. University of Illinois at Chicago, PhD dissertation.

"Understanding the Stress Response." *Harvard Health Publishing,* 18 March 2016. www.health.harvard.edu/staying-healthy/understanding-the-stress-response.

End Notes

[1] This story is my version of the delightful explanation of the stress response offered by Robert Sapolsky: Sapolsky, R. (2004). *Why Zebras Don't Get Ulcers: a guide to stress, stress-related diseases, and coping.* 3rd Ed. New York: Henry Holt

[2] Field responders also struggle with a lack of closure: a medic may work furiously to help stabilize a patient in shock after a major accident then lose contact with him once delivered to the emergency department, with no idea whether he lived or died. So, lack of closure in the general sense is not unique to the 9-1-1Pro. Both the medic and the telecommunicator would benefit greatly by knowing the end of the story in which they have invested themselves emotionally. Yet in my view, the difference is that the medic may have the opportunity to seek that closure by direct contact with receiving facilities; the 9-1-1Pro is "stuck" in the comm center moving on to the next call with fewer breaks and bound by policy restrictions that disallow re-contacting involved field team members for outcomes.

CHAPTER 4
Facing the Impacts of 9-1-1 Stress: The Reality of PTSD and Depression in the Comm Center

Michelle Lilly
Interviewed by Jim Marshall

Editor's Introduction

9-1-1 telecommunicators have something in common with law enforcement officers, medics and fire-fighters (as well as crisis therapists, emergency room doctors, nurses, and others): they face a greater likelihood of exposure to traumatic events in the line of duty than other workers. So, they may be at higher risk of stress-related conditions, including post-traumatic stress disorder (PTSD). For this reason, I call this group, including 9-1-1Pros, Extraordinary Care Givers (ECGs, see book Introduction). Since 2005, I've been urging our Public Safety Answering Points and all 9-1-1 stakeholders to recognize the stress impacts among 9-1-1 telecommunicators, and work strategically to prevent them to the greatest extent possible. *Extraordinary stress requires extraordinary attention and support.* But what evidence do we have about the extent of the risks faced by the 9-1-1Pro? More than ever before.

These dispatchers, their agency leaders, and all 9-1-1 stakeholders must be empowered with this knowledge to assure the wellbeing of the Very First Responder and the future viability of our 9-1-1 centers. In this chapter, researcher Dr. Michelle Lilly (Northern Illinois University) teaches us about the findings of her ground-breaking research revealing the high rates of PTSD and clinical depression she has discovered among telecommunicators. Yet her research also helps reveal some of the key factors driving these high rates. So, Michelle's work points us toward strategies to prevent and heal PTSD and depression in the 9-1-1 family, as we'll discover in the remainder of the book.

JM

Post-Traumatic Stress Disorder and Clinical Depression

Jim: I think the story of how your 9-1-1 research originated is really fascinating, and key to this chapter. You and I have something in common with perhaps all of our mental health colleagues—we didn't recognize the crucial role of 9-1-1 telecommunicators, or the risks to which they are exposed, until a telecommunicator helped us see it. It was my sister, Debbie Achtenberg who opened my eyes, and your eyes were opened by a student. Can you tell us this story?

Michelle: Heather Pierce, a former 9-1-1 dispatcher, was my student at Northern Illinois University. She wanted to study how much PTSD might exist among her former colleagues in the 9-1-1 industry. Having been a telecommunicator for seven years, she was able to tell me first-hand about 9-1-1 work and all it entailed. My eyes got big and my jaw dropped. I just couldn't believe it—I really had no perception about what 9-1-1 telecommunicators did or how taxing their work could be. Heather wanted to do a project with this population and I immediately agreed to join the effort.

Jim: That was my reaction to my first sit-along with my sister in 1986. We're not alone in this reaction. In 2011, Sara Gilman and I presented a session at a conference to over one hundred trauma therapists entitled *EMDR and Treatment of First Responders.*[1] By a show of hands, nearly all of these clinicians had treated our law enforcement officers, fire fighters and or medics, but only seven of them had treated 9-1-1 dispatchers. It was a massive "Aha!" moment for this group. Mental health professionals generally do not recognize telecommunicators as first responders unless they are brought into the invisible 9-1-1 world by one of its members. So, once Heather opened your eyes, and you conducted this first study, what did you expect the results to be?

Michelle: I anticipated the rate of PTSD among telecommunicators would be in line with the rates that we have seen from firefighters and police. For example, the prevalence of duty-related PTSD has been shown to range between 7% and 35% for police officers (Marmar 6), and between 17.3% and 22.2% in Canadian and American samples of firefighters (Corneil 134), respectively. These numbers are notable given that epidemiological research has shown a lifetime PTSD prevalence rate of 7.8% in the US general population. Since telecommunicators aren't physically on scene, I anticipated the rate of PTSD among telecommunicators would be in line with the rates that we have seen with firefighters and police…On the one hand not being on scene was anticipated as being a protective factor, Yet, on the other hand, having only auditory exposure to a call without knowing how it ends could actually enhance their risks.

After Heather compiled the data from our study, I was shocked at the results. We found that nine to ten percent of the telecommunicators in our sample group acknowledged symptoms consistent with a diagnosis of PTSD (Lilly and Pierce 135). While this rate was high, we had several reasons to believe that the actual rate was even higher: there were a number of limitations in the way that we measured PTSD in that first study; it was a small sample, mostly from Illinois or New Mexico; and, we asked dispatchers only about the stress impacts related to one critical incident. So, this was a preliminary study; more research was needed.

Jim: Michelle, I remember when those preliminary findings came out. Your study became national news. Clearly, it wasn't just clinicians who had underestimated 9-1-1 risks. The media and the public had, too. Then, in 2015, your second study was published and these findings were even more extraordinary. Can you tell us about this second study: first, how was this study different, then tell us what you discovered?

Michelle: In the second study, I recruited over eight hundred telecommunicators from across the country. (The first study involved 197 participants within the state of Illinois.) In the first study we asked dispatchers questions related only to the stress effects of one particular 9-1-1 incident. But this time we used a different PTSD screening tool asking additional questions about PTSD, and we did not ask respondents to think of just *one duty-related event* while answering questions; instead, we asked them to consider whether they had symptoms resulting from duty-related exposure over the course of their *career* as a 9-1-1 profession.

Jim: This is an important change in your study approach, because now you could directly correlate 9-1-1Professionals' *cumulative* stress experience at work and its impacts on them. What did you discover?

Michelle: The rates were much higher in the second study (Lilly and Allen 262). Using self-report measures of PTSD that were scored using military cut-offs, we found an estimated 17.6% of our telecommunicators endorsed symptoms severe enough to meet criteria for PTSD. However, using civilian cut-off scores, the rate was 24.6%. That's about 18 to 25%, almost four to five times greater than what we would see in the general population. Therefore, the first study underestimated the extent of PTSD in telecommunicators. I can't say I was that surprised.

Jim: This finding is remarkable, especially since 9-1-1Pros are still often not considered to be emergency responders. Let's take one quick science moment for our readers' sake: could you clarify what it means when we say "military cut-off scoring." Can you clarify the distinction between military and civilian cut-offs?

Michelle: In this second study, we used the Posttraumatic Check List (PCL) which is a measure developed by the National Center for PTSD. Their work has historically been with combat veterans. They found that it makes more sense to use a higher cutoff score for PTSD with combat veterans (versus civilians) because they have such high exposure to traumatic stressors through combat. The goal was to make this screening tool as accurate as possible in identifying probable PTSD compared to a clinician conducting a full clinical interview. The folks at the National Center found that creating these higher cut off scores was the only way to achieve diagnostic results in accord with what a clinician would reach (whether concluding a person does or does not have PTSD).

Jim: *Thank you.* Now about this finding of high rate of PTSD among our 9-1-1Pros. This could be very discouraging news, yet you and I both know that there is much that can be done to improve this problem if we, as an industry, face it head on. Can you offer some hope here?

Michelle: This rate is not a locked-in PTSD rate for the future, only between ten and twelve percent of the telecommunicators in our study had received mental health services. I can also assure our readers that *PTSD can be fully or significantly resolved with today's evidence-based treatments* (EBT). I'm teaching graduate and doctoral students how to implement these therapies and they are very effective in treating PTSD. So, even if someone has the diagnosis, it is not a life sentence to suffer from this disorder.

Jim: This is a vitally important message because many of our veterans and emergency responders with PTSD still believe there is no healing for this problem; and this fuels a feeling of hopelessness and probably contributes to depression and suicide among these populations.

Michelle: The more people think PTSD is something they're going to have to struggle with for the rest their lives the more likely they are to avoid seeking help, which certainly can prolong symptoms. We also know symptoms can be prolonged when people avoid memories, thoughts and things that remind them of upsetting events. Our 9-1-1 professionals are going to be much better off if we can get them to start talking about their experiences and their symptoms and reduce the culture of stigma associated with mental health struggles.

Clinical Depression Among 9-1-1 Pros

Jim: This point about the negative power of avoiding seeking help is crucial. So, I want to ask you more about that; but you also studied depression among 9-1-1 Pros, and it would be valuable to hear about those findings first. Can you tell us what you found?

Michelle: Sure. We used a tool to screen for depression among those same eight hundred telecommunicators and we found that about 25% reported symptoms severe enough to warrant a diagnosis of major depression. That too is very remarkable, especially when taken as a full picture: about ¼ of our sample reported a problem with depression or PTSD, and in some cases, both. The prevalence of depression in that sample was about *double* what we see in the general population.

Jim: These findings about the 9-1-1 experience of depression and PTSD, are definitely striking, especially when taken together. They merit very careful reflection for all of us who are stakeholders. Your data powerfully reinforce the need for the 9-1-1 industry to aggressively work towards assuring the best resources and most supportive working conditions for these professionals. What do you propose we do about these challenges as an industry?

Educational Information

Michelle: As we discussed earlier, knowledge is power. I think by acknowledging this reality about PTSD and clinical depression among our telecommunicators, we can create an environment where people feel more capable to talk about their struggles and they are more apt to seek help. This is a very good first step.

Employee Assistance Programs and Evidence-Based Treatment

I also think employee assistance programs (EAP) are very important. Most employees of call centers have access to an EAP; these programs are valuable in providing help with basic emotional and relationship struggles. Seeking treatment early through the assistance of an EAP can help prevent development of more serious problems like clinical depression and PTSD. That is, early treatment when one is initially struggling can help build resilience against the effects of later exposure to distressing events.
I have also tried to emphasize the importance of having 9-1-1 centers establish connections with clinicians in the community who are qualified to provide empirically supported treatments for PTSD or depression. Note here

that people often use the terms "empirically supported treatment" *and* "evidence-based treatment" interchangeably, since they mean roughly the same thing. Evidence-based treatments are those treatments shown to be effective when evaluated, using strong, robust research designs and a high level of burden of proof. That is, one cannot claim that a particular therapy approach is effective to treat PTSD after just one study showing that some people got better after treatment. To claim that something is evidence-based, there must be evidence across multiple studies, and study populations, showing that a particular approach helps reduce suffering in regard to a particular disorder (e.g., PTSD or depression).

The Veterans Administration (VA), after reviewing the treatment literature and evaluating the many findings related to PTSD, endorses the use of several evidence-based approaches. One is eye movement desensitization and reprocessing (EMDR; see Chapter 9). Other approaches, with a robust literature supporting their use, include cognitive processing therapy (CPT), and prolonged exposure (PE). These three approaches are considered the gold standard in the treatment of PTSD by the research literature and VA. It may be particularly beneficial to 9-1-1 professionals if call centers can help them identify practitioners in the local community who offer these treatments. If center leaders can provide this direction or seek assistance of the EAP, they may help employees who would not otherwise seek or find these practitioners.

Jim: Michelle, these are such important points: helping our 9-1-1Pros get educational information, access to their EAPs, and to find evidence-based clinical care for PTSD and depression. In Chapter 9, Sara Gilman and Reannon Kerwood will fully explain EMDR and share cases in which 9-1-1Pros were successfully treated with this "gold standard" therapy. As you imply, most of our EAP providers are equipped to provide a basic level of care that does not include treatment of more serious clinical issues such as depression and PTSD. Yet, as you also suggest, the EAP can play a vital role in bridging 9-1-1Pros to these specialists. In Chapter 17, EAP provider Randy Kratz explains the role of EAPs at their very best in service to 9 1 1. And, since finding a truly qualified therapist can be a daunting task, the 911 Training Institute is building a free Registry of EMDR Therapists for 9-1-1 (see Additional Resources at the end of this chapter).

Michelle: Finding the right therapist can be challenging, for sure. It is crucial to have therapists in the community who are interested in serving and learning more about 9-1-1 professionals and their particular struggles, and who use empirically supported treatment skills to intervene. I think sometimes we just say to a person who is struggling, "Go get therapy," but they don't know what they're looking for, or where to look. That's why I am always happy to help people find individuals in the community who do that kind of work.

Jim: It is tremendous that you're willing to personally help 9-1-1Pros reach the care they need, Michelle. Our telecommunicators desperately need guidance. At most 9-1-1 training sessions I've conducted since 2005, at least one dispatcher has privately asked me to help bridge them to a qualified therapist. This leads us to another key point, though. For many of our 9-1-1Pros, therapy is essential to do deep healing work. Yet, many will never go to treatment unless they are encouraged by their peers.

The Role of Peer Support

Michelle: Right. I think that 9-1-1 peer support programs, as you are working on, Jim, have a lot of promise (see Chapter 16). Certainly, these programs help reduce stigma about mental health in the PSAP. They create an environment where people can talk about, rather than *avoid,* their inner struggles. This is really important because avoidance is a really problematic approach to dealing with stress. (We'll talk about that more in a bit.) As a result, I think those first few things hold a lot of promise: providing educational information about 9-1-1 stress risks and resources, working to target qualified mental health treatment providers in the community, and preparing peer supporters in the 9-1-1 center.

Critical Incident Debriefing

Jim: As you know, for many years, our law enforcement officers and fire fighters have been provided critical incident stress debriefing sessions after their exposure to traumatic events. Yet, even today, the telecommunicators who handled those same calls are often not invited to participate in those sessions. This has fueled resentment among our dispatch personnel since they were often psychologically impacted as much as the involved field responders. Did your study explore the value of debriefings in preventing PTSD?

Michelle: I know that a lot of call centers pursue participation in Critical Incident Stress Debriefing (CISD). But the jury is a little bit out on debriefing. There is some evidence that supports it, but a lot of evidence against debriefings. In our research study I did ask people if they were debriefed after their worst call. Some were and some were not. The study found that there was no correlation between their participation in CISD and prevention of PTSD. But we did find that those who had the opportunity to be involved in debriefing felt more job satisfaction.

Jim: This finding (increased job satisfaction) really reinforces how important it is for leaders to be sure 9-1-1Pros are invited to debriefings when they were involved in the incident being addressed. Through the years in my classes, telecommunicators have stated that they feel more respected and valued as fellow responders when included in these sessions. In my resilience classes, though, I also strongly emphasize that such participation should never be mandatory. Your thoughts?

Michelle: I certainly think 9-1-1Pros *should not be forced* to participate in them. In some cases, if you require somebody to go through a debriefing against their will it can have negative effects, possibly including an enhanced risk for PTSD. Yet, again, having those resources available for people is great. They represent the first pieces of the puzzle we need to put in place to help prevent PTSD and depression. We need more research to learn how they pan out-- what impact they can have.

Telecommunicators are a long-ignored population in need of help. My goal and hope are that if I were to do a similar study in five or ten years, the PTSD rate among 9-1-1Pros will actually have gone down. The more I speak with people across the country, the more emphasis there is on doing resilience training and implementing peer support programs, which show tons of promise.

Mixed Feelings about Facing the 9-1-1 PTSD Problem

Jim: I once had a national leader express concern that my educational work about PTSD in the 9-1-1 industry could encourage employees to fake the disorder (a behavior called *malingering*) to gain disability pay, paid leave or to justify abuse of sick leave. In my view it is highly unlikely that our 9-1-1 professionals would seek to be falsely labeled with PTSD to gain such unfair advantages. It betrays their core identity as responders. And frankly, as the brother of a dispatcher, I was a bit offended when this leader made that statement. Yet, it would be ironic if I judged this person since they too may have learned to survive by following that old "suck-it-up" emotional code. I explained that the clinical process of diagnosing PTSD includes safeguards to prevent successful malingering. What would you say to this concern?

Michelle: There are now good tests, and good clinicians, who can identify people who are malingering. Leaders should support employees struggling with PTSD by encouraging them to get the help they need. If one of my people were suffering with a serious problem with really bad asthma or some other problem, I'd want them to seek help. As a citizen, when I call 9-1-1, I want the person at the other end of the line to be as healthy as possible. If they had experienced trauma but had not gotten treatment, they might be more easily triggered by details of a call than if they had they been treated. Therefore, if telecommunicators are battling symptoms of PTSD, their struggle needs to be addressed and resolved to assure that they can do the job effectively.

Overcoming the Negative Power of Avoiding and Stigma

Jim: All of your recommendations here are fully in accord with the National Emergency Number Association (NENA) *Standard on Acute/Traumatic Stress Management*. Later in the book, we'll provide more information about this standard and help our readers build Comprehensive Stress Management Programs consistent with your recommendations (see section 3 of this book). Your message about how effective therapy can be in resolving PTSD is so important. As you said, if folks don't think there are solutions to these problems they are apt to avoid facing them. In your study, you learned more about the negative power of avoiding. Can you unpack this for us?

Michelle: Sure. Let's say you experienced some very distressing event in your life and you choose to avoid talking about it. That avoidance doesn't help you. It actually has the inverse effect. Instead of the distress actually going away, avoidance likely produces and prolongs symptoms over time. That's because it doesn't allow you to process the distressing experiences or integrate the related thoughts, emotions and sensations into your autobiographical memory—the story our minds write about ourselves to help us make sense of our lives and function well. The traumatic experience just gets stuck inside. Fortunately, when folks learn that avoiding doesn't work, they are more willing and able to spot early warning signs of PTSD and seek out the assistance they need to heal. How you cope with those early symptoms can have an effect on whether or not you go on to develop PTSD.

If you look optimistically at our research, more than three quarters of the participants in the study, even if they had acute stress reactions shortly after traumatic calls, did not develop PTSD. My point is that recognition of those early symptoms can play a big part in prevention. Some folks may become distraught when diagnosed with PTSD, due to the stigma surrounding it. That is very unfortunate. I tell people with untreated PTSD: "This is not a weakness; we're here to help you recover." The diagnosis can be very challenging, but by learning this information we can empower them to help themselves and help each other.

Jim: I absolutely agree. And I hope our readers can really tune into your bigger message here about the costs of avoiding our distress and seeking needed help. I teach my 9-1-1 students that, historically, military personnel and emergency responders share the same *Emotional Code* (Chapter 5). That is, they share a similar belief about what they should do with their distressing emotions. The avoidant emotional code can often be summed up in three words: suck it up. In other words, this group has been inclined to avoid their feelings as a way of survival because they didn't know what else to do. I hear you saying that avoidance (which is driven by this emotional code) perpetuates PTSD and depression. In your study you discovered a trait shared by the 24.6% who scored consistent with PTSD: you call it *psychological inflexibility*. It has a lot to do with this whole avoidance struggle. Can you unpack this critical concept for us?

Michelle: Psychological inflexibility has been a subject of a lot of research in the last ten to fifteen years. Before I define it, it will help to first define psychological *flexibility*. It is the extent to which a person can *adapt to fluctuating situations and demands* by rallying their mental resources to think as a given situation requires. It also involves the ability to shift and think differently as another situation may demand; and to shift your perspective of a situation in the moment as you take other people's perspectives into account. The final piece of psychological flexibility is being able to balance your own competing desires and needs in different areas of life to succeed. We know that having greater flexibility in how someone manages their emotions and behaviors in response to any given situation has a profoundly positive effect on one's health.

Jim: I'm struck that Psychological Flexibility as you define it, is one of the key characteristics of a successful telecommunicator! It also sounds like a first cousin to *resilience* (Chapter 6). Now, let's define psychological *inflexibility*. I have a hunch it may be a first cousin to the suck-it-up emotional code.

Michelle: Okay. So, psychological *inflexibility* is being very rigid in how one approaches situations and demands in the environment. It's an inability to take on new perspectives, and a tendency to deny one's own emotional experiences rather than being open to them. If a person struggles with this inflexibility they may try to always deny their emotional experiences and avoid thinking or feeling a particular way. This inflexibly is connected with a whole host of negative outcomes: depression, PTSD, anxiety disorders, eating pathology, and personality disorders. We know that if we can enhance flexibility we can enhance resilience and reduce negative outcomes for people. In the 9-1-1 study we found psychological inflexibility was the strongest predictor of PTSD. It was stronger than any other variables such as high levels of negative affect, anger, basic emotional regulation skills, and the amount of distress a person expresses on the job.

Jim: Michelle, this last finding about psychological inflexibility points us clearly to the solutions offered in this book. We need to respect the traditional ways that 9-1-1Pros and other first responders have dealt with job-related stress (typically by "sucking it up"). Yet, as you have taught us, we must help them see the power of facing their battle wounds and rally to prevent and heal PTSD and depression. Your research not only helps us reckon with the realities of these stress-related risks. It also reinforces the call for us as stakeholders to come alongside our Very First Responders, devoted to helping protect their resilience and mental health. Like you, I'm optimistic that we, joined by our readers, can help them safeguard their future wellbeing and the performance of our 9-1-1 centers. Now it's time to build on this knowledge you've provided and explore the solutions in the pages to come.

Thanks so much for your contributions to the 9-1-1 industry, and to the mission of *The Resilient 9-1-1 Professional* project!

Questions for Reflection

To get the most from this chapter, you are encouraged to write your reflections here (in both the Kindle and paperback versions of this book).

- What was your main take-away from reading this chapter?

- What specifically made it valuable to you?

- How can you apply this take-away concretely to improve some aspect of your personal life and or efforts to support the wellbeing of 911Pros?

Additional Resources

- See Seeking Personal Help: **www.911training.net**. This page connects 9-1-1Pros to crisis help customized for first responders, and provides information about EMDR therapy, with links to learn more. It also provides questions you can ask to help choose therapists.
- See *List of EMDR Therapists for 9-1-1*: **www.911training.net**. This page guides 9-1-1 Professionals in finding an EMDR therapist who is a member of the Registry of EMDR Therapists for 9-1-1.

Works Cited

Corneil, Wayne, et al. "Exposure to Traumatic Incidents and Prevalence of Posttraumatic Stress Symptomatology in Urban Firefighters in Two Countries." *Journal of Occupational Health Psychology*, vol. 4, no. 2, April 1999, pp. 131–41, PsycINFO, doi:10.1037/1076-8998.4.2.131.

Lilly, Michelle M., & Allen, C.E.* "Psychological Inflexibility and Psychopathology in 9-1-1 Telecommunicators." *Journal of Traumatic Stress, Advanced Online Publication,* 2015, pp 262-266, doi: 10.1002/jts.22004

Lilly, Michelle M., & Pierce, H. (2013). "PTSD and Depressive Symptoms in 911 Telecommunicators: The Role of Peritraumatic Distress and World Assumptions in Predicting Risk." *Psychological Trauma: Theory, Practice, and Policy*, vol. 5, no. 2, 2013, pp 135 141,doi:10.1037/a0026850.

Marmar, Charles R., et al. "Predictors of Posttraumatic Stress in Police and Other First Responders." *Psychobiology of Posttraumatic Stress Disorders: A Decade of Progress*. Ed. Rachel Yehuda, Blackwell Publishing, 2006, pp. 1–18.

End Notes

Michelle Lilly

[1]*EMDR and Treatment of First Responders.* With Sara Gilman. Annual EMDRIA National Conference, Long Beach California, August 13, 2011. (Selected for EMDRIA Approved Continuing Education filming/archives)

CHAPTER 5

Building the Resilient 9-1-1 Mindset, Part 1: The Power of Your EmotionalCode

Jim Marshall

Editor's Introduction

In Chapter 4, Dr. Michelle Lilly revealed the truth about the very high rate of PTSD that she identified in her study of over eight hundred 9-1-1 professionals throughout the United States. Yet, Dr. Lilly didn't simply drop those sobering statistics in our lap and say, "Have a nice day." She emphasized that there is now healing help available. There is also a great deal that you as a 9-1-1Pro can do to *prevent* these conditions and safeguard your future wellbeing and your quality of life. It all comes down to building what I call the Resilient 9-1-1 Mindset.

JM

ଓଃ୫୦

The Resilient 9-1-1 Mindset

The Resilient 9-1-1 Mindset has two parts. Part 1 is a healthy Emotional Code, which is the topic of this chapter. Part 2 is the ChoicePoints™ strategy, which we will explore in Chapter 6. To help you get the most out of these chapters, let me briefly introduce you to both parts and how they are related.

Your Emotional Code shapes your mindset about dealing with emotions. In other words, it is what you believe you should do with what you feel. For example, when a family member, dear friend, or colleague dies, this code will determine whether you're inclined to just push through and never look back, or if you're able to feel the grief and accept support.

A healthy Emotional Code serves as the foundation upon which you can build Part 2 of the Resilient 9-1-1 Mindset: the ChoicePoints strategy. This strategy helps you recognize moments in which it is wise to deploy resilience skills empowering you to:

- *Prepare* for stressful events
- *Reset* your mind and body during and after these events, and to
- Sustain your "inner battery" to safeguard your resilience (McCraty 44).

Figure 1 summarizes the roles of your Emotional Code and the ChoicePoints strategy in achieving the Resilient 9-1-1 Mindset.

The Resilient 9-1-1 Mindset

PART 1. Build Healthy Emotional Code	I CAN... A) Deal with Emotion wisely B) Seek the Support I need
PART 2. Build ChoicePoints	I AM... A) Attuned to Stress Cues B) Able to use skills to Prepare, Reset & Sustain

Figure 1

Practicing both parts of the Resilient 9-1-1 Mindset can pay-off in great ways for you, including:

1) More success in moment-to-moment, day-to-day management of distress and that means...
2) More enjoyment of daily life
3) Improved personal health, performance and relationships
4) Stronger protection against developing serious stress-related emotional and physical conditions
5) More positive influence on the morale of your 9-1-1 squad and comm center culture.

So, let's get started building Part 1 of the Resilient 9-1-1 Mindset: a healthy Emotional Code.

Understanding the Power of Your Emotional Code: Vernors and the Golden Frog

The Resilient 9-1-1 Mindset, Part 1

As a kid growing up in Michigan we drank "pop." Where you live they may call it "soda." Well, it's pop! Anyhow, I learned the hard way that one particularly delicious brand of pop, Vernors Ginger Ale, was extremely carbonated. When you hold a can of Vernors even six inches from your head you can hear the bubbles roaring like fans at a college football game. I made the mistake of attempting a sip at the same moment I was breathing in through my nose. An army of bubbles charged up my nostrils and into my sinuses, and a series of massive sneezes followed. It's wiser to let Vernors rest a couple minutes before you drink it. This potent pop is the first ingredient in a bizarre experiment I'd like to propose related to our Emotional Code.

Imagine you and I are now joined by eight 9-1-1Pros on a hike with a guide through the rain forest on the Pacific coast of Colombia. We're searching for our second ingredient for the experiment: The Golden Poison Frog. Its venom has been used for centuries by hunters of the Emberá tribe. The poison of a single frog is so deadly that, if you subdivided it onto the tip of ten blow darts, you could kill ten men (National Geographic).

After capturing this little amphibian, our Columbian expedition heads back to the U.S. We join together in the classroom, all ten of us seated in a circle with tables, ready to begin. I fill up a large balloon with three gallons of Vernors, carefully extract and pour the venom of the Golden Poison Frog into the opening of the balloon, then tie a tight knot in its top. Now I plop the balloon down on the table in front of me and explain our objective, "We want to see how many times we can bounce this balloon from person to person around the circle before it explodes. Who'd like to go first?"

I know; absurd, right? You might wonder, *who in the world would be foolish enough to be part of an experiment that could lead to their demise?* Fair enough. Yet, very smart people may actually enact this experiment every day, psychologically. Here's how.

In my experiment, the balloon represents the human body, the Vernors is the emotions we are filled with as we experience stressful life situations at work and home, and the poison is the traditional paramilitary Emotional Code most 9-1-1Pros have learned: "Suck-It-Up!" In Chapter 3, I emphatically pointed out that stress alone can't kill people; however, what we do (or fail to do) with it can do big damage.

We can effectively release our emotions along the way using many strategies: recognizing our distress and managing our thoughts (as I'll teach you here); seeking support from others; exercising; and through other mental and spiritual disciplines. These proactive strategies improve the likelihood that we may have no negative fallout from most stressors. But, if we just stew in irritability, frustration and resentment, or we keep avoiding and bottling up our emotions like hurt, fear, anger, sorrow, or grief, we may eventually "explode" like the balloon.

The explosion we experience if we stew in and 'suck up' emotion for too long might begin with pressure leaks: irritable attitude; outbursts of anger; isolating; depression; or chronic health problems. We may try to fix those leaks on our own by self-medicating and addictions. Or we might push ourselves even harder, trying to outrun the distress. Of course, the more you run, bouncing that balloon along the way, the greater the risk of a negative fall-out. That may include greater relationship conflicts, worsening mental state, or in some cases, violence towards others or ourselves. Sometimes when we keep stuffing stuff and there is no blow-*up* or blow *out*; sometimes the frog poison just kills the fizz and erodes the balloon—we get progressively sicker physically and or emotionally. So, what's the option?

Changing an Emotional Code, we've lived by for years isn't easy, but the good news is that it's totally possible. Our success will begin by *wondering compassionately* about why we may have adopted this toxic mindset about emotion management in the first place. So, let's imagine a scenario, though fictitious, that captures the very real experiences of many of our emergency responders involving their Emotional Codes.

Wondering Compassionately: How do We Carry Our Pain?

Bradshaw and Telgman are two dedicated officers who have been partners on the road for over fifteen years. They consider each other 'brothers from another mother'. Their agency's 9-1-1Pros have dispatched them to countless tragic scenes over the years. Yet, neither of them has every really 'broken down', 'fallen apart', or 'really lost it'. Until today, when they arrived on the scene of a bad domestic violence call where shots had been fired. No one died. However, the mother was in serious condition after sustaining a gunshot wound from her husband, who then passed out drunk. He posed no threat to the officers when they arrived. Bradshaw searched the house. He found two little boys huddled and shaking in a closet. Sadness flooded him, but he blocked it to comfort the kids and arrange a plan for their care.

Medics entered the house, cared for the mother and then took her to the ambulance. They cuffed the suspect, secured him in the back of the police car, and took him to the station for processing.

Finished, Bradshaw and Telgman headed back to their car to continue working;

The Resilient 9-1-1 Mindset, Part 1

Telgman was cracking jokes, but Bradshaw was quiet. When he sat back in the car, Bradshaw dropped his head on the wheel and his emotions broke open. For the first time in two decades on the job, he started to cry. His own boys at home were the same ages as the two children in that house and this scene had triggered a flood of other calls involving children he had suppressed. Telgman was taken totally off-guard and reacted automatically. He reached over and grabbed Bradshaw by his shoulder, yelling, "What the hell is happening to you? We've been through this shit a hundred times, and suddenly you're freakin' out! Get your crap in a row, buddy!" Bradshaw complied, wiped his face, turned the key and they drove off as if nothing had happened.

This was definitely not the kind of supportive response he needed from his partner. But we need to wonder compassionately what might have driven Telgman to react as he did. What do you think?

Respecting the Old Emotional Code & Weighing the Costs of Keeping It

As close as these two officers are, when one of them hurts, the other will likely feel it too, right? Perhaps Telgman did for a split second. Maybe he didn't at all. As with many of our responders, it is possible that these partners had learned over their years together how to become highly desensitized to human suffering as a survival strategy; similar to suiting up in an emotional Kevlar vest. It's certainly not wrong to protect ourselves. We guard ourselves from physical threats, and we are neurologically wired to defend against emotional threats the same way. After all, who could endure feeling all the suffering of every caller on every scene over a full career as an emergency responder? Some emotional distancing is essential to emotional survival.

By the way, Bradshaw wasn't the only officer on scene that day that had children the same age as those boys. So, did Telgman. When he saw his partner's deep pain, it may have triggered his own sorrow too: for those kids on scene, for his friend, and even for himself. Ironically, even if only for a split second, this means that Telgman may have actually felt deep *empathy* (a sharing in, and understanding of, someone's feelings). That may be precisely why he reacted so harshly. All that emotion may have made him feel too vulnerable, as if he could feel cracks in his Kevlar. All he probably wanted, when they cleared that scene, was to file the report, forget the faces of those two little kids, and go home to enjoy his own family. Now that Bradshaw had opened him up, that would be far more difficult.

Sure, it would have been good for Telgman to *show* some empathy to Bradshaw in this scenario. But there are at least two factors we've got to respect that made this difficult. As many of our responders, Telgman (or

Bradshaw) may have received little or no training in stress management or in peer support. He may not have known that by supporting and joining Bradshaw for just a few minutes to feel and release some of this sorrow, his friend could have felt huge relief. And Telgman may have felt empowered as a friend. Even as vital as basic stress training is for responders, they must also be part of a work culture led by leaders who fully recognize how critical such emotional caring and support is. But their department has always followed the 'old school' paramilitary mindset about dealing with emotions. Their culture was driven by adherence to the Suck-it-Up Emotional Code.

Bradshaw and Telgman's organization was just one of among many in the country whose leaders had yet to change their culture. Again, we are not judging here. We are wondering compassionately, because if we can gain new insight, we may recognize that change is needed and possible. When, for example, police suicides have occurred, I have known agencies that struggled for survival in two very different ways, both deserving empathy. The devastation of the tragedy may trigger a group reaction to hunker down and keep low, governed by the Suck-it-Up Emotional Code. The emotional landscape in the department then becomes eerily 'normal', as everyone tries to go about their way as if nothing had happened. Inside though, many are tangled in profound grief, remorse, anger, helplessness, and feeling very much alone. Sadly, this is precisely the emotional state and group disintegration that refills the balloon.

9-1-1 as Part of the First Responder Culture

Did you notice as we've explored the concept of our Emotional Code that I didn't feature a scenario between 9-1-1 professionals?

I chose to focus first on our officers to make an important point. The vast majority of our comm centers in the United States have traditionally been operated by Law Enforcement Agencies (LEA). LEA's have been predominantly staffed by males. It is a fact of history that males, more than females (with exceptions based on family culture and personal differences) have been inclined to embrace the Suck-it-Up Emotional Code. This style of emotion management is part of the traditional indoctrination of men, "Little boys should not be 'sissies', they should be 'big boys' who don't cry." While the majority of our nation's telecommunicators are female, the Suck-it-Up mindset prevails among responders of both genders. Why? All of us want to fit in and be accepted by our peers and our culture. We adapt and assimilate to survive.

Breaking Free to Build a Healthier Emotional Code

We know from Michelle Lilly's research that the more prone our dispatchers are to avoid feeling and seeking help for emotional distress, the greater their risk of PTSD. She called this bent toward stuffing and avoiding, *Psychological Inflexibility*. Strikingly, about three quarters of the eight hundred and eight dispatchers in her study were females. Had they adapted to the LEA culture in a way that was now damaging their wellbeing? There's a point at which members of a comm center, whether operated by an LEA or other traditionally minded responder agencies, must evaluate the impact of the Emotional Code they are living by. This change is hard to make because we get so entrenched in the stuffing/avoiding pattern.

Redefining our Emotional Code in the Face of Tragedy

Dispatchers, in the aftermath of a co-worker's suicide, strain to understand the factors driving their peer's death. But too often they do this on their own, without support from each other. They may lay blame on themselves for failing to do something they think could have made a difference in the person's outcome. Then they suck up this distress, carrying it as a heavy, toxic load inside. This is not productive. There is no guarantee a deceased peer would still be alive if others had done more or less of one thing or another. Guilt and remorse carried too long only worsen our mental health and ability to make a difference for others. If we want to be at our best, we must choose to get the help we need to heal, and to stop destructive self-blaming. If you have lost someone to suicide, I urge you to practice compassion, not only for others involved in the tragedy, but for yourself.

The fact is this: we usually do the best we can with what we know at the time. We default to what we have found that helps us feel safe, and we honor what our culture expects of us—until we recognize new options. It can be incredibly fruitful to break free from blame and the old allegiance to sucking up sorrow; to resolve as an individual and as a PSAP that you will embrace a healthy Emotional Code. One PSAP team in my Survive and Thrive class defined the code they want to follow this way: "We don't talk about our pain around here. That's got to change. In the future, I'll seek help when I need it. Let's be sure that everyone knows we're willing to hear each other out, to listen, and be supportive."

You may already manage difficult emotion well. Or perhaps you recognize the need to try living by a new Emotional Code. In either case, consider adopting the following healthy Code, which has three important parts:

- I'm going to explore how I've dealt with my emotions up to this point in my life. (Wonder Compassionately)

- I'm going to try to acknowledge when I'm struggling and seek the support I need. (Commit to Self-Care)
- I'll try to keep an eye out for those who might also be struggling and offer them support too. (Commit to Peer Support)

In the last section of this chapter, I'll offer you concrete steps you can take to begin practicing the three elements of this healthy Emotional Code. But first, did you notice the key word in each of these sections of this Emotional Code? *Try!* It may not be easy to let go of the Suck-it-Up Emotional Code when it is deeply engrained. When stuffing your distress has been your primary emotional survival strategy for a long time, you're not going to just start spilling your stuff to everybody. In fact, that's not a great idea for any of us. But you can make immediate *progress!*

Respecting and Managing Vulnerability

A healthy Emotional Code doesn't push us to feel everything all the time with everybody. We've already established that this is just not practical. I, for one, am very careful who I confide in. If we are wise, we'll balance our privacy with seeking the support we need. We'll pick our times to open up, and carefully pick the people we open to. For many folks, it's not hard to allow emotion or seek out others for support. Yet for others, like Telgman, even when we resolve to seek support wisely, this can feel very risky. Take a look at Figure 2: The "V."

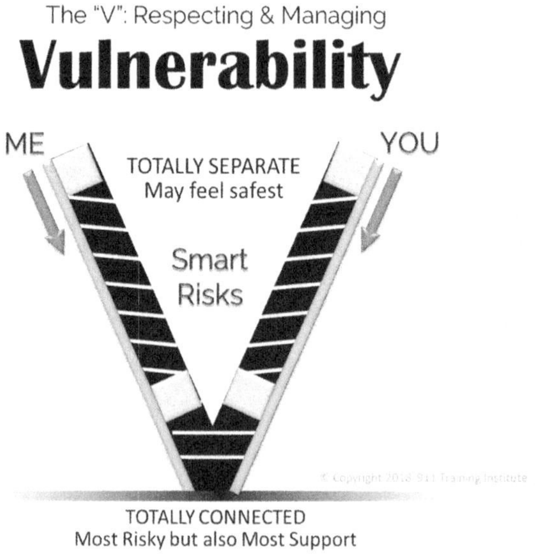

The "V": Respecting & Managing
Vulnerability

ME — YOU
TOTALLY SEPARATE
May feel safest

Smart Risks

TOTALLY CONNECTED
Most Risky but also Most Support

Figure 2: The "V"

The "V" concept helps clarify several important points that are keys to building an Emotional code that's wise to live by:

- *We all need emotional safety.* The more we've been 'burned' by others, the less we are apt to trust, and the more we are inclined to avoid opening up, to stay safe. Also, if we are inclined toward shyness, or if we struggle with depression, this is especially hard. We all need people who 'get us' and who can reach in respectfully.
- *Seldom is the solution in the extremes:* Being totally isolated from others fuels depression and makes support impossible. Yet, opening up too freely to others can lead to violations of our trust and may put too much burden on others.
- *No one else can or should tell us* how much we should open up to others. We each must take Smart Risks, by deciding with whom it is safe to share difficult emotions. The "V" is a staircase with handrails. We may need to take just one step at a time building relationships with peers to establish the trust it will take to open up when needed.

So, take a couple minutes and reflect on how you can personally relate to the "V" and these key points. Hopefully, this concept will help you feel a sense of balance as you strive to improve your Emotional Code. Let's wrap up the chapter by looking again at the three parts of this code and real steps you can do to walk these out in daily life.

- *I'm going to explore how I've dealt with my emotions up to this point in my life.* This is about Wondering Compassionately how you currently relate to your own emotions and arrive at your own code to live by. To help you take this step, I've prepared *My Emotional Code Screening Tool.* You'll find it at my website (see *Additional Resources* at the end of this chapter).
- *I'm going to try to acknowledge when I'm struggling and seek the support I need.* This is about taking steps of commitment to Self-Care. Consider these steps (be sure to read all three, since some may not fit for you right now):
    - Think of one person at your PSAP or in your personal life that you trust and you know cares about you. If you have access to a peer support team, consider one of its members, too.

- o Even if you're not currently struggling with an issue, consider going to this person and being direct about your decision to practice better self-care; see if they will agree to meet you for a soda or a beer to talk about this chapter, and any insights you have gained. Offer to provide informal peer support to each other. If you are struggling, just open up to the extent that feels manageable but make the effort. No risk, no reward (but respect your vulnerability in accord with the "V" in Figure 2).
  - o If these first two suggestions feel too difficult, and you feel stuck in the Suck-it-Up Emotional Code, don't judge it. This is common among emergency responders. Rally courage and give serious thought to sitting with an EAP counselor for a couple sessions. This can really help you to explore your code and gain the help you may need moving toward a healthier relationship with your emotions. This step, in and of itself, is great start!
- *I'll try to keep an eye out for those who might also be struggling and offer them support too.* Your agency may not have a Peer Support program. But even without one, or formal training, you can make a potentially life-saving difference in your comm center by deciding you will proactively reach out to your peers when you are concerned for them. If you're not certain that they already know it, be sure to let them know clearly that you don't want to live by the old Suck-it-Up code anymore and that you want to be there for them. Don't underestimate your power to come alongside a peer. If your gut says they may be struggling, err on the side of asking them if they are okay. Even if they say "yes" (which responders usually do, regardless of the truth), check your internal B.S. meter and be persistent. And remember this thought, however cheesy it may sound, *you already are the somebody that someone needs.*

Conclusion

You may already practice a healthy Emotional Code. If you do, I hope this chapter has given you more insight to strengthen it even more and help build a healthier emotional culture on your shift and in your PSAP. If reading the chapter has made it clearer that your Emotional Code is unhealthy, please don't beat yourself up about it. Remember the "V;" respect your right to go slowly, one step at a time in improving the way you relate to yourself and others emotionally. But definitely seek professional help right away if your gut tells you you're at risk of worsening depression, suicide or if you're experiencing any other major struggles. Go for some EMDR therapy (Chapter 9) even if you're not in a major crisis! Get a few sessions of EMDR if you simply realize you could benefit from unloading some emotional baggage. Free yourself up to travel light and more able to enjoy your life! Explore the other chapters in this book for support, ideas and for more information about resources.

Questions for Reflection

To get the most from this chapter, you are encouraged to write your reflections here (in both the Kindle and paperback versions of this book).

- What was your main take-away from reading this chapter?

- What specifically made it valuable to you?

- How can you apply this take-away concretely to improve some aspect of your personal life and or efforts to support the wellbeing of 9-1-1Pros?

Additional Resources

- Complete My Emotional Code Screening Tool at **www.911Training.net** under the Resources tab.
- Consider reading *Emotional Survival for Law Enforcement: A guide for officers and their families* (2002). Kevin M. Gilmartin. This book has become a classic and provides more insights that support what you've learned in this chapter.
- Try the free exercises and guided meditations to support Self-Compassion offered by Kristen Neff, PhD. Her perspective on this topic, and these resources, are encouraging especially if you struggle with shame. **http://self-compassion.org/category/exercises/**

Works Cited

"Golden Poison Frog." *National Geographic,* www.nationalgeographic.com/animals/amphibians/g/golden-poison-frog/

McCraty, Rollin and Mike Atkinson. "Resilience Training Program Reduces Physiological and Psychological Stress in Police Officers." *Global Advances in Health and Medicine,* vol. 1 no. 5, November 2012, pp 44-66, **https://www.ncbi.nlm.nih.gov/pmc/articles/PMC4890098/**.

CHAPTER 6
Building the Resilient 9-1-1 Mindset, Part 2: The ChoicePoints Strategy

Jim Marshall

In Chapter 3, I set the table for this next discussion about stress by telling you the story of Momma Z, who narrowly escaped the jaws of Leo the Lion. We defined *Stress, Stressors, The Stress Response*, and *Homeostasis*. (You can flip back to that chapter for a quick refresher if you'd like.) Now we need to build on that fundamental knowledge about stress, by exploring how to equip our 9-1-1Pros with the resilience they need to protect their health and enjoy a great quality of life. So, let's start by defining our key terms.

Resilience: The Essential Mojo to Survive and Thrive!

I'm glad the word resilience is spoken a lot more these days. The only problem is that the common definition--"the ability to bounce back"—is puny; it radically trivializes how important resilience is to your life, one heart beat at a time. So, let's cut to the chase and explore why resilience is so important, using an analogy from my life as a family guy (not *that* Family Guy).

I'm going to spare you the details, to protect the privacy of my loved ones. But here's the bottom line: my cell phone is very important to me, not because it is a Samsung or an I-Phone or because it does cool things. My phone is important because it is a lifeline. One of my family members whom I love greatly has severe medical problems that have placed them near death's door many times. I'm not their primary care giver, but if it weren't for my phone, their cry for help would never have reached me. I would have failed to be there for this precious person and the rest of my family when they needed me most. That's why I keep my phone plugged into a wall or a car almost constantly: it must always be charged and on-duty. Knowing it's on and ready enables me to relax, confident that if another crisis comes, I'll be in position to assist. Here's a key in this analogy: if I don't do my job charging my phone, it can't do its job either.

With this in mind, consider how Rollin McCraty, a pioneer in psychophysiology (how the mind and body interact) and his colleagues at the Institute of HeartMath define human resilience:

> *The capacity* or ability to prepare for, recover from and adapt in the face of stress, adversity, trauma or tragedy. *The energy* you have available to use for physical, mental and emotional needs…like a battery to draw upon to handle your daily challenges and duties, and to: remain calm, think clearly and be in control of your emotions…rather than become stressed out, which further drains your energy reserves (44).

According to Dr. McCraty, developing and sustaining this kind of resilience is essential to survive and thrive in every major area of your life. This is the resilience we need to be fully alive, to be present, and able to come alongside our families with the love and support they need, and to serve the 9-1-1 Family. And our well-charged inner battery may be the most crucial factor in determining our health, longevity, and quality of life—especially as Extraordinary Care Givers! (As defined in the Introduction, ECGs are those exposed to inordinate amounts of human suffering on a regular and unpredictable basis in the line of duty). So how do you and I charge our inner battery, to be on the ready like this? All humans need water, sunlight, sleep, nutritious food, exercise, and love. But if you're an Extraordinary Care Giver, you need to do even more to recharge because your work requires huge emotional labor. So, you've got to be more strategic in how you spend and recharge your own resilience batteries.

Have you ever started out a day and you're already toasted, spent, got nothing left in the tank? A majority of our 9-1-1Pros nod *yes* when I ask that question in the classroom. They push themselves extremely hard to manage and balance the demands of their console work and their home-lives. Most dispatchers usually operate on a serious sleep deficit (see Chapter 11 for help), relying on sheer grit and big caffeine. So, may the mighty hand of God help me if I try to take away a 9-1-1Pro's coffee! But the problem with relying on it as our number one source of mojo is that it blocks the brain's fatigue signals and enhances dopamine production (Caffeine Metabolism).

"Wait, Marshall, that's exactly why we use it, silly man: it's a solution, not a problem!"

Yep, I get it: it solves the *immediate* problem of feeling our exhaustion, so we can push on. But that also produces a big problem in the *bigger* picture. If we aren't in touch with our mind and body's fatigue, we can drive our health and our performance into the ground. This is hard for me to say, dear 9-1-1 Family, but you need to hear this loud and clear: you need far more than caffeine and determination to survive and thrive. You need genuine resilience.

The Resilient 9-1-1 Mindset

In Chapter 5, I stated my strong belief that, to rock the console and your personal lives, all 9-1-1Pros need to develop the *Resilient 9-1-1Mindset*. I explained that this mindset is comprised of three elements: strategic self-care, a healthy Emotional Code, and attunement to 9-1-1 stress cues. By practicing this mindset, the telecommunicator is positioned to apply proven skills and use great resources to advance their resilience in the face of extraordinary demands. This chapter is about helping you develop the third component of the Resilient 9-1-1 Mindset: *attunement* to, and strategic use of, stress cues.

Let's start by clearing some debris out of our way--some of the discouraging misinformation about stress you may have bought into, that could program you for failure.

Does Stress Really Kill?

The Iatrogenic Effect! Sounds like the title of a vintage Matt Damon movie, right? Actually, *iatrogenic* refers to a pretty disturbing phenomenon: it means that behavior of well-intended healthcare professionals can mess you up pretty badly, and not just by leaving scalpels in your gut after they sew you back together. Doomsday health predictions from the mouths of health authorities can actually make you sick. Here's one of those lovely messages, *"Stress is gonna kill you…"* Okay, well thanks much, Doc, and you have a nice day too! This has actually been a popular message about stress from physicians and psychologists to the public for decades.

Extremist stress messages like this have also been delivered to us by journalists who pounce on the data from preliminary studies and serve it up as absolute truth. But the phrase "stress kills" is way too black and white. I too have warned my 9-1-1 audiences about the dangers of stress for their health. Why? Because there *are* risks associated with stress, and this book is dedicated to helping you avoid and manage them. But there's more to the true story about stress, and it is actually very encouraging, if we'll take it to heart and apply it. Otherwise, yes, we're all gonna die. (Well, not really. Well, actually eventually, yes. But not everyone will die because of stress.)

An Accurate Look at Stress Risks

It is true that a person's repeated exposure to stressors can trigger a pretty ugly cascade of psychological and biological impacts that *may* lead to many conditions including tooth and gum disease, death, and even worse…erectile dysfunction. And yes, as we saw in Chapter 4 and will see in later chapters, there's no doubt that 9-1-1 stress can be very dangerous. But stop right there, take a breath (really, take a nice deep breath) and listen closely to what may be one of the most important sentences you'll ever read. Read it, and then repeat it to yourself out loud. Stress *itself* does not kill anyone.

Sure, if I am subjected to extreme, sustained, and inescapable demands, like weeks of Chinese water torture, it'll eventually get the best of me. But in general, the impact that stressors have on a person are determined by how our minds lead our bodies in relating to them. In one fascinating study of 38,000 Americans, researchers discovered an extraordinary fact, "it wasn't stress alone that was killing people. It was the combination of stress and the belief that stress is harmful. The researchers estimated that over the eight years they conducted their study, 182,000 Americans may have died prematurely because they believed that stress was harming their health" (McGonigal xii).

Gulp. Listen up, 9-1-1Pros: the belief that stress is a killer, that it is always bad (as killers usually are) is actually more dangerous than stress itself. How could that be? In the last chapter, we defined your Emotional Code as, "what you believe you should do with what you feel." If the mantra you recite in the face of big loss or trauma is just "suck it up," you're more apt to stuff your distress, carry your pain, and end up seriously depressed. Likewise, if we believe stress kills, our minds convince us we are powerless in its force field, as if we must drop to our knees and bow at Lord Vader's feet so he can behead us with his stress saber. In essence, we feed our brains the code and it becomes the software we live by, for better or for worse.

But wait a minute. If the mind can so powerfully influence our health in such potent negative ways, can't it conversely be used as a stress-subduing saber? The answer to that is, absolutely! You can rally strategic thinking to defend yourself from the ridiculous onslaught of acute stressors you face as an Extraordinary Care Giver. Fortunately, it's not hard to learn how to sharpen and wield that stress-saber. So, let's get equipped right now.

Control is Not the Solution

What do you do with what you cannot control? Even if you and your PSAP managers do all you can to optimize work conditions, you still won't be able to avoid stressful circumstances. If we must totally transform these conditions to find peace, we're all screwed. We'll become victims of one circumstance after the next for a lifetime. And no one hates feeling like a victim more than a dedicated 9-1-1Pro. But you don't need to.

By definition, victims lack the resource to overcome this force. But we are not victims when we can access means to influence our experience (even if we can't change our circumstances): we're *survivors*.[1] That is precisely why this book's subtitle is *Surviving & Thriving Together in the 9-1-1 Center!* The Resilient 9-1-1 MindSet is a strategic way of thinking about and responding to those stressors in your 9-1-1 and personal worlds you can't change, to protect your resilience and quality of life. This mindset, will help you to activate what I call *The Resilient 9-1-1 Skillset.* You will be able to:

- *Notice the cues to do something smart for you*
- Create *ChoicePoints*, to recognize your mental and behavioral options in real-time
- *Activate a skill* that will quickly change your biochemistry, and in turn…
- *Recharge* and sustain your battery charge (your resilience) which, empowers you to…
- Optimize your behavior and performance

While this combined mindset and skillset are very useful for how we manage the big (potentially traumatic) stressors, they are easier to master, and super helpful, when applied first to the everyday stressors that often drain us the most. Which reminds me of a Buick.

Reckoning with Buicks. Stop the Self-Torture!

Have you ever been upset driving in traffic? "Um, Duh, Marshall!" you might say. For the sake of your optimal learning experience, I'm going to confide in you about my own driving story[2]. (This is very embarrassing, so it must stay strictly between you and me.) One fine morning, I hopped in my car, heading for Lansing, Michigan, about an hour and a half away from home. I was on a mission to train 9-1-1 professionals. And as you may well know, a session with 9-1-1Pros means (besides guaranteed absurdity and fun), if you're less than a half hour early, you're late! The traffic heading west on I 94 was moving at a nice clip as the sun rose behind me, setting the morning sky aglow. I was relaxed, centered and grateful.
I arrived in the hotel parking lot and strolled inside, pulling my bag on wheels, with plenty of time to set up my gear, then greet my students as they arrive. Walking towards my classroom I noticed the door was closed, it was still dark inside, and there were no tables set up. *What the…* That's when reality struck like someone had just tossed a running blow dryer into my tub full of water: *It's the right day…the right time…But I'm in the wrong hotel in the wrong city!* It was 7:20, my class, the one I was supposed to teach, was to start at 8:00 sharp, and it's an hour and a half away in Southfield! *Shit! I can't believe I did this!* That was

the raw, uncensored thought that burst out of this fine Christian man's mouth. Cognitive scientists call this an *Automatic Thought*. Have you ever said something you wished you hadn't said, but it was too late to take back? (Oh, the regret!) Well, that's an example of an Automatic Thought that just happened to slip out of your mouth before you could take your foot off the gas! (Plenty of dispatchers have more than one digital recording of such blurted messages that earned them love letters from their supervisors.)

Anyway, my emotions were a combo of panic and anger at myself for this colossal mistake. I hauled my wheeled bag back out of the hotel whispering like Rain Man, "shit, shit, shit, shit;" and dragged my sorry butt back into my car. I powered up the GPS *again*, set the new destination, careened out of the parking lot, and pointed the vessel due east. Suddenly, Google turned miles of my route bright red, adding a sweet little symbol of a traffic accident and the note, "17 min Delay." My heart was beating fast and heavy like a big mallet on a bass drum. Staring at the cars ahead of me, the muscles in my right leg were tight as the head on a snare drum, and the cascade of self-flagellating thoughts crashed in my ears like cymbals:
How...Could...You...Have...Done...THIS?

As we've already established, being late to a 9-1-1 event is sinful enough. But being absent for the entire morning—of the class I was supposed to *teach*–I was quite certain that should bring the death penalty.

Part of me was saying, *Marshall, you need to settle down, this isn't' helping*, but the other part of me, the part that felt it was essential to freak out, took over. I heard myself say, "To hell with this! I'm taking matters in to my own hands." I swung off the highway at the first exit, reset my GPS to *Avoid Highways*, and grit my teeth. Soon I was on a fifteen mile stretch of a secondary road with a 55 mile an hour speed limit. But there was a long line of traffic full of wise guys like me trying to beat the system; and somebody at the front of the pack had apparently set their cruise control to an agonizingly geriatric 38-miles-per-hour! I was working to keep cool, but my grip on the wheel was tightening. I was crazed, bending my head to the left, looking around cars for my first opportunity to pass. I was channeling the frenzied Richard Dreyfuss as the psychiatrist in the classic movie, *What About Bob?*

The Power of Noticing

That's when I *noticed* the real problem. It wasn't the traffic, and now, it wasn't even that I was late. My core problem was being stuck in my mammal brain, the limbic system; obeying its fire alarm, the amygdala; reacting with a pure Fight response to a circumstance I could not change. I was going to be late no matter what, and this approach was accomplishing four things—all bad. I was:

- Draining my internal resources, my resilience battery (McCraty)
- Compromising my ability to think and act wisely in the moment (potentially with deadly consequences if I chose to pass unsafely)
- Locking into that frenzied state of mind that would impair my ability to serve and teach the 9-1-1 family when I finally arrived on-site. And, last but most importantly, I was
- Setting myself up for future health problems (if I let myself practice a life pattern of being yanked around by my primitive stress response like this).

Marshall, the irony of it! You're on your way to teach dispatchers how to manage stress and you're not applying one bit of it when you need it for yourself! That too was an *Automatic Thought*. My objective was to get back into my cortex as fast as I could, to do my best thinking and safest driving. But how? By taking a few basic steps to activate the Resilient 9-1-1 Mindset. (I'll explain how to do this in a minute, but let's get back to my story. Dispatchers need closure!)

So, there I was, blazing down the road at less than forty miles-per-hour, so tempted to jam on the gas, swerve out into the other lane, and pass as many cars as I could. My eyes were bulging, the size of billiard balls. After all, a classroom of tired, over-spent dispatchers would soon be sitting and waiting when they could be home sleeping, because of my screw-up. I lamented, *these guys have told me how they often feel under-valued as professionals. Arrrrgh! This will never happen again.* This was justification to put the pedal to the metal. But there's a time when it's far wiser to take our foot off the gas, and downshift from the sympathetic nervous system to the parasympathetic nervous system, to shut off or change the mixture of the stress hormones we're releasing, to reset all of our systems for the good of all involved (Chapter 3). It was definitely time to *Shift* and *Reset!* Time to create what I call a ChoicePoint.

ChoicePoints: A Key to the Resilient 9-1-1 Mindset

In essence, a ChoicePoint is an intersection you create when you notice your raw stress response and before you mess up your future with unmanaged stress hormones. But here's the secret: you can only create the ChoicePoint in that moment if you *realize* you've experienced the Stress Response. To make my point, let me ask you the same question I asked earlier: have you ever said something you wished you hadn't, and then it was too late? [3] That's the equivalent of blowing through a ChoicePoint, blind to the potential costs of blurting out that Automatic Thought. Then you're looking back at the wreckage in the intersection. It would have been great if we'd pulled into the proverbial Walgreens parking lot before we entered that intersection, to reset and identify our best plan of action.

Noticing the Cues to do Something Smart for You

So, help me help you by trying a little experiment of sorts. Without judging yourself, recall one of those moments when you blurted out those regrettable words (or when you failed to say or do something you later regretted). Seriously, try this right now. Once you have this memory clearly in your mind, zoom in so you are up close, right in the middle of that experience. *Notice* what you're seeing and try to reconnect with the distress. Now, answer the following questions impulsively; as quickly as you can without thinking:

- What was your automatic thought in that moment when the stressor happened? (Remember, this is the raw, uncensored thought. It may be the same thought you blurted out of your mouth; or it may be the thought that energized those words.)
- Notice your *emotion* in that same moment. What was it?
- Do a quick body-scan: where did you feel the distress? It could be anywhere from the bottom of your feet to the top of your head.

If you were able to answer even one of these questions, congratulations! These are the three elements of our stress response that occur automatically when our brain perceives a threat to our physical or emotional safety. I call them our Automatic Cues: Auto-Thoughts, Auto-Emotions, and our Auto Body (sensations). When you notice one or more of these cues, it's time to create a ChoicePoint and spare yourself avoidable energy drains and mistakes. Now, let's bring it all together. Take a moment to study Figure 1 below, then we'll unpack this concept more.

The Resilient 9-1-1 Mindset, Part 2

Creating ChoicePoints
To Activate The Resilient 911 MindSet

Moments Past	Present Moment: Now	The Future
(You've experienced...)	(You near the intersection...)	(Results follow Choice)

Incoming Stressor → **Acute Stress Response**

3 CP Options
1. Notice Cues to Use Skills → • Optimize Perf. • Prevent Drain
2. Don't Notice/Ignore Cues → • Impair Response • Chronic Stress
3. Notice but React Anyway → • Impair Response • Relationships Suffer

Example: Any "Buick" Or Potentially Traumatic Event (PTE)

3 STRESS CUES: Automatic...
- **Thoughts** & *Images*
- **Emotions:** *Fear, Anxiety, Worry, Frustration, Anger, Impatience*
- **Body** *Sensations*

© J. Marshall, The Resilient 9-1-1 Professional, 2018

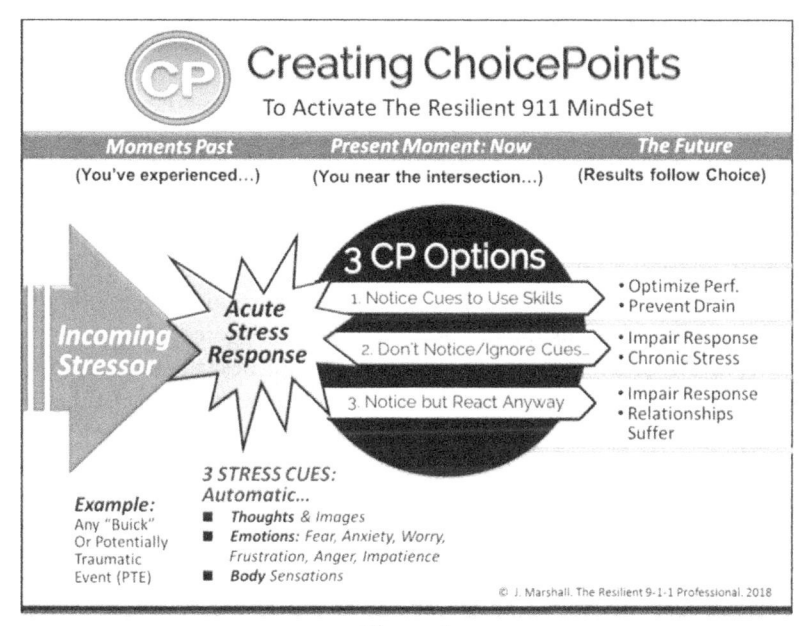

Figure 1

My Stressor, being terribly late to my own 9-1-1 class, was totally self-induced: I drove to the wrong city. When I realized the error, I had an *Acute Stress Response* as shown in the diagram. I was a bit of a mess until I *noticed* the cues. This is the recognition I needed to create a ChoicePoint. If I had just ignored the cues (Option 2), my response would have still been impaired. And stuffing my distress in blind obedience to the old Suck-It-Up Emotional Code would have set me up for more stress-related fall-out.[4] If I had "believed" and obeyed my automatic, raw, uncensored thoughts (Option 3) I'd have continued beating up on myself. I may have also driven like a wild man taking risks that placed everyone around me in peril. (And, as Figure 1 shows, when we give ourselves permission to react to anything we feel without using the cues to do something smart, our relationships will suffer sooner than later.)

That day, by noticing the cues (Option 1), I created the chance to pause mentally for a moment and use a quick resilience technique to reset my psychophysiology. I took a few deep breaths, imagining I was breathing in and out of my heart area, about five seconds in, then five seconds out, and repeated this for about a minute or two. That technique, called Heart Focused Breathing (HFB), was developed by Rollin McCraty, the scientist mentioned earlier. It's based on his groundbreaking research on Heart Rate Variability (HRV) which he describes as, "a measure of the beat-to-beat changes in heart rate." It turns out that your HRV has a powerful effect on your mental, emotional, physical, and spiritual wellbeing.

By doing a few moments of Heart-Focused Breathing, I was able to optimize my brain and body's response to the stressors I faced that day. Specifically, this technique changed my heart rhythm from *chaotic* (where the speed varies erratically) to *coherent* (where the speed steadily increases, decreases, then increases, etc.). This smoother rhythm is called *heart coherence* (McCraty).

Here's why this matters so much. When we produce chaotic heart rhythms, our heart sends messages to the amygdala triggering the fight-or-flight responses by flooding us with stress hormones. To respond to something major, we may need all this mojo, but this response triggered when not necessary, or too often, impedes our ability to do our best thinking, depletes our reserves, and is toxic to our systems. This excessive triggering of the unmanaged stress response (and the bad biology it produces) is called Chronic Stress and is also bad for our health. But when we notice the cues and activate coherent heart rhythms, using Heart Focused Breathing, for example, the heart sends signals to the thalamus. The thalamus is an important relay station in the limbic system that sends stress information from our senses to the cortex. When our heart and brain sync up this way, we can optimize how we process and respond to stress. We're producing Grade-A Genuine Mojo with no bad side effects!

The Rest of my "Wrong City" Story

That day in the car, it took about a minute or so of Heart Focused Breathing before I felt calmer and more in charge of my thinking again. Now I was able and willing to ask the key question at the ChoicePoint that leads to the best possible outcomes, "What's the smartest thing I can do right now in this situation?" After a few moments, a couple ideas came to my mind, and I did both. First, I called the hotel and arranged for my students to enjoy a full complimentary breakfast. Then I asked to be patched into my training room since, surely, by then, a couple early bird 9-1-1Pros would be there. Sure enough! Kelly, from the local PSAP, answered. I sincerely apologized for running late and asked her to tell the class to enjoy their breakfast, and I'd also have lunch catered so we could make up all our lost minutes and get them home on time. I also resolved to put my cortex in charge of my right foot, send my amygdala on a time-out, and pass only when safe to do so. Eventually I made it to the front of the slow-moving traffic. And then I saw *the* car. It was a Buick! It's always a Buick! I leaned forward and twisted my neck, because I was dying to see who was driving that car. You might be picturing a little blue haired lady. But no, he was a 20-something hipster. It's the Buick curse: whoever inherits a Buick from her will drive just like her!

When I arrived, the dispatchers were chatting with each other and smiling as they finished their bacon and eggs. That may have been the first breakfast in a long time they ate during work hours while it was still hot!! These 9-1-1Pros were incredibly gracious and forgiving. We ended up having a great day together. As regrettable as this mistake was, it was not a catastrophe; I wasn't running for my life from Leo the Lion. The stressor I faced that day on the road was not a life-threatening stressor. It was a friggin' *Buick*.

What are Your Buicks?

Are there Buicks in your life at work or home, important but not life-threatening, that you tend to get too jacked up about, like I did? 9-1-1Pros in my classes can make a very long list of Buicks that may get the best of them: callers abusing the 9-1-1 line in many varied and sundry forms (we won't even go there!); field responders that are under-appreciative and over-demanding; a new policy flung wide and far, leaving all employees to pay for the sins of the few; expired food in the breakroom refrigerator (threats of bodily harm have been levied for this crime). The list is nearly endless. Then there are the Buick stressors you face in your personal life. But here's the million-dollar question that your health, peace of mind, and a decade of your life may depend on: how many of these stressors actually represent a threat to your ultimate security or safety, such that we need to activate Momma Z's full-blown stress response?

Speaking of Momma Z.: she, along with baboons, and other mammals may lack our fancy cortex that enables us to do all our complex, analytical thinking. Yet, as Dr. Sapolsky says, these critters tend to be far more accurate in perceiving when a stressor merits a full-blown stress response. So, they are far more efficient than us in their activation of stress hormones that place huge demand on all their systems. And that's "why zebras don't get ulcers" (Sapolsky).

My intent here isn't to pick on people for how we respond to stress. I just want you to recognize the toll excessive under-managed distress can take on us. Think about this in relation to your work in the comm center, and ponder a potent question: how many times in a week do you think a 9 1 1 telecommunicator gets seriously frustrated at a caller, a field responder, or (act shocked) a co-worker or manager? Five times? Ten? Twenty? A hundred. Maybe even more? We've got to create ChoicePoints so our reactions are proportionate to the actual degree of threat we face.

Identifying When You Need a ChoicePoint

So how will you know you've just activated the stress response and need to activate a ChoicePoint? Notice the cues. For example:

- Your raw, uncensored thought in reaction to those daily 9-1-1 "stresspasses" might sound something like *How could you be so #@!$%# stupid?... Are you #$@!' serious?*
- You're super frustrated, annoyed or irritated
- Your face feels like a stove burner
- Your chest is pounding like the bass drum I was thumping in the car
- Your jaws are squeezed tightly together like a pond alligator clenching a snack poodle

Creating ChoicePoints during "Hot 9-1-1 Calls"

Hopefully, the steps I took in my story to practice the ChoicePoint strategy, along with Figure 1, will help you follow suit. But, can you use this strategy if you're in the middle of a hot call? I sure don't expect you to say the inconsolable caller, "Please hold while I do Heart Focused Breathing. Yet, is it possible to take a deep breath during a crisis call? Most all dispatchers train distressed callers to do it. So, when could you "steal" deep breaths yourself? Veteran 9-1-1Pros affirm you can take that breath when the caller is talking, as you're entering data into CAD. I call this *CAD Breathing*. You may not get the complete benefit of Heart Focused Breathing, but it will still help a lot. Telecommunicators are amazing multi-taskers. As many of my students who've been using this technique will attest, you *can* do this!

Then, in between calls, whenever you have a spare minute, you can take a few Heart Focused Breaths to more fully reset and recharge your resilience battery. And keep this important factoid in mind: every time you do a few deep breaths like this during moments in between the craziness of life, you're recharging and sustaining your inner battery and boosting your resilience. When could you create intersections preventively? As you get in your car to leave work and before heading home; literally, while you're sitting in traffic; when you change your clothes. Any moment in between life events. Heck, I've even hidden in the bathroom to steal a few deep breaths and reclaim my sanity. Think about it this way: you have to breathe anyway, every moment of your life, right? So why not breathe with intention--in a way that optimizes your mental and emotional functioning. And, no one needs to know you're doing it. It's something you can do anywhere at any time.

To maximize the effectiveness of Heart Focused Breathing, practice it at bedtime. Most all humans lay in bed awake for at least a few minutes before falling asleep (or much longer), and HFB has been shown to *improve* your quality of sleep. This makes bedtime the perfect chance to practice it. Until it becomes a habit, you're not likely to think about strategic breathing in the middle of your busy life. But by practicing HFB at bedtime you will engrain the skill, like writing brain software. So you'll be more apt to think of taking helpful CAD breaths when you need them most at work.

Practice Time: Create a Choice Point!

To practice creating and using a ChoicePoint, identify one stressful situation you've experienced at work or at home which you will likely experience in the future. Begin to walk through that situation in your mind. Do this right now. Now, go through these quick steps just as you will in real-time when the event occurs:

- Notice the cues from your stress response (the Automatic Thoughts, Emotions, and Body Sensations). What are they?
- Now, acknowledge (rather stuffing) them. For example, "Yep, this is a tough experience. These feelings and thoughts are normal."
- To shift and reset, take a couple Heart Focused Breaths (or, if you're in the middle of a hot call, just steal a couple CAD Breaths).
- Now, ask yourself: *What's the best way for me to handle that situation?*

By noticing the cues, and activating this ChoicePoint strategy, your heart and brain will be synced to enable your best thinking and guide your best response. Now your behavior choice is apt to have a positive impact on you and others rather than a regrettable one.

Frontloading ChoicePoints for Future Stressors

To prepare in advance for any future event you dread, bring it up in your mind; then make a genuine attempt to connect with the related Automatic Thoughts, Emotions, and Sensations. Notice these cues to create your ChoicePoint, and then follow these steps:

- Take Heart Focused Breaths for a minute or so
- Visualize yourself traveling through the experience with calm and confidence

- If you get distressed again while doing this, just reset by taking a couple of Heart Focused Breaths, then re-enter the scene, confidently, through to the end of the event (McCraty).

9-1-1 Pros Need the Power of The Challenge Response!

As you can see, once we notice our stress cues and reset by using Heart Focused Breathing (or CAD Breathing), we can activate some pretty amazing and beneficial changes in our biochemistry. One of those changes is called the Challenge Response. I'll let Kelly McGonigal describe what she has discovered, in her own words:

> When your survival is on the line…biological changes come on strong, and you may find yourself having a fight-or-flight response. But when the stress situation is less threatening, the brain and body shift into a different state: the challenge response. Like a fight-or-flight response, a challenge response gives you energy and helps you perform under pressure. Your heart rate still rises, your adrenaline spikes, your muscles and brain get more fuel, and the feel-good chemicals surge. But it differs from a flight-or-flight response in a few important ways. You feel focused but not fearful. You also release a different ratio of stress hormones, including higher levels of DHEA which helps you recover and learn from stress. This raises the growth index of your stress response, the beneficial ratio of stress hormones that can determine, in part, whether a stress experience is strengthening or harmful (52).

9-1-1 Pros who feel properly prepared for the tasks they face, are more apt to produce the Challenge Response, which gives them full "access to their mental and physical resources, and the result is… enhanced concentration and peak performance" (McGonigal 51). In summary, the Challenge Response can save your butt at work and help you rock your future! But wait, there's more. McGonigal goes on, "…a challenge response, rather than a threat response [which triggers basic fight-or-flight] is associated with superior aging, cardiovascular health, and brain health. Middle aged and older men who have a challenge response to stress are less likely to be diagnosed with metabolic syndrome than those with a threat response" (111).

Holy hormones, Batman! And did you get this part of McGonigal's message: when you activate the Challenge Response you're not only more apt to peak perform, you'll produce more DHEA, enabling you to recharge your resilience battery even as you're facing a big stressor. That's why DHEA has been dubbed *The Vitality Hormone* (111-12).

How to Activate the Challenge Response in 9-1-1 Work

Okay, so let's say I've convinced you the Challenge Response can radically transform your risks into gains that help shape your best future. How do you actually produce this powerful response in real time at the console (and at home)? Achieving it is a team sport in the comm center. You and your leaders share responsibility for your ability to produce the Challenge Response: its power requires your sincere belief that you are prepared for the challenge you're facing. So, it's an immense help when your leaders provide you with the training you need to gain competence in performing your core duties at the console, whether call-taking or dispatching, or both. And, of course, you must invest in your training, ongoing professional development to build mastery in your work, and use these resilience skills.

McGonigal found out that the more prepared we feel to face a challenge, the less threatening it is. In other words, if we feel the resources we have to do our job meet or exceed the demands of that job, we'll be able to shift from our initial, "Oh crap!" response and tap into a confident self-statement, "Yep, this is scary stuff, but I'm equipped to manage it. So, bring it on!"

But what if your agency doesn't provide you the formal training you need to build the confidence you need, upon which the Challenge Response depends? Do your best to augment your formal training by taking every chance you have to optimize your abilities and boost your competence. When you can, observe and seek out a senior dispatcher you respect and trust: confide in them about what you fear, ask questions, take notes, and replay and discuss your calls. In essence, you'll be writing more great brain software to optimize performance and prevent energy drains.

But, imagine that a new telecommunicator is cut loose from training before he is equipped to perform Emergency Medical Dispatching. He answers one of the hardest 9-1-1 calls; the screaming mother whose baby isn't breathing. The 9-1-1Pro's first automatic thought may be, *Oh Crap! I'm not prepared to do this. Help!* His heart is pounding, and fear floods his stomach and he's more apt to stay stuck in this basic fight-or-flight response because his automatic thought is accurate. He's not prepared. When this call ends, even if the child survives, this telecommunicator will be more greatly drained, more apt to be traumatized (see Chapter 10) and more apt to leave the profession.

If our young telecommunicator had been trained to use emergency medical dispatch protocols, and he had read this chapter, he would likely be able to reset, rally confidence, and turn on the Challenge Response. By the way, this response not only activates cortisol and DHEA, it adds a third compound, called oxytocin. This helps us become more empathic and connected in all our relationships. It is a great asset to protect and enrich the personal lives of 9-1-1Pros, and critical when striving to help callers in crisis such as those suffering with suicide or PTSD. Now you know why at the 9-1-1 Training Institute I repeatedly say that telecommunicators need training both in resilience and in call mastery dealing with the call types most likely to activate the fight-or-flight response. Your ability to take the next call and activate that "Bring it on!" attitude depends on being properly prepared: both by believing the good news about stress and by being trained to deal with high-stress call types. [5]

So, imagine you're at the console, and one of the calls you most dread (but are capable of handling) comes into your headset. Your objective will be to shift from the fight-or-flight response to the Challenge Response as quickly as possible. So, using the ChoicePoints model, you'll use these steps:
1. *Notice* your Automatic Cues (thoughts, emotions, or body)
2. Acknowledge these as normal, "Yep, this is scary…"
3. Take a Quick CAD Breath as you mentally Affirm your ability, "…But I'm equipped to do this. Bring it on!"

That's it! Notice you're not following the old "Suck-it-up" Emotional Code by just stuffing the distress and pushing through. You're respecting your natural human response, which helps it pass through you rather than lock in place. And that makes the rest of this technique more effective.

Conclusion: Sharing Responsibility

The Resilient 9-1-1 Mindset, Part 2

Earlier I said that producing the Challenge Response and its benefits is a "team sport." In addition to the responsibility that you and your 9-1-1 leaders take to provide and use good training, other stakeholders in our industry who influence standards and funding for training must also do their parts. They include our state and national 9-1-1 offices and government officials. Fortunately, these folks are working hard and doing their best to fulfill their end of this bargain.[6] (See Chapters 15 and 16 for in-depth discussion about national standards and essential training.)

The knowledge you've gained from this chapter about resilience, the ChoicePoints strategy, and resilience techniques are all part of building The Resilient 9-1-1 Mindset. Now, in Section Two, you'll enter the lives of several Extraordinary Care Givers who battled though "Big T" stressors to gain greater resilience. Before you dive into their stories, pause for a few minutes to reflect on all you've just read, by answering the question below.

✼

Questions for Reflection

To get the most from this chapter, you are encouraged to write your reflections here (in both the Kindle and paperback versions of this book).

- What was your main take-away from reading this chapter?

- What specifically made it valuable to you?

- How can you apply this take-away concretely to improve some aspect of your personal life and or efforts to support the wellbeing of 9-1-1Pros?

Additional Resources

- Visit the Institute of HeartMath for extensive and fascinating information about coherence and resilience.
  https://www.heartmath.org
- Read Kelly McGonigal's *The Upside of Stress* (2015) for a great exploration of how stress impacts people and many outstanding exercises you can do to improve your mindset and boost your ability to manage and excel when faced with stressors.
- See also the Recommended Minimum Training Guidelines for 9-1-1 Telecommunicators (endnote 6 below).

Works Cited

McCraty, R., Atkinson, M., 2012. Resilience Training Program Reduces Physiological and Psychological Stress in Police Officers. Global Advances in Health and Medicine 1 (5), 44-66.

McGonigal, Kelly. *The Upside of Stress.* Avery, 2015.

"Caffeine Metabolism." *Caffeine Informer,* 9 November 2017, www.caffeineinformer.com/caffeine-metabolism.

Sapolsky, Robert. *Why Zebras Don't get Ulcers: a Guide to Stress, Stress-related Diseases, and Coping.* 3rd Ed. Holt, 2004.

Endnotes

[1] There are true victims—those who are trapped at the low end of a power imbalance in which somebody is abusing their power to do harm of some kind. In such cases, they need help from the outside to escape. A partner trapped in domestic violence (DV) under the threat of death if they escape is an example. While 9-1-1 dispatchers can become cynical about DV calls because of abuses of the 9-1-1 system, as a 9-1-1 Family, we must be careful not to judge the caller reporting DV, for their sake and for the sake of the 9-1-1 peer who may be sitting at the next console, secretly struggling

with DV too. I address this extensively in the course, *Why Do They Stay?* See **www.911training.net**.

[2] The first part of my story happened just as I reported it here. The second part of the story involving a Buick actually didn't happen on that particular day; but it has countless other times! Still, the inclusion of the Buick in the episode helps to capture my very real challenge that day en route to training: to move from a super-distressed state (while caught in slow traffic) to a much healthier, more effective one.

[3] We often regret not just what we have done, but moments that passed us by, in which we *should* have said or done something. We could say the first blunder is a "sin of commission" while the second is a "sin of omission." These are both regrettable situations in which it would have been better to create a ChoicePoint in response to a Stressor.

[4] In Chapter 5, we discussed how the Emotional Code (what you believe you should do with what you feel) drives our management of emotion as we travel through stressful time. The problem with the Suck-It-Up Emotional Code traditionally embraced by our military and emergency response personnel, is that it labels their distress as weakness, something to be avoided. So, these folks have been more apt to select *option 2* at the ChoicePoint: disregarding the cues of anger, sadness, frustration or irritability, because they have believed they must do so to get the job done. Unfortunately, without noticing these cues, we're apt to blow through the moment complicating the situation and missing the chance to optimize our response to the stressor.

[5] This is also why the NENA Standard on Acute/Traumatic and Chronic Stress Management (Chapter15) stipulates that all 9-1-1 centers provide training in such high-stress call types as part of their Comprehensive Stress Management Programs. (See the Standard at: https://nebula.wsimg.com/711721acb5a76c6e020996ba09a3dfd4?AccessKeyId=3210927A8AD89F7745AA&disposition=0&alloworigin=1

[6] Many states have established 9-1-1 training standards with associated funding sources to assure basic training for all telecommunicators. In addition, Laurie Flaherty, director of the National 9-1-1 Office (National Highway Traffic Safety Administration), the National Association of State 9-1-1 Administrators, and other stakeholders have established *Recommended Minimum Training Guidelines for the Telecommunicator*. All 9-1-1 directors are urged to fully comply with existing state standards and do their best to follow the national guidelines. To download these guidelines visit:
https://www.911.gov/pdf/Minimum_Training_Guidelines_for_911_Telecommunicator_2016.pdf

SECTION II

WHEN 9-1-1 PROFESSIONALS HIT THE WALL: OVERCOMING STRESS-RELATED CONDITIONS

CHAPTER 7
The Kevlar Couple's Journey: Courage to Heal & the Power of a New Emotional Code

Jan Myers

Reader Caution: this chapter contains a story involving struggle with suicide. There are no gruesome details and there's great cause for hope in this story. Still, if you've been personally touched by suicide, have yet to heal, and know you're easily triggered by such stories, this could be very tough reading. We advise you to pass over this chapter; or at the very least, "buddy up" with a peer to read it, stay attuned to how you're impacted, and seek professional support as needed. Whether you read this chapter or not, be sure to read Chapter 9: *Does Your Console Need a Reboot?" 'EMDR Therapy for Healing Traumatic Stress & Self-Care*. If you are considering killing yourself, please just set down the book and give a call to the National Suicide Prevention Life Line, a fully confidential 24/7/365 helpline. Their number is 800-4273-8255. Or text HOME to the Crisis Text Line at 741741 in the United States.

Editor's Introduction

Most of the world's 9-1-1 telecommunicators and other first responders, along with military veterans and active duty personnel still believe there is no cure for Post-Traumatic Stress Disorder (PTSD). Some live in, or are destroyed by, despair, driven by the misconception that their best hope is to "gut it out" the rest of their lives just "managing" PTSD symptoms. They have no idea that this is a "disorder" with a cure! Jan Myers knows this good news because she has experienced it. As a veteran 9-1-1 professional she quickly became known as what emergency responders call the "shit magnet" of her comm center: several callers completed suicide in her headset during the first couple years of her career.

In chapter 5, I wrote that our Emotional Code—what we believe we should do with what we feel—will have a major impact on our wellbeing and quality of life. In this chapter, Jan, now a licensed mental health professional, courageously shares her story about a lifetime process breaking free from an old emotional code that began with childhood traumatic stress. She tells how this early trauma was reactivated by exposure to her 9-1-1 work, leading to

PTSD. I first heard her tell this story while sitting among my 9-1-1 students when Jan first brought me to Oregon to teach my resilience course. It was a story she knew those new responders needed to hear; and it's one I could never forget. Jan weaves this remarkable story together with the story of her husband Mike, a career detective whose own untreated PTSD nearly led to suicide. Jan and Mike's courage, combined with the extraordinary support they received, paved the way to healing and a powerful shared life of service to their peers. In these pages Jan delivers the encouragement and insights all 9-1-1 professionals need to hear—not only to save their own lives, but to also help save their colleagues!

JM

⁂

I was recently asked what it takes to be a 9-1-1 Emergency Dispatcher. It wasn't the first time I had been asked that question, nor will it be the last. After working as a front line First Responder for a long time, there are three things about which I am 100% certain. First, each responder has a shelf life, an expiration date, so to speak. Mine was January 21, 2001. Second, we didn't find the job, the job found us. (I'll get back to that in a bit.) Last, no matter what we do for a living, we are not put on Earth to handle this life on our own. Others support and help us along the way as we try to overcome and achieve, yet, in the end, it is up to the individual to meet their desired goal. As Lily Tomlin once said, "We're all in this together, alone."

My Roots

Be assured, I'm not going to launch into a sad diatribe about how I was wronged as a child, nor how I continued to feel wronged as an adult. In fact, just the opposite. I didn't discover until much later in life that things were not "normal" growing up in my Irish Catholic, military, alcoholic household. Times were occasionally tough. But my normal drove me to become an assertive and independent being. Chaos and dysfunction is generational in my family. So, as an adult, I didn't hesitate when offered the opportunity to work in an environment that included organized chaos, "family" members with whom I could hang out and drink, and hot guys in uniform. What more could a girl ask for?

After working initially as an emergency room (ER) admitting clerk, I moved on to police and fire records, and then 9-1-1 dispatching (to include tactical dispatch and training). Along the way, I met and married an outgoing, funny, smart, and good-looking paramedic; that lasted for about three years. Neither of us was ready to deal with the stuff from our upbringings, let alone be partners in a relationship. Then, not surprisingly, I fell in love with a co-worker. You know, another guy in uniform. We'll call him "Mike," because that's his name. Mike was a cocky undercover narc, full of piss and vinegar. I can still remember the first time we spoke on the phone at work. When I asked what he wanted, he copped (no pun intended) an attitude. I put him on hold and asked a sergeant standing nearby, "Who is this asshole, Mike Pool?" Eleven years later I married him. Even today I refer to him as the 'nicest asshole I know.'

When Mike and I first met, he was a bit more of a mess than I was, though neither of us knew it at the time. The city we worked for was a "bedroom community" in Marin County, CA, where the likes of Sean Penn and George Lucas reside. It's not a place in which a majority of its First Responders could afford to live. And because of crime, it was also a city in which you could never really relax on duty. Just as you began to take a deep breath and settle in, another takeover robbery, home invasion, or triple homicide/suicide with an AK47 occurred. The "Oh shit!" factor kicked in, and you quickly got back to work.

Our Responder Lives and Losses

Mike and I had our share of nasty calls and life experiences prior to meeting, but more difficult calls quickly came our way after we started seeing each other. There was the sixteen-year-old who shot himself in the head after unsuccessfully begging Mike to shoot him. I was on the line with the reporting party, listening to the gun shot in the background. Then there was the triple homicide/suicide, two elderly women savagely beaten to death by a mentally ill neighbor...you get the gist. But the circumstance that challenged Mike the most was the suicide of one of our co-workers whom we'll call "Paul," because that's not his name.

Paul was a tall guy with great thick brown hair, blue eyes, and a smile that took up most of his face. He wasn't your average detective. He was always kind, said hello and thank you, grinned nearly all the time, and just made you feel good when he was around. Twenty years later I can still hear his voice. Very little was said about his suicide. We knew only that he went to the east side of the Golden Gate Bridge, handed a citizen his wallet with his badge, and then calmly jumped over the railing. Just prior to his death, some of us had inquired about where he was, because he had been off work for a while.

We were told he was experiencing stomach problems, and no one was to contact him.

Later, we later found out that Paul had been suffering from depression and was seeing a psychiatrist who had prescribed an antidepressant. This was in the early 1990's; taking antidepressants was stigmatic for anyone, let alone a cop. It was an issue no one would talk about. Back then agencies and administrators didn't know much about what to do with a depressed cop. In California, if an officer was placed on a fourteen day hold due to mental health issues, they lost the ability to carry a firearm. That was a key reason why so many of them would not report their struggles.

It still pisses me off we were all ordered not to speak to Paul. It's painful to consider how lonely he must have been. Mike and I would give anything to have gone against the order, to simply sit and talk with him, especially Mike. Paul was one of his closest friends. Believe it or not, we still hear agency leaders telling their employees to refrain from contact with a peer who is struggling emotionally. So, these suffering responders are apt to sit and stew in it alone, sometimes until it's too late. How sad is that? Fortunately, many agencies are becoming more understanding about what can happen to folks in this business; attitudes are getting better.

When Mike Hit the Wall

After losing Paul, and so much more trauma from nearly thirty years in the business, Mike was a mess, to the point he was suicidal. He had the gun in his mouth twice. In those moments, he truly believed we would all be better off without him. That's the thing about folks who think they want to end their lives, they are literally, yet temporarily, out of their minds. Please never forget this reality. Sometimes all anyone need is someone to listen to them, sit with them and feel their pain with them. Fortunately for Mike, on the second occasion he had a flash vision of his daughter that provided a quick glimpse of reality. Even though his pain felt unbearable, he simply could not end his life.

After the second near attempt, a few of Mike's friends and I decided it was time to make a drastic move. As Mike recalls, a couple of us drove him to San Francisco International Airport under the guise of going out for a group dinner. I only remember thinking that we needed to get him on a plane headed to the On-Site Academy, in Massachusetts. This is a facility which specializes in treating First Responders suffering from Post-Traumatic Stress Disorder (PTSD) and whose lives are in jeopardy. And Mike's life was definitely in jeopardy. His job was on the line, his relationship with his daughter was slipping away, and ours was struggling. I had basically washed my hands of him. He needed to fix his shit, and I needed to fix mine. However, regardless of all of his perceived faults, one thing was certain, I loved Mike. Underneath his gruff exterior, he was kind, compassionate, confrontational, curious, able, and quick witted: a nice asshole. But right now, he was enough of a mess for the two of us!

Mike's Recovery

When Mike flew home after six days of treatment at On-Site, I was there at the airport to meet him. He was expecting one of his best friends, not me. However, I had called that friend the day prior, asking if I could pick Mike up. I needed to see if something, anything had changed in him. This was pre-9/11, when you could meet people at their gate. Without knowing I was there, Mike walked right in my direction. I could see the spring in his step and the spark in his eye. He was full of piss and vinegar again. There was the guy I knew, the guy I fell in love with; not the suicidal, hopeless shell of a man he had become the last few years.

When he finally saw me, he fell into my arms and cried for what felt like an eternity. This burly, strapping, SWAT cop cried with relief that, despite all of his transgressions, faults, and mistakes, I still loved him. I just held him, waving-off those who felt a need to stop and stare for a moment or two. Move along … nothing to see here…

How Mike's Healing Happened

When the dust settled after his return, Mike and I sat down for a long and intense conversation. Referencing the spring in his step and the spark in his eye, I asked him what exactly those people at On-Site did for him; because whatever it was, it worked! He explained that the program was developed by, and staffed with, First Responders who "get it." They didn't judge him when he explained his story, or question why he did or did not do what he did or did not do. They simply asked, "And then what happened?" They didn't cringe when he spoke of blood and guts. Unlike a few other therapists in the past, they didn't pat him on the shoulder and cry, saying, "I can't help you." Mike explained the different care and treatment approaches On-Site applied with clients: peer support, group critical incident debriefing, and a therapy called Eye Movement Desensitization and Reprocessing (EMDR).

Now understand, Mike is not a therapy-friendly, "touchy feely" guy. He's a cop's cop; a man's man. My mouth literally dropped when he spoke of how much these supportive and therapeutic processes helped him. At that time, I didn't know anything about EMDR, and I didn't really care. What I knew was that the guy I fell in love with was back; he wasn't perfect, and his nightmares hadn't gone away, but he was about eighty-five percent back. As Mike and I finished our discussion that day, I recall asking him, "Why is there only one facility for First Responders like this in the entire country?" He shrugged his shoulders. We realized then the need for a program like that in every state.

My 9-1-1 Traumatic Experiences

Back in the day, I was the shit magnet for nearly every suicidal person in my jurisdiction. I joked once to a co-worker, as a 9-1-1 line rang, "I bet this is a suicidal subject." Then I picked up the line and asked, "9-1-1, what is your emergency?"

The caller responded, "I'm going to kill myself."

I replied, "How do you plan on killing yourself?"

My co-worker heard my question and shook her head in disbelief.

I swear, people who struggled with suicide knew my schedule! I listened to grief-stricken family members upon the discovery of their loved ones who had ended their lives, to co-workers, and poor unassuming passersby who were suddenly pulled in to the hell of an unknown person's world. I tried to decipher the words of a fifteen-year-old that had shot himself in the chin with a revolver, as he calmly told me what he had done. And I've talked with countless souls battling hopelessness, negotiating with them to put the gun down, or lay down the machete, or step back from the ledge. Many did. Some did not.

January 21, 2001 was the day the straw finally broke this camel's back. At 3:23 a.m., one of my officers clearly and succinctly transmitted the words, "Radio, I think I'm being shot at." And indeed, she was. A pissed off drunk guy, who just had a beef with his common law wife in another city, decided he wanted to die. He exited the freeway and stopped his truck in the middle of the intersection where my officer was patiently waiting for drivers to blow through red lights. The driver jumped out of his truck and started firing, striking my officer's car, windshield, and literally burning a hole into the left shoulder of her uniform as the bullet flew by.

Rick, another cop was a short distance away. He arrived quickly, and ultimately shot the suspect using his night vision scope. Although this incident was actually over in seconds, we all had to proceed on the premise of an active shooter because we were not certain that the threat had been neutralized. It wasn't until later, when the sun began to rise, that we were able to confirm that the solo shooter was in fact dead, lying next to his truck.

A few hours later, long after I originally had to pee, I was finally relieved from the radio. I robotically walked to the restroom. But by the time I reached the stall, I was sobbing. I had never cried after a call. I wondered, What the hell is going on? The voice in my head was screaming, Suck it up! Move on! Deal with it! Get over it! I finished my business, threw water on my face, and walked out of the bathroom as if nothing happened...until I saw Rick. There's a phenomenon that occurs between dispatchers and street responders who work a shitty call together. However unspoken, we're bonded for life. When I'm teaching today I refer to these experiences as "shit sandwiches." No matter how much we would like to avoid them, we are forced to eat them, and we'll never forget who we were with the day it happened.

When I saw Rick, I started saying wonderfully supportive things like, "I'm so sick and tired of this shit...I'm sick of listening to my officers screaming for their lives!" Real supportive, right? Rick and the agency 'Cop Doc' (police psychologist) decided it was a good idea to take me for a walk. We walked out to the parking lot, where I saw both patrol cars involved in the shooting. They were riddled with bullet holes. I nearly dropped to my knees and vomited. Shit just got really real.

All of us working that early morning were put on administrative leave and sent to the police psychologist for evaluations—yes, including dispatch! Can you believe it? Our psychologist was the late great Al Benner, a San Francisco cop who started one of the first (if not the first) law enforcement Behavioral Science Units (BSU) in the country. When I saw Al, I told him I couldn't do it anymore; my shelf life had expired. He simply replied, "Okay. I suggest you keep talking with someone, preferably a female therapist who gets law enforcement. Want a cup of coffee?" Al didn't judge me, question me, or doubt me. With those words, he just showed that he understood what I was saying, why I said it, and that I meant it. One human to another. How refreshing.

As I'll share later, Al, Mike and I would eventually become business colleagues, working on a life-changing project. He was one of the good guys who helped so many people in his lifetime, including Mike and me.

My Turn at On-Site

After that January 2001 suicide-by-cop call, I began having nightmares that Rick was doing horribly violent stuff to his own family—things that were horrific which he would never really do. When I finally asked for help, I didn't care how much it would cost, or what I had to do. I'd do anything to stop those nightmares. So I plunked down my credit card and took my own plane ride to On-Site. It was finally my turn. Earlier I shared how Mike had received EMDR therapy there, and that it was super helpful. It was for me too. I won't try to offer a full description of EMDR or explain the science of how it works. (Sara Gilman and Reannon Kerwood do that in Chapter 9.) But, I will share the highlights of the results I experienced after taking part in this therapy. Keep one thing in mind: while the healing that Mike and I experienced happened rapidly, every person's experience varies, depending on a lot of personal factors. Be skeptical. But this is my story.

Let me emphasize that before we started doing the actual EMDR, my therapist helped me prepare so that I'd feel safe traveling through the traumatic stuff. The treatment work began with a therapist asking me questions about the suicide-by-cop incident that led me to seek help. After the assessment phase, we began the treatment. The therapist instructed me to keep my eyes on his fingers as he wagged his hand back and forth from right to left and asked me questions about my trauma. What I didn't know then is the "wig-wagging" stimulates the right and left hemispheres of the brain. That's called "bilateral stimulation." I know, I know. It sounds like weird "voodoo" shit, but it worked. The eye movements the wig wagging activated helped open the lines of communication so that different parts of my brain could "talk" to each other. This kind of inner-brain activity allowed me to process overwhelming traumatic incidents that couldn't otherwise be processed.

In laymen's terms, the EMDR experience is like sitting on a train, recollecting the brief snippets of a traumatic event as a scene in photographs or videos pass by. Sometimes this mental processing leads you to the next train station—to a similar event when you had similar feelings. I began by discussing and recalling the events of the suicide by cop. But as the process progressed, my mind shifted to an earlier memory: I saw myself pounding the walls inside a walk-in closet. When the clinician asked about that memory, I revealed this is exactly what I did—pound on the walls of a walk-in closet—immediately after learning that my older brother was killed in a helicopter crash.

As the clinician and I talked through that event, I was suddenly seeing snippets of an even earlier memory: I was about five years old, walking to the store with my father. As I took his hand, he collapsed to the sidewalk. In my little five-year-old mind, all I knew was that I took my father's hand, and suddenly he was lying on the ground. So, I must have done something bad to cause him to collapse. I must have killed him. I walked home alone. When my mother saw me re-enter the house, she asked where my father was. She knew the two of us had left for the store only minutes before. Because of my ill-conceived guilt about what I believed I had done, all I could conjure up in that moment was, "I don't know."

I still don't know what happened to my father that day, but I do know I didn't kill him. He lived to be eighty-four years old. However, I grew up the day he collapsed, taking the weight of the world onto my shoulders. During my EMDR process, I realized my experience at the age of five led me to become a caretaker working tirelessly to assure no one else would ever again "drop to the sidewalk." The burden of responsibility I took upon myself as a child led me to become an ER admitting clerk, a police and fire records clerk, a 9-1-1 dispatcher, and now a mental health clinician.

I'm not saying that other responders' paths to their professions were led by their traumatic experiences as mine was. But it really is no wonder I became a 9-1-1 dispatcher. If I believed I killed my father when I was five, why wouldn't I try to ensure that others were not going to die on my watch? But EMDR, amazingly, put all of the pieces of my life's puzzle together in one flippin' ninety-minute session more than thirty years after his collapse. (Let me emphasize again, the more trauma you've been through, the longer EMDR can take. So, others may have different experiences.)

I've had one other EMDR session to get over my fear of flying that developed after 9/11. Of course, that piece of work led me back to my brother's traumatic death in the helicopter. Everywhere we go, there we are carrying with us whatever is not resolved. There's that damn shit sandwich again. Bad things happen to good people. Accidents happen. Crimes happen. I couldn't save 'em all, Mike couldn't save them all, and neither can you. Sometimes we have to eat the shit sandwich, whether it's a psychotic drunk guy with a gun, a hopeless man on a bridge, or a little girl on the sidewalk with her father. The good news is EMDR can help bring resolution.

Self-Care & Giving Back: Part of Healing and Recovery

Bessel van der Kolk, an expert in trauma, states that when working your way through trauma, it's also super helpful to do journaling, exercise, meditation, hypnosis, and to "give back" (van der Kolk). After my intensive treatment at On-Site, I continued individual therapy, practiced yoga, journaled, put aside alcohol, attended CoDependents Anonymous (CoDA) meetings for nearly two years, volunteered for WCPR (more on that later), and exercised. I never became very good at meditation but the other activities were amazingly healing for me and didn't cost a dime.

Now, Mike and I destress by talking, walking, going to the movies and comedy shows. We spend time with our chronic attention-seeking dogs and spoil our grandkids. When he begins to act like an icky asshole, I call him on it. When I start to act co-dependently about a situation or person, he calls me on it. My nightmares were gone right after I attended On-Site; his nightmares show up every now and then, but much less frequently. We give each other space to be individuals before we focus on being a couple. We're all in this together, alone. I am not proud of some of the things we did together or apart; I am proud of who we've become together and individually because of those experiences. Somehow, after the darkness of PTSD, we were able to focus on post traumatic growth, and move on with our lives, focusing on "paying it forward."

Our Turn to Help: Paying it Forward

After two years of planning and developing, about a dozen dedicated, compassionate and driven First Responders, including Al Brenner, launched the West Coast version of the On-Site Academy. The West Coast Post-trauma Retreat (WCPR) was located in the very county in which Mike and I had worked. Most of us who brought the plan to fruition had experienced trauma long before we started our responder careers, and then experienced more of it on the job. WCPR held its first retreat in May 2001, three years after Mike's initial treatment (he would go through the program twice) and just months after I put myself through.

Mike and I believed there were a few key healing components of the On-site program that were integral to our own post traumatic growth (PTG, which is growth that folks can experience as a result of how they travel through trauma: more wisdom, life-meaning, and mental toughness to face the future). One healing component is reaching out to First Responders in need before they attend treatment. Initially, they are usually scared shitless they're losing their minds that no one can understand them, certainly not the public—and God forbid if their co-workers know they're struggling. To hear another person supportively commiserate and share stories (like my horrid nightmares) is, for a First Responder, like handing them a wrapped gift of undeniable and non-judgmental understanding. Someone gets me. I'm not losing my mind. I am not a freak. I am not alone. Following up after they've completed the program is equally important to assure they experience the same support as they work to re-enter their demanding lives once again.

Mike and I worked feverishly with WCPR for over fifteen years. We lost count of how many suicidal First Responders we sat with, talked down, cried and sympathized with, as well as yelled at over the years. Yes, you read correctly, yelled at. Folks in our business are tough cookies. They're apt to wait until they are at their worst to finally ask for help. Sometimes, hell oftentimes, they need a verbal "brick to the forehead" to snap out of their stinkin' thinkin'. We got calls at our home in the middle of the night, on holidays, Sunday mornings, and wherever we were on vacation—Hawaii, Alaska, Tahoe, the Oregon coast…Our goal has been, and will likely always be, for others to have someone they can talk openly with, because it was so hard for us to find the help we needed when we needed it the most. If we had received training to understand serious stress reactions before and while we were on the job, we may have both lasted longer in those jobs.

From 2007 to 2013, I worked for Oregon Public Safety Academy (OPSA) as a Class Training Coordinator (ranked as a Lieutenant per my twenty plus years of law enforcement experience). One of the many blessings I have received from my own difficult experiences was the opportunity to teach a resilience course at OPSA for hundreds of new recruits in various roles: police, corrections, parole/probation, and 9-1-1. Many of them had served up to five tours in Iraq and or Afghanistan.

The course objective was to better prepare these recruits to manage their experiences of traumatic events on the job. I was grateful to be able to offer immediate support to students as they recognized and connected with their own traumatic experiences.

In 2012, I decided I needed to learn and do more in order to better serve those who had served this great nation of ours, whether in the military or as First Responders. So, I went back to school to study Mental Health Counseling and received my graduate degree in June of 2015.

Today, I'm a behavioral health clinical intern with the County of Sonoma (CA), working with mentally ill clients as they enter the system. I have a caseload of over fifty, many of whom sit in front of me and tell me about how they attempted or want to kill themselves. The anonymity of a 9-1-1 phone line no longer protects me.

As I finished my graduate internship at a local substance rehab program serving clients that included many addicted First Responders, my best friend said to me, "Jan, do you realize you keep serving the same people? You're doing the same job, but just in a different setting?!"

I replied, "Yes, but now, I'm much more prepared, experienced, and healthier to handle it. I've walked through my pile of shit; I stopped dancing around it."

Just a final word about Mike and what he's up to these days? He is the best grandfather that three beautiful kids could have. He teaches Simunitions to law enforcement agencies across the country, and he consults with groups or agencies interested in developing peer support teams, training or intensive post trauma recovery programs.

Applying Our Story to Your Story

Our story resonates with countless others who've also saved their own lives. Through it all, he and I have leaned on the advice of Winston Churchill who once said "If you're going through hell, keep going." Don't linger in it, don't malinger in it, and don't get lost in it. Fight like hell to save yourself. Put aside the notion that you will get your 'old' normal back. Fight like hell to find and develop a "new" normal: new ways to help you cope, grow, and heal. This may cost you. My agency refused to pay for my treatment at On-Site. So, I did. I needed to regain control of my life, no matter the cost. Did I eat bologna for a while? Did I lose some friends who wanted me to stay unhealthy? Was I vulnerable in this process? Was I uncomfortable? Was I scared? Yes, to all the above. Do I regret getting the help I needed and certainly deserved? No. Life is short. This is not a dress rehearsal. Do what you gotta do, now. Do it regardless of what society (or your coworkers) think you should or shouldn't do or feel.

I don't know how or why Mike and I survived. I do know that we leaned on each other, even when we were emotionally and physically miles apart. There was no way we could have gotten through our situations without the support of others. Still, we each had to choose to save our own lives. Others bore witness to our journey by listening to, sitting with, crying with, even yelling at us to save our own f*#<ing lives. We can't do it alone, but no one can do it for us. That's why I say we are all in this together, alone. Thanks, Lily.

My goal is to continue my work with First Responders bringing to bear all my own experiences with this population: as a 9-1-1 professional, and living life alongside responders as a wife, daughter, and sister. (My other brother is a retired police officer and firefighter and my sister was an ER nurse.) Now as a licensed clinician I'm equipped to work clinically within our unique responder culture. I've also been blessed to serve on several amazing projects advocating and educating to promote 9-1-1 resilience and prevent PTSD (see About the

Contributors). I mention these activities not to brag, but as an example of what is possible for any of us as we pursue healing from PTSD.

Life is hard—whether you're a first responder or not. In the end, it's all about perspective. I'd rather go through shit with others, than sit in it alone. I am grateful for those who stuck it out with me and yet I can appreciate those who threw up their hands and walked away. I always look forward to sitting down with someone in need, whether they're in uniform or not, even if I'm scared or feel like I have nothing intelligent to say. Sometimes simply sitting with the person is enough. I'll end with a few words from Carl Jung that have become my own mantra: "I am not what happened to me, I am what I choose to become" (Flavia).

Conclusion

My hope is this chapter will support your aspirations to become a 9-1-1 professional who is emotionally and physically well, as well as ready and prepared to handle the caller's worst day. The choice is yours. I was taught to suck it up and move on. You don't have to do that. Get up and fight back. Wipe the sweat from your brow, the tear from your eye, put aside what others may say or think about you, and regain your life. I can't say with certainty what will or won't work for you, so try different things until you find what helps you regain your life balance and allows you to become resilient again. Through your career as a 9-1-1 professional, you will likely experience one or several calls for service that may rock your world, emotionally, mentally, physically, and/or spiritually. There are many ways to prepare for these events as well as counteract them. Keep reading to learn more!

Questions for Reflection

To get the most from this chapter, you are encouraged to write your reflections here (in both the Kindle and paperback versions of this book).

- What was your main take-away from reading this chapter?

- What specifically made it valuable to you?

- How can you apply this take-away concretely to improve some aspect of your personal life and or efforts to support the wellbeing of 9-1-1Pros?

Additional Resources

- Viktor Frankl - Man's Search for Meaning
- Gifts of Imperfection – Brene Brown
- Bessel van der Kolk – The Body Keeps the Score

Works Cited

Medrut, Flavia. "15 most enlightening Carl Jung quotes." *Goalcast*, 23 January 2018. www.goalcast.com/2018/01/23/15-enlightening-carl-jung-quotes/.

Van der Kolk, Bessel. *The Body Keeps the Score*. Viking, 2014.

CHAPTER 8
Recovering from the Loss of a Peer's Suicide: My Path through Trauma into Resilience

Ryan Dedmon

Reader Caution: this chapter contains a story involving struggle with suicide. There are no gruesome details and there's great cause for hope in this story. Still, if you've been personally touched by suicide, have yet to heal, and know you're easily triggered by such stories, this could be very tough reading. We advise you to pass over this chapter; or at the very least, "buddy up" with a peer to read it, stay attuned to how you're impacted, and seek professional support as needed. Whether you read this chapter or not, be sure to read Chapter 9: *Does Your Console Need a Reboot?" 'EMDR Therapy for Healing Traumatic Stress & Self-Care*. If you are considering killing yourself, please just set down the book and give a call to the National Suicide Prevention Life Line, a fully confidential 24/7/365 help line. Their number is 800-4273-8255. Or text HOME to the Crisis Text Line at 741741 in the United States.

※

My Friend Kathy

Like many people who work in law enforcement, I wanted to be a police officer since I was a kid. That is probably thanks to my upbringing, and Hollywood. My parents instilled in me a servant's heart from a young age. While all of my friends growing up were watching cartoons, I was watching television shows like *Perry Mason, Murder She Wrote, Matlock, Hunter,* and *Law & Order*.

Many years later in 2002, I was working to find an internship in the field of criminal justice for an educational requirement in my final semester at Biola University. I found the Gang Division at the Anaheim Police Department (CA), where I met Officer Kathy Johnson.

She was slender in build, but physically fit. The stride in her step had a purpose unlike any I had ever seen but was not so intent that she passed coworkers without saying "hello." The tone in her voice was the type that demanded respect, but not from a lofty arrogance. She spoke with a gentle directness, never condescending. Kathy was the type of officer who had been around the block more than once, with the stories to prove it.

She was a new Background Investigator in the Personnel Division, and I was the first applicant she was assigned to handle. As a result, she spent much more time with me than was necessary - specifically to complete a background interview for a college intern. Her passion for law enforcement was evident from our first meeting. She was so interested in my dream of a career in police work, she helped set up a timeline of small goals for me, until it came to fruition.

After completing my internship, Kathy convinced me to apply as a Police Cadet; a goal on my timeline. Once hired by the department, Kathy spent much of her personal time mentoring me, along with a handful of other cadets. She went above and beyond her duties to ensure we succeeded in becoming officers. We studied radio codes, reviewed case law, and practiced scenarios. It was during this time Kathy was diagnosed with breast cancer.

A Dream and a Nightmare

Anaheim promoted me to Police Communications Operator in dispatch. However, in 2005 my dream came true. I left Anaheim to work for a neighboring city as a police officer. Yet, after just four months, I decided the job wasn't for me. I returned to the Anaheim Police Department to work in dispatch. During my brief absence, Kathy's cancer had progressed rapidly, and her overall physical condition had deteriorated. The chemotherapy treatments caused her hair to fall out, her weight to fall, and she lost that commanding voice. Even the way she walked and moved made her appear so fragile. As a result, she was switched to light-duty in dispatch. We often sat at consoles next to one another. We handled calls, had legal debates, discussed tactical scenarios for training, and told stories of funny calls. It was tremendous fun working alongside my mentor.

Then, one day four months later, I received one of the worst phone calls imaginable. Scheduled to work the graveyard shift that evening, I was asleep when my phone rang. With a somber tone, a supervisor advised me the department received notification from a neighboring agency that Kathy killed herself at her home. She called 9-1-1, but hung up when the dispatcher answered, and didn't answer when the dispatcher called back. Officers were sent to her home on a welfare check. When the officers arrived, they found a letter from her on the front door. She gave instructions for special notifications to her family, and to our department. The supervisor wanted those of us scheduled to work that night to know about Kathy before we arrived.

Like a dog paddling in the open ocean, I did my best to stay afloat in the sea of emotion flowing through me. I was closer to Kathy than most others at the department and her death troubled me deeply. I had so many questions. At the time of her death, the department didn't have a "Peer Support" program; there was nothing specifically implemented to help employees process and cope with our loss. Our debriefing that night consisted of seven dispatchers sitting around a table staring at each other in complete silence before we started our shift. I tried coping by my own version of "occupational therapy": keeping myself so busy with work, and related projects, I didn't have to introspectively examine all I was thinking and feeling.

No one spoke about her death; no one broke the silence to say they were troubled by it. To me, that meant I would look dysfunctional, or weak, if I admitted I was so disturbed and needed help. So, I did what I do best: work, work, work. In chapter 5, Jim Marshall explains that each of us has an Emotional Code we live by. This code is "what we believe we should do with what we feel." He notes that most emergency responders, and military personnel, were trained on the job to internalize an emotional code that can be summed up in three words, "Suck it up." Yes sir, that's exactly what I did.

How Bob Brought Back Kathy

Before I knew it, seven years had passed since Kathy's death, and it became something like a distant memory. Almost as a subconscious goal, I detached from it, dissociated my feelings and maybe even blotted her death from my memory. It couldn't bother me if I didn't remember or think about it. So, I continued to self-medicate through workaholism, as I suspect many other employees at the department did. Little did I know at the time, my heart and mind were like a slumbering volcano, ready to erupt under the right conditions.

As a police telecommunicator, I spoke to a lot of people. After only a year working at a busy agency, I had heard it all: shootings, stabbings, rapes, robberies, assaults, domestic violence, and very interesting combinations of all of these. They became routine. However, suicide calls were always the toughest.

Some folks who call 9-1-1 are struggling with pain in their lives that may prompt them to think of suicide. They don't have the intent, a plan, or the means to carry it out, but they're in pain and they're reaching out. Others who call mentioning suicide are at immediate risk. When I answered Bob's call, on a Saturday afternoon in the early spring of 2013, I could tell by the tone in his voice; he was at high risk.

"9-1-1 Emergency."

"I need the Anaheim Police Department."

"This is the Anaheim Police Department. Where are you?"

"I'm at a warehouse in Anaheim."

"What is your emergency?"

"My name is Bob. I have a handgun, and I am going to shoot myself. Don't bother hurrying, I will already be dead by the time police get here. You'll find me outside, in the rear parking lot, next to my car. There's a handwritten note to my wife in my back pocket. Please make sure she gets it. I'm so sorry you're the person who answered the phone. Goodbye."

Those were the last words Bob spoke. He hung up, and my callbacks went straight to voice mail. I entered the information into the computer, then stood up and shouted for the radio operator to send officers right away. Our department's helicopter spotted Bob within two minutes. Officers arrived on-scene shortly thereafter. The note was in his back pocket.

There was tightness in my chest, my throat constricted, I couldn't breathe, and my heart raced, but I made it through the rest of my shift. This call bothered me, which I thought was strange. Since Kathy's death in 2006, I had handled plenty of suicide-related calls: hangings, overdoses, people who jumped, and others who injured themselves.

To cope over the years, I developed a strong mental detachment from work, desensitizing myself from most of the trauma I was exposed to while handling calls like these. Later I realized why Bob's call was different; he was my first gunshot victim - since Kathy.

Bob called late on a Saturday afternoon, from a vacant warehouse, located in an industrial area of the city. No one was around to hear the gunshot. He called 9-1-1 so police could find his body. He wrote a note with instructions to notify his family. He had developed a detailed plan before killing himself. This was something he had thought through and planned out accordingly. It eerily resembled Kathy's death. She was home alone when she shot herself, no one heard it. She also called the police to advise them, and she wrote a note with instructions to notify her family and our department. Sadly, it was also something Kathy had thought about, and planned. The similarities were striking.

Reckoning with The Impacts of Tragic Loss

I called out sick the following day. I didn't tell anyone that handling Bob's call disturbed me. As I learned when Kathy died, our peers didn't usually acknowledge when they were bothered by a call. In accord with my Emotional Code at the time, neither could I. We were tough. We had thick, calloused skin that hardened to armor, which protected us from the terrible things we hear. We punched our timecards, hit the "Answer" button when the phone line rang, and we went home at the end of our shift.

So, there I sat, surrounded by peers, but not talking about Bob (or my dear friend, Kathy). I reverted to working excessively to self-medicate and submerged in projects to distract myself from Bob's call; it reminded me too much of Kathy.

Time passed. Days turned to weeks, and weeks to months, until Halloween 2013 - when I handled the last 9-1-1 call I would ever answer.

The graveyard shift relieved us early, but it was busy. I picked up the phone at 5:52 a.m., "9-1-1 Emergency."

"My daughter just shot herself", an elderly male said.

"Ok." I had to pause for a second. The mental and emotional walls I had worked so hard to erect the last few months crumbled. Trying to regain my composure I asked, "Where is your daughter?"

"She's on the bed in the bedroom."

"Where is the gun?"

"It's on the bed next to her."

"Ok, pick the gun up for me, and move it away from her and put it away somewhere safe. Is it just you and your daughter inside your home now?"

"Yes. I left the house about ten minutes ago because she asked me to pick up a couple of items from the liquor store just down the block. When I came back home, I set the items on the kitchen counter and saw a handwritten letter that was not there when I left. I started reading it and it was from my daughter, and I... I... I went into the bedroom and found her."

"Is your daughter conscious now? Is she awake?"

"No."

"Is she breathing?"

"Sorta."

"I'm sorry, sorta?"

"Yeah, but it's like she's got some fluid in her throat or something, like gurgling."

The officers had just arrived outside.

"Sir, I want you to put the phone down, without hanging up, and walk out the front door of your house, with nothing in your hands. I have police officers outside waiting for you. Do you understand?"

"Yeah, I'm setting the phone down now and walking out."

The caller did exactly as I instructed and set the phone down without hanging up; he set it on the bed right next to his daughter. As the caller had described, I could hear his daughter gurgling as she struggled to breathe in the background. I listened to this on an open phone line for fifteen to twenty seconds while police officers cleared the interior of the house to make sure it was safe. When officers came into the bedroom, I disconnected. She was still alive. They transported her to a local hospital, where she would later succumb to her wound.

Ever have a song stuck in your head? The top-hit single from your favorite artist playing over and over? No matter what you do, you just can't seem to shake it. At first you gladly sing along "la-la-la-laaa." But, soon, the constant playback of that song becomes a torment, as it consumes everything you think and do. This is what happened with the father's call on Halloween. I remember every word of that conversation. It kept playing in my head and took me back six months earlier to my conversation with Bob. That led me back to Kathy. Like a cascade, one event triggered the next. I don't remember walking out of the station that day; I don't remember driving home. But when I got home I felt overwhelmed in every way imaginable. I was not sure if I wanted to hit something or curl up in the fetal position. For the first time, I was forced to examine Bob's suicide call, and Kathy's death ... and I cried hard and long.

I never realized how angry I was at Bob. The conversation had only lasted about a minute. He had prepared himself with the information he knew I needed, and it was so well-rehearsed that he didn't give me a chance to talk. Like many telecommunicators with several years of service, I was damn good at my job. I would like to think, if given the chance, I would have been able to talk Bob down, or at least stall him long enough for officers to arrive and help. He never gave me that chance. It wasn't fair, and as a result, I felt a heavy guilt. As if, somehow, I was responsible for failing to help Bob, thereby causing him to follow through with his act of suicide.

"Perception is Reality": Guilt that Isn't Ours

It may be easy for you to recognize my thinking as irrational. But perception is reality, and prior to healing, that's what I believed. And I'm not alone. There are members of our 911 family out there who still struggle with this kind of guilt.
The feelings of responsibility also transferred to Kathy. Suddenly, I felt responsible, in a way, for her death, too. When she took her life, it came as such a surprise. I knew her so well. So, I started asking myself the hypothetical question, "What if...?"

As a 911 telecommunicator, you know that no one is more self-critical, or beats themselves up more than we do. I obsessed over the *what ifs*. *What if* I had seen warning signs in Kathy? *What if* I would have interrupted Bob during his rehearsed script? Would that have helped me save their lives, or changed the outcomes? I constantly thought about the things that Kathy did and said that might have warned me of her desire to end it all. I thought about Bob, replaying his conversation over and over in my head. If you have experienced a similar "what if" battle, you now know you're not alone in the struggle. But, please, keep reading, because there's good news on the way!

A few days went by after my Halloween shift, and I was having trouble sleeping, something highly unusual for me. I am the type of person who needs nine to ten hours of sleep to feel good, and function well. I lost my appetite and was having trouble eating even when I wanted food. This was also highly unusual for me. I am built like a greyhound; I can eat whatever I want all day long, and still not gain a pound. After a few more days of constantly thinking about these incidents, and not eating, or sleeping normally, I knew something was wrong.

I had worked in law enforcement for eleven years, and had plugged away alongside my coworkers, handling countless emergency incidents from highly distressed callers. None of these peers ever appeared to need help because they had trouble coping with a call - *at least none I was aware of*. Again, I felt the stigma; I might be labeled as defective if I asked for help. What would my coworkers think of me? How would supervisors judge my performance? A week went by, and I hadn't returned to work. Two weeks, then three weeks, went by and I still hadn't returned to work. I was voluntarily burning sick leave and vacation time. I knew I needed professional help, but I wasn't even sure how to ask for it.

Reconciling Perceptions with Reality

When I finally went back to work, I met with my manager. As I paced back and forth in his office, he evaluated my performance handling the suicide call. I was surprised to learn he gave me a very favorable evaluation. I had handled the call according to policy: gathered necessary information for a call to be entered within X-number of seconds, added supplemental updates to the call within another X-number of seconds, and got medics on the phone to assist with pre-arrival instructions for first-aid. I explained to my manager how this call reminded me of Bob's suicide earlier in the year. He said he remembered me handling that call, and found I had no fault there either. I had completed my duties within department policy. That was unacceptable to me. What good was it that I handled the call within policy, and had no fault, if the caller still shot himself and didn't survive? Wouldn't it have been better if I'd gone beyond policy, and the caller had lived? These are the questions that haunted me. That's when I realized I needed a break from the job.

With no additional civilian positions available at the time, I was told I was unable to transfer out of dispatch. So, I was offered disability. Disability? I was 32-years-old at the time. I still had at least 30 years of work to do before retirement. What would I do with disability? That label would follow me the rest of my life. I made a personal decision, and voluntarily resigned from my position.

When I started my career, I discovered I had been adopted into a family of six hundred brothers and sisters, who accepted the same call to public service. There is an indescribable family tie in public-safety that intimately bonds coworkers together. This bond gave me self-confidence and transformed my identity. I was mentored by so many who helped mold me into an upstanding public servant. Yet, ironically, despite that strong family tie, I never felt more alone than the day I walked down the stairs of the communications center for the last time.

I always thought I would be the person to have thirty years of service in law enforcement. I imagined on my last day of work all the officers would line their vehicles up, flip on their overhead lights and I would get a final "sign off" over the radio as I headed into retirement. Instead, my last day was just the opposite. I hope none of you, my fellow dispatchers, ever have to feel the way I did that day.

Battling Demons through Self-Medicating

Three months later, I was not in a good place. I was now self-medicating with excessive running. I had been a competitive long-distance runner for several years in high school and college.
I had extensive experience using running as a coping mechanism. I pushed myself longer and harder than I should have in my condition, because I was still not sleeping or eating normally. Sometimes, I ran multiple times a day. I ran to physical exhaustion. Alcohol became my other "medicine." I drank… a lot. I thought the numbing effects of alcohol would help quiet the voices in my head. Instead, it just slurred their speech.

I never wanted to hurt myself in any way, yet I was on a very self-destructive path that would've ended in a dead-end sooner or later. Thankfully, a couple of members from the department's Peer Support Team checked in on me, even after I resigned. Then, out of the blue, I received a phone call from Dr. Heather Williams, a mental health professional. She was employed by a non-profit organization contracted by the police department to help provide support services to victims of crime, as well as department employees.

The Clinical Calvary Arrives: "Well, of course you are."

Dr. Williams said, "Hey, I happened to come across an article on the Internet and it made me think of you, so I just wanted to call, and see how you're doing."

I began to cry. I was so tired, so angry, so exhausted. I didn't want to live like that anymore. I summoned the courage and told Dr. Williams I needed help.

Dr. Williams referred me to Dr. Deborah Silveria, a clinical psychologist, who specialized in working with first-responders battling work-related stress issues. I pictured her in this dark office, candles burning, and "Sounds from the Rain Forest" playing softly overhead. She'd sit behind her giant desk, all her degrees hanging behind her, with a couch on the other side of the room. Oh, yes, the couch, where I'd be forced to lie down to discuss all of my problems, while Dr. Silveria would write cryptic notes on a legal pad. Ah, the stigma of mental health! Following this line of thinking, it is no surprise why dispatchers are so afraid, and hesitant, to seek out professional mental health help. Dispatchers don't ask for help; they *are* the help! However, when I rallied the courage to go, and I walked into Dr. Silveria's office for the first time, I found my imagination couldn't have been farther from the truth.

During our first meeting, Dr. Silveria asked me what brought me in to see her. I talked about Kathy's death, about my conversation with Bob and his death, about the cries from a father, and the last breaths of his daughter. I spoke about my perceived failure in each incident, and that I was running excessively, and abusing alcohol, in my attempt to cope.

"Well of course you are," she said.

I will never forget that response. Again, I cried. Those simple words brought me so much comfort, because Dr. Silveria validated my struggle, and withheld all judgement. She made me feel like my reactions to the traumatic incidents were normal, considering all the circumstances. She recommended several sessions of counseling to include a specialized therapeutic process called Eye-Movement Desensitization and Reprocessing (EMDR).

The Whacky Eye Movement Treatment

During the EMDR treatments, I would sit in Dr. Silveria's office holding a small paddle in each hand. The paddles would alternately light up and vibrate, creating a sensation in each of my palms as I talked about my thoughts and feelings regarding the suicide calls I handled. The relief came immediately. The anger, guilt, shame, and helplessness faded more and more with each session. I felt distinctly different when I thought about each of the suicide incidents. It was remarkable. I'm aware that results don't always happen this quickly, but they can, and they did for me. (In Chapter 9, Sara Gilman and Reannon Kerwood will explain more about EMDR and how it can help dispatchers.)

Aside from the trauma, it took a lot of talking in therapy for me to understand the identity crisis I was experiencing from not wearing a uniform anymore. I spent enough time in the industry that many of my friends knew me as "Dispatcher Ryan." Professional colleagues from other agencies knew me as "Ryan from Anaheim." The old saying "Your job is what you do, not who you are" sounds cliché, but rings true. I spent so much time, and made so many sacrifices, creating my professional identity, that it was more difficult than I ever imagined to leave it behind. I finally realized the uniform did not make me, I made the uniform.

My original diagnosis was Post-Traumatic Stress Disorder (PTSD). After several EMDR and counseling sessions, I am completely healed today. The voices of those I lost to suicide no longer haunt me. When I think about those incidents today, I sometimes feel the sadness, but I no longer feel the anger, guilt, shame, helplessness, and responsibility. I recall those incidents as memories now, instead of reliving them. EMDR helped my mind reprocess those events into a healthy form, allowing me to regain control of my emotions and find healing. I am forever grateful to my family, friends, and those who came to my rescue in my darkest hours.

The Courage to Seek the Help You Need

Understanding your need for professional help and finding the courage to ask for it may be the hardest decision you make in your career. Many of you, as 911 professionals on the frontline, may still suffer in silence, because you feel helpless about what you can do to heal. But, please believe me when I say *you are not alone*. Many in the 9-1-1 field have walked down that path of self-destruction as I did. My life is proof that we need professional mental health services in the 9-1-1 industry, and that those services work. So, if you are suffering, don't be afraid to make the choice to ask for help. Extraordinary healing *is* possible.

Thank you all for your service. Be brave, be safe, and carry on your good work. We never walk alone.

☙❧

Editor's note

In Chapter 9 you'll learn a lot more about EMDR. Then in Section III, the authors will introduce you to a full menu of supports and services you can put in place at your PSAP to help prevent and heal serious fallout of 911stress. There is plenty of cause for hope if you'll take this vital information to heart and use it to shape plans for your personal healing--and for your comm center.

JM

Questions for Reflection

To get the most from this chapter, you are encouraged to write your reflections here (in both the Kindle and paperback versions of this book).

- What was your main take-away from reading this chapter?

- What specifically made it valuable to you?

- How can you apply this take-away concretely to improve some aspect of your personal life and or efforts to support the wellbeing of 9-1-1Pros?

Additional Resources

Save-My-Life-School: A First-Responder's Mental Health Journey, by Natalie Harris. Natalie Harris is an advanced care paramedic in Ontario, Canada. Her book is a memoir based on her lived experiences surviving PTSD, suicide attempts, and addiction.

After the Call: Mental Health Awareness for Families of First-Responders, by Nick Halmasy. Nick Halmasy is a firefighter and registered psychotherapist in Ontario, Canada. His book uses his experiences as a firefighter and a clinical practitioner to help first-responders and their families begin conversations about mental wellness.

CHAPTER 9
Does Your Console Need a Reboot? EMDR Therapy for Healing Trauma & Self-Care

Sara G. Gilman and Reannon Kerwood

Editor's Introduction

Sara Gilman is the past president of the international association of therapists who are trained to conduct Eye Movement Desensitization and Reprocessing (EMDR International Association). She is also a former firefighter and emergency medical technician with a big heart for her fellow first responders. Since we met in 2010, "Dr. Sara" has tirelessly worked with me to educate our EMDR colleagues about the role of emergency telecommunicators as the Very First Responder. She has co-presented with me at our annual conferences on the topic and joined me in writing a chapter in a textbook for therapists on understanding and customizing treatment for 9-1-1 Professionals.

In this chapter, joined by her EMDR colleague Reannon Kerwood, Sara reaches directly to you. Sara and Reannon don't get bogged down in theory or academic explanations about EMDR; they share as real people about their experiences treating your 9-1-1 colleagues; so, you can fully understand this extraordinary therapy. I will let these authors speak for themselves but know this: I have used EMDR since 1990 and there is no way I could have remained in my profession as a trauma therapist without it. The healing it has produced countless times for people I love and care about (including family, closest friends, and many 9-1-1Pros) has been a source of hope and empowerment for them, and for me as a therapist.

Now, enjoy!
JM

✥

Part 1. 9-1-1 Traumatic Stress: Meet Caroline

Another day, another shift. Long-time Dispatch Supervisor, Caroline, filled in for a peer who took a personal business day.

Does Your Console Need a Reboot?

A report of a stolen vehicle came across the morning report. Her good friend, Officer D., called in to report that he pulled the vehicle over. As she said, "Copy" and repeated his location, she was blasted with the sound of rapid gun fire. There was no response when she called her officer's name over and over. She then heard her own voice shout through the radio, "Shots Fired! Officer Down! Shots Fired! Officer Down!"

Life would never be the same for her (or anyone else in the department) following the murder of their beloved brother. Caroline showed tremendous courage and stamina that day, staying 'in charge' as the gunmen took off to kill other officers. In the following months, she continued to provide leadership and compassion to her struggling team. Yet she suffered silently. She was determined to find help for her co-workers. Their pain, grief, fear and sadness were palpable. As she sat at her console, she could see her officers as they walked by the glass wall of dispatch. They glanced at each other with an unspoken sense of hurt and pain they were all experiencing.

She continued to push the department to get help for everyone. Yet, no one seemed to know what to do, where to look, or even what they needed. Not even Caroline. Little did she realize, but she too needed the help she was encouraging others to get.

A year after the incident, an officer attempted suicide, which shocked everyone. Finally, a counselor was brought in to provide services. When Caroline was initially offered the opportunity to see the counselor she said, "No thanks, let my team go first." So, they did. Guess who covered their shifts? Yep, Caroline.

Throughout treatment sessions with the dispatchers and officers, the counselor kept hearing about Caroline. They told her how Caroline took the call, how she kept going for hours, days and months as the manhunt ensued. She heard about Caroline covering shifts when the others were either too upset or too exhausted to come in. Everyone was grateful that she was so helpful and strong. However, the counselor became quite concerned about Caroline's wellbeing. This type of pile-up and exhaustive schedule could pull even the most resilient dispatcher headlong into trouble. In an attempt to learn more about her, the counselor did a "sit-along" during one of Caroline's shifts. After some time together, she encouraged Caroline to follow her team's lead and seek assistance. She offered several appointment times and Caroline bravely, but hesitantly, accepted.

As evidenced in the story above, the nature of 9-1-1 work guarantees you will experience exposure to traumatic stress. It is not a matter of *if* you will experience negative consequences of this occupational hazard, it is a matter of *how much and how often*. The question is, will you be able to recognize it and know what to do about it? Fortunately, there are now evidence-based stress management interventions that have consistently shown to produce positive outcomes over time (VA/DoD, Foa). This chapter explores how Eye Movement Desensitization and Reprocessing (EMDR) therapy is one important component of your success in maintaining well-being throughout your career (Adler-Tapia). We will share EMDR cases involving dispatchers, so you can get a sense of how powerful this approach can be in helping you to reset your stress load.

Part 2. EMDR: *What it is and How It Can Help You*

Eye Movement Desensitization and Reprocessing (EMDR) Therapy is a specialized integrative psychotherapy approach that has been extensively researched and shown effective in reducing the negative effects of traumatic stress exposure (Shapiro). This is not a new therapy, it has been around for over twenty-five years and has been designated as an effective treatment by the World Health Organization (WHO), American Psychiatric Association, the U.S. Department of Veterans Affairs and Department of Defense, and the U.S. Department of Health and Human Services (HHS), among others. This powerful psychotherapy approach has helped an estimated two million people around the world. We mention this because when you see how EMDR therapy works in a session, you may think, "this is ridiculous. It must be some weird form of psychological 'voodoo'." Well, it does seem like that at first, we agree! Yet, when you talk to other dispatchers who have experienced EMDR they most often say, "I don't know how or why it works but I feel a lot better; back to myself. And I'd do it again."

When something seems *magical* it is often because we simply don't understand how it could work the way it does. Yet, we've seen it with our own eyes, or experienced something in an undeniable way that defies explanation. After over twenty-five years of extensive and continual research, along with intense intellectual debates, the scientific community has developed theories of how EMDR therapy produces the reduction in posttraumatic stress symptoms including: hypervigilance, irritability, cynicism, chronic fatigue, visual or auditory flashbacks, and sleep problems. There are also many books and articles that provide in-depth information on the neuroscience of EMDR.

Does Your Console Need a Reboot?

The reference list for this chapter is a starting point of resources if you would like to learn more. You can also go to the EMDR International Association web site, which provides additional information for the public. For the purposes of this chapter, we offer an analogy of how EMDR works that dispatchers have told us makes the most sense to them.

Eye Movement Desensitization & Reprocessing (EMDR) is a psychotherapy that allows people to heal from the distressing symptoms that emerge after they experience disturbing life events. One of the reasons people talk so much about their experience with EMDR therapy is due to the significant results achieved in a much shorter time than traditional talk therapy. EMDR therapy has shown, time and again, that the mind can heal from significant pain, just as the body heals from injury.

EMDR Therapy is thought to activate the natural healing process in the brain. After a few processing sessions, many clients say things like, "I slept through the night for the first time in a year," or "I feel so much lighter, I can breathe easier," or "Wow, I can think about that situation and it just doesn't bother me." EMDR has given them a natural jump-start to healing.

To make sense of EMDR, it can help to think of it this way; *our brain and nervous system are, in combination, like a super-computer.* This super-computer downloads data from life each day (thoughts, emotions, sights, sounds, and physical sensations). The brain's information processing system is an innate operating system that naturally moves toward mental health, by storing all of this data in the best and most organized way possible. When information is stored in an organized and efficient manner, we tend to sleep well and be in a positive mood more easily. Yet the system may get stuck, blocked or imbalanced by the impact of a disturbing event or a pile-up of multiple experiences; so, the download does not occur efficiently. In this case, the system may struggle hard to regain balance. This struggle is similar to how our computers behave when they are buffering and can't seem to sync up properly. When your brain's operating system is overloaded with trauma, everything is slowed down or you simply can't operate well at all…system overload! When this happens, you may experience: increased irritability, inconsistent sleep pattern, feeling jumpy, or being startled easily. Physical symptoms may include headaches, declining vision, and increased hunger.

If these symptoms progress over time you could be suffering from what is known as Posttraumatic Stress Disorder (PTSD). As Jim Marshall explained in the Introduction to this book, PTSD is now also often referred to as Posttraumatic Stress Injury (PTSI).

Responders who have been exposed to trauma will hopefully be more apt to seek help for an 'injury' that can heal, than if they think they have a 'disorder.' You can find out more about these types of symptoms and descriptions on the Global PTSI Foundation web site. You can also learn more about PTSD by reviewing information from the National Center for PTSD. Both websites can be found in the Additional Resources at the end of this chapter.

Through the treatment steps in EMDR therapy, the 'reset' button is switched on and the system which is stuck gets a reboot. It then continues to file the information (memories) in a place that enhances meaning. This brings relief to the taxed system and order to the information. In other words, this process heals the injury. Another way to think of it is EMDR processing is that it activates what we call, the *innate wisdom* of our internal information processing system; it re-organizes the information in a way that supports and builds psychological resilience and promotes posttraumatic growth. This type of reboot allows thoughts and feelings to be re-digested. Then what is no longer needed is discarded. The system is restored and can continue to process future experiences. This type of intervention assists the mind and body to work at its best and is a key component to maintaining mental toughness and resilience throughout the 9-1-1Pro's highly stressful career.

When our super-computer is running efficiently, it is easier to be our best selves: happier, sleeping well, and more easily productive. We are no longer stuck 'buffering' to find peace and calm. Life is easier. People who have been through significant life events and have posttraumatic stress symptoms are not broken or weak, they are just stuck. EMDR therapy helps to get things moving again in a healthier way.

What does an EMDR session look like?

Your first meeting will be a time to share your story and some of your history, both professionally and personally. The therapist will ask you a variety of questions about your life and health to get an idea of how best to proceed. You will describe what types of stress reactions you are having and how they are affecting you. Don't worry if you aren't sure about how things are affecting you. The therapist will help you clarify this. Depending on how many sessions your insurance covers (or personal finances can afford) with your EMDR therapist, the first meeting will also include an explanation of the EMDR therapy process.

In the first session, you will also discuss treatment goals, strategies and the length of treatment.

Your Employee Assistance Program (EAP Chapter 17), or other insurances, may only allot for about three to six sessions, which may not seem like enough. However, you will be surprised about the relief and progress you can make with an experienced EMDR therapist in a relatively short amount of time.

The sessions which follow, will focus on processing the emotional distress that brought you in for treatment. You will also learn skills to help soothe your mind and body, such as breathing techniques and visualizations. Stress management strategies will be discussed and practiced. The therapist will then use EMDR processing to reset your system.

The Mechanics of EMDR

The EMDR processing is done by prompting 'bilateral' activation of the brain—alternating stimulation of the right and left hemispheres using any one of several approaches: the therapist can wave a pointer across your field of vision guiding your "eye movements" left and right repeatedly. Bilateral activation can also be prompted with two gently and alternatingly vibrating 'tappers', one held in each hand, or through headphones emitting alternating tones in the right and left ears. All three of these methods 'wake up' the whole brain and activate the re-filing system. This manually prompted bilateral activation is similar to Rapid Eye Movement (REM) patterns we naturally experience during sleep.

Part 3. Up Close and Personal: Examples of EMDR's "Magic"

In this part of the chapter we will share stories of 9-1-1Pros who have experienced repeated exposure to traumatic events and who sought out EMDR therapy. Their experiences demonstrate how this intervention can help reboot your over-taxed system. These stories are a combination of various cases, with names and certain information changed to maintain confidentiality.

Case Study #1
Here Comes my First Dispatcher! "I was fine, until I wasn't."
Reannon and Sandy's Journey Together

Although I have been a therapist for a long time, with thousands of client hours under my belt, Sandy was my first dispatcher. She was forty-four years old and had been doing 9-1-1 telecommunicating for nine years when we began working together.

She had never had any work related 'issues', as she put it, until after the death of her father. Sandy knew her department offered a program she could access to see a counselor with no questions asked. Still, she was reluctant to make the call. She wanted to believe that her overwhelming sense of loss would go away on its own. Who could blame her? Sandy had suffered several weeks: she was easily irritated at work; couldn't sleep when she was off; and, she felt really lonely.

One day a co-worker asked Sandy if she was okay. The co-worker had noticed Sandy didn't seem like herself lately. When asked this question, she felt embarrassed and responded with, "Sure, I'm fine, just tired lately." Soon after that she decided she wasn't able to shake it off, so she made the call for an appointment. Then she promptly cancelled it. Yet I knew she had good reason to call for help, so I was persistent in getting her scheduled for an appointment. I knew once she came in she would be feeling better sooner rather than later.

Sandy eventually made her way through the door. We discussed how hard it was emotionally for her get to my office, even though she fully knew how much she needed help. She had always been supportive of peers taking advantage of the EAP but going herself felt far more difficult. In our first session we discussed her Dad. She recalled what she would miss most about him, as well as some things that occurred while he was dying. We then practiced some skills to help her navigate through the irritated feeling which would pop up at work. At the end of the session, I asked Sandy if she thought therapy was as awful as she imagined. She laughed, said "No," and asked for another appointment. I felt relieved that we had begun her reboot.

Sandy was adamant that what she was experiencing had nothing to do with work. She was just sad and moving through her grief. Work was just something which interfered with the process. So, we decided to focus on grieving the loss of her father. However, during the EMDR processing, in between the sets of bilateral activation (administered through the alternating buzzing of the tappers—much like the vibration from a cell phone), she spontaneously remembered a call from earlier in her career. She remarked, "I don't know why I'm thinking about this now, but I remember a call from years ago." I encouraged her to follow that memory. The sounds and pictures in her mind of an elderly man bubbled up; thoughts and feelings of sadness about what he and his family had been through also surfaced. Once these memories came up, they quickly passed through her mind and the feeling of sadness dissipated—as if the air in a balloon was released.

As Sandy's shoulders dropped, her chest loosened and she was able to breathe easier. She said, "Now I understand what that family went through. I miss my Dad." Sandy started asking questions about "that cumulative career stress thing" I had explained to her earlier. Her nervous system, mind and body, had been managing to keep things filed away for years. It wasn't until she had something terrible and unexpected happen in her own life that a similar human experience in her memory bank was brought up. While her grief about her father appeared to have nothing to do with her 9-1-1 work, they shared something in common which soon became apparent. These experiences were filed together in her brain because they both involved unexpected and sad moments over which she had *no control*.

EMDR processing jump-started her system, enabling her to refile these connected experiences. So, it came as no surprise to me that soon after this session, Sandy began to feel like herself again. She reported sleeping better, smiling more and was less irritable and preoccupied with negative thoughts. With a big focus on improved self-care in and out of work, she felt like she had a renewed energy to do more for herself. She became more social, developed a sleep routine, joined a book club and went for walks during her lunch breaks at work. Her co-workers mentioned that she, "sure seemed happier lately."

Sandy will be the first to tell you that she was *fine, until she wasn't*. She loved her job and she was really good at it. Through her EMDR work, she discovered that a 9-1-1Pro doesn't have to be totally debilitated by a massive critical incident or other traumatic event for this treatment to be helpful. She now knows her own red flags and early warning signs of a stress pile up and is quick to take action. With a maintenance session every now and then, Sandy stays healthy and emotionally solid. She is able to do her best work without it taking such a toll on her energy, sleep and joy in life.

Case Study #2
Dr. Sara Reaches out to Dispatch supervisor Caroline: "Shots Fired, Officer Down… I've got this… Now it's got me"

At the beginning of this chapter, I introduced you to Caroline. I was greatly impacted by her story. This woman's courage, endurance, depth of silent suffering and then profound healing, is etched in my heart with the clear message that dispatchers truly *are* our very *first* First-Responders.

Caroline was a twenty-year veteran dispatch supervisor. She was under the headset when her good friend, Officer D., was gunned down. Twelve months following the incident, with the sound of gunshots stuck in her head, she startled at the littlest noises both at work and home. She was an avid hunter, yet now found it intolerable to be out in the open. She felt vulnerable, and the sound of the gun firing made her nauseated. Many nights she would wake up, sometimes in a pool of sweat, unable to shake the images of her friend's death. The slightest change in the tone of an officer's voice over the radio would cause an immediate adrenaline rush. She would be full of fear and become hyper-vigilant.

She also noticed over those months that her eye-sight and hearing got progressively worse. She had been an accomplished nature photographer; then she just couldn't do it anymore. It felt like too much work and it frustrated her. Her growing sadness was evident to some, yet she did her best to hide it. The things she loved—being in nature, hunting, photography, being with friends—were fading away. Everything just seemed too hard. She found herself wanting to be alone more and more. Yet, she continued to take on extra shifts. When I asked her why she voluntarily took on so many overtime hours she said, "To spare my team...just in case something bad happens. I'll be the one there to take the call. I don't want anyone to go through what I've been through."

In our first session, Caroline told me what the last year had been like for her. I could hear her sense of purpose in wanting to support others at work. Yet, I also heard the progressive isolation and significant symptoms of posttraumatic stress overload. I explained to her that the things she was experiencing were all due to an overloaded system, full of stuck information. I explained how EMDR worked and how it might help her rebound from this tragedy. She was skeptical, yet open. She said, "I just figured that this is how I will always feel after such a horrible experience." I assured her that once her system was operating more efficiently, her life would be easier and happier.

We began EMDR processing as she told me the story of what happened on the day of the shooting. With each set of eye-movements we activated, she moved through the memories of her experience with tears and frequent deep sighs; as if her body and mind were letting go of piled-up energy blocks. There was one particular looping thought she had been telling herself: *I should have found out more about the vehicle and the men who stole it. Then maybe I could have told him to stand-down. I didn't protect him, it's my fault.* Caroline had not told anyone she struggled with this thought. She had held on to it for a year; suffering in silence. It caused her to believe that she had to protect everyone, thus the hypervigilance and over working.

Through the EMDR processing, these thoughts were re-digested and their painful emotional charge dissipated. This allowed a new, healthier thought to emerge; during this EMDR session she spontaneously said, "Everything happened so fast. There was nothing I could've done for Officer D. I was able to stay focused to help save the other officers…no one else died. Officer D. would've been proud of me for being able to do that." With her confidence in these new thoughts, Caroline was able to forgive herself. She reconnected with positive memories of her relationship with Officer D., which restored her connection to his life, not just his death. This was only the first session…

The stuck belief, "It's my fault," had impacted her in many ways throughout the year. We discovered other circumstances in her life where she experienced a similar sense of shame and self-blame. Working through this helped bring her previous thoughts, feelings and memories into a current, healthier understanding. This helped to jump-start her healing.

Following the first session, she began sleeping better, no longer jolted awake by distress. This is so important because when someone starts sleeping better, they can clock more REM sleep, which naturally supports efficient filing of information from memories and experiences. This, in turn, helps the super-computer get un-stuck so it can stop buffering and start filing.

By the third EMDR session, she asked me if my 'magic wand' (a pointer I use to prompt clients' eye-movements) could improve eye-sight and hearing? I asked her to tell me what prompted this question, what she was noticing in herself. She said, "I forgot to tell you. My hearing had been getting so bad that I went to the doctor a few months ago. They said it's declining, and I might have to get hearing-aids. Also, I've had to get two new vision prescriptions in the last year, because my eye-sight was getting worse. I just thought it was an aging thing. Since we've been doing the EMDR, everything around me looks brighter. It's easier to read and my eyes don't get so tired as fast. I've even been taking *off* my glasses to do things. I noticed the other day that I actually turned *down* the radio, which I've only been turning up in the past year. So, I decided to pick up my camera and go take some shots. It was amazing how I was able to see things and enjoy my photography again." Tears were rolling down her face, as they were mine. Caroline was able to regain parts of herself and her life that she loved. She started feeling like herself again.

While I don't know if the 'magic wand' actually restored her hearing and seeing, what I believe is that her system reboot through EMDR restored her mind and body systems to a more efficient way of operating.
This may have allowed her sight and hearing to be restored as well. When we are overloaded with stress, grief, negative thoughts and exhaustion, it is hard for our mind, body and soul to do its best job.

Caroline's recovery was remarkable. It pained me that she had spent a long year of suffering before getting help and healing. Caroline may have begun to bounce back much sooner if her department understood the keys to mental health and resiliency and provided easy access to counseling and EMDR services. This is not a criticism of our emergency response agencies; it is recognition of the need for this chapter and this book. Caroline is my reminder to keep educating these agencies about the importance of helping their employees reboot mentally throughout their careers. Such regular rebooting can produce great gains: a much healthier and happier work force, in turn yielding better efficiency, higher productivity, less sick time and improved retention. This all translates to a cost savings to the agency. It is important that 9-1-1 centers and their clinical providers gather data to show such positive outcomes of providing mental health services to dispatchers (and all first responders). Research is already showing positive outcomes of early EMDR intervention with rescue workers, yet there needs to be more specifically related to outcomes with dispatchers.

Part 4. Hello 9-1-1 Professional...What's Your Emergency?" Knowing When to Call for 'Back-Up'

In this part of the chapter, we want to help you identify stress *pile-ups* that may occur in yourself and others, and how to pursue self-care when these pile-ups happen. This ability will be important to prevent worsening struggles. Still, despite your best efforts, you might suffer significantly from a *single call* that would normally be no big deal. And in some cases, even without any apparent connection to a specific call, you may begin feeling like you're *not yourself*. However the onset of your struggle may occur, you're more apt to recognize the need for help when any of the following signs arise:

- You struggle with deeply troubling self-doubts. In the privacy of your own self-talk, you may hear yourself say things like, "*If only* I would have gotten the address faster, they would have survived" or "Why didn't I say it another way so I could keep them on the line?" or "My officer got hurt because I didn't act fast enough."

- You suddenly wake up and you're upset; having nightmares or night terrors
- You can't stop thinking about or hearing a portion of an incident, replaying it over and over.
- You're over focused on something in your personal life and can't let it go,
- You find yourself really pissed-off about something that generally wouldn't get you so riled up.
- You feel tightness in your chest, or are now routinely holding your breath when you put your headset, or when a particular call type comes in.
- Your stress management and self-care tools just don't seem to be helping the way they usually do. For example, exercise or a walk has become exhausting rather than reviving you.
- You don't want to do things you normally enjoy.
- You experience changes in sleep pattern: insomnia; broken sleep; sleeping too much or not enough; and, not feeling rested upon awakening.
- You find yourself using some unhealthy coping mechanisms like drinking more alcohol than you have in the past, or more than you expect to drink on more than one occasion.
- You minimize and push through serious distress that deserves support, saying to yourself, "It's just part of the job. I'm fine."

If you can relate to these signs of serious struggle, please don't wait to get help. You may find relief with a couple EMDR sessions. A qualified therapist can help you look at your situation and help you release the grip that your distress may have on you and your nervous system.

How EMDR Therapy Builds Resiliency

Recent neuroscience research shows that getting this super-computer reboot sooner rather than later may improve how your experiences and memories are filed. So, rebooting sooner after critical incidents may prevent a stress pile-up, possibly even posttraumatic stress disorder.

The Webster Dictionary defines resilience as, "The capacity to recover quickly from difficulties; toughness." Sustained resilience is the goal for 9-1-1Pros: to continue building resilience throughout your career. EMDR is one important ingredient in achieving this goal. It keeps your mind and body in the best shape possible, while you are continually exposed to traumatic experiences and human tragedy on the job. A quick recovery is the first thing on everyone's mind when they are physically injured. Dealing with post-traumatic stress injury is no different.

EMDR jump-starts quick recovery mentally by hitting that reset button we spoke of earlier. As you move through EMDR therapy, you reduce the number of distressing files that can get triggered by your current life experience. When your brain has less pile-up of historical data to sort through, it can resolve distress more quickly. When that pile-up is not resolved, responders are more inclined to stronger stress reactions (with unproductive anger and anxiety). These reactions often lead to emotional shutdowns, the urge to binge eat or drink, or other forms of self-medicating. But, following EMDR processing, this chain reaction is prevented. Imagine something going completely wrong, and instead of freaking out, you can breathe and problem solve, without having to work at it. This is resilient behavior, and it boosts your ability to reset after stressful events, prepare for upcoming stressors, and sustain your energy for increasing resilience capacity. (See Chapter 6.)

EMDR therapists – How do I select one?

Before you select an EMDR therapist, it is important that you speak with them ahead of time to assure the best fit between your needs and their qualifications. Here are some questions we think are important for you to ask your potential therapist:
1. Are you EMDR certified? How long have you used EMDR Therapy?
2. How much experience have you had working with trauma?
3. What experience have you had with the first responder culture?
4. Have you treated first responders with EMDR?
5. Have you ever done EMDR with a 9-1-1 dispatcher?
6. Have you ever done a "Sit-Along" in a dispatch center? Would you be willing to?

Resources to Locate an EMDR Therapist

- *911 Training Institute* - **www.911training.net/list-of-emdr-therapists-for-911**. The clinician's on this list have taken special steps to learn about the 9-1-1 profession for best results. Since the list is new, therapists are not yet cited for many areas, but clear instructions are offered to most effectively find a qualified EMDR therapist in your area. The list also provides a link to the EMDR International Association (EMDRIA, see below).

- *EMDR International Association* – has a directory of trained therapists. When you look on a profile, look for whether they have listed 'first responder' as a population they work with. **http://emdria.site-ym.com/general/custom.asp?page=findatherapistmain**
- *Coherence Associates, Inc.* **www.CoherenceAssociates.com**

Thank you for taking time to read our chapter. We sincerely hope you have gained the knowledge you need to wisely pursue EMDR yourself and to help your 9-1-1 colleagues seek this healing help too. Before you move on to the next chapter, take a few moments to review the Questions for Reflection and the Additional Resources below.

Questions for Reflection

To get the most from this chapter, you are encouraged to write your reflections here (in both the Kindle and paperback versions of this book).
- What was your main take-away from reading this chapter?

- What specifically made it valuable to you?

- How can you apply this take-away concretely to improve some aspect of your personal life and or efforts to support the wellbeing of 9-1-1Pros?

Additional Resources

- To learn more about efforts to advance the concept of Post Traumatic Stress Injury, visit: Global PTSI Foundation **http://globalptsifoundation.org/**
- For the most trustworthy, up-to-date information on PTSD, visit the National Center for PTSD **https://www.ptsd.va.gov/public**

- To explore using EMDR for personal healing, consider reading Getting Past Your Past, the book by EMDR's originator, Francine Shapiro (see more information in the Works Cited section below).
- The following documents expand on discussion in this chapter. You will notice the chapter for therapists written by Jim Marshall and Sara Gilman; it is included on this list to inform our readers about our efforts to educate clinicians about the role and needs of the 9-1-1 Professional. Their ability to effectively provide treatment to 9-1-1Pros depends on their understanding of the telecommunicator's work life and related stressors.

Bisson, J., Roberts, N.P., Andrew, M., Cooper, R. & Lewis, C., "Psychological therapies for chronic post-traumatic stress disorder (PTSD) in adults (Review)". *Cochrane Database of Systematic Reviews 2013,* DOI: 10.1002/14651858.CD003388.pub4, 2013

Jarero, I., & Uribe, S., Artigas, L., Givaudan, M. "EMDR protocol for recent critical incidents: A randomized controlled trial in a technological disaster context." *Journal of EMDR Practice and Research, 9,* 166–173, 2015.

Marshall, J., and S. Gilman (2015). "Reaching the unseen first responder: treating 911 trauma in emergency telecommunicators." In M. Luber (Ed.), *EMDR Scripted Protocols: Treating trauma- and stressor-related conditions (pp. 185-216).* Springer Publications.

Shapiro, E., and Laub, B. "Early EMDR intervention following a community critical incident: A randomized clinical trial." *Journal of EMDR Practice and Research, 9,* 17-27, 2015.

Shapiro, E. "EMDR and early psychological intervention following trauma." *European Review of Applied Psychology, 64*(4), 241-251. doi:10.1016/j.erap.2012.09.003, 2012.

Works Cited

Adler-Tapia, Robbie. "Early Mental Health Intervention for First Responders/Protective Service Workers Including Firefighters and Emergency Medical Services (EMS) Professionals." *Implementing EMDR Early Mental Health Interventions for Man-made and Natural Disasters: Models, Scripted Protocols and Summary Sheets.* New York: Springer Publishing Company, 2013.

Department of Veterans Affairs & Department of Defense (2017). "VA/DoD Clinical Practice Guideline for the Management of Post-Traumatic Stress." *U.S. Department of Veteran's Affairs*, 2017.
www.healthquality.va.gov/guidelines/MH/ptsd/

Foa, Enda B. et al. *Effective treatments for PTSD: Practice Guidelines of the International Society for Traumatic Stress Studies.* Guilford Press, 2009.

Shapiro, F., *Getting past your past: Take control of your life with self-help techniques from EMDR therapy.* Rodale Press, 2013.

CHAPTER 10
When Your Give-A-Damn is Busted: Rebuilding Your Life After Compassion Fatigue

Jim Marshall

A Student I Could Never Forget

I've never forgotten Greg, or the first day he spent in my classroom. I'd been asked by Jan Myers (Chapter 7) to bring my comprehensive resilience course, *Survive and Thrive in 9-1-1 Together*, to Oregon. He strode into the room a few minutes after the other thirty 9-1-1Pros. He made his way to the back of the room in long, slow steps with a John Wayne swagger: head high, chest out, and shoulders rolling. It was hard not to assume he was cocky before he even said a word. He chose a seat amidst a couple of dispatchers he seemed to know well.

Throughout the morning, as I worked to help the class recognize the risks of unmanaged stress impacts, Greg rolled his eyes, tapped his pencil on the desk, and frequently leaned into the peers on his right or left whispering comments, with a big smirk on his face. He rarely made eye contact with me. He was disruptive, to say the least. He lacked respect for both his classmates and me. Who knows, someone's future in that class could have depended on learning about the stress risks and preventive care we were trying to discuss, and he was interfering with that. He was beginning to get under my skin. I gave him a stern look and he settled down a bit, but his pencil kept tapping away. Something was going on with that man.

Then the thought struck me: *Marshall, you clod, who do you think might need this class most?*

Beware the Horns of the Bull

As my psychology colleague, Frank Campbell warns, "beware the horns of the bull." It is so easy to judge, and the vast majority of the time, when we do so in reaction to being offended, we are at risk of being gored by our own assumptions.

When we judge, we miss the opportunity to learn who the person really is. I knew better. The attitude Greg seemed to display is common among those struggling with the very topic I would present in the next moment of class! I began by asking my students to draw an umbrella with two handles. "Now, in the body of the umbrella, write the phrase *Compassion Fatigue*…Then, under the left handle, write *Secondary Traumatic Stress (STS)*."

STS is what can happen when you as a caregiver are exposed to another person's traumatic event—an event during which they were at risk of serious injury or death. Even though your involvement didn't place you personally at physical risk, your secondary exposure to their trauma can lead to struggles later: difficulty sleeping, fear, unwelcomed images of the upsetting event popping into your mind or avoiding things that remind you of the event. That's STS. Then I told the class my own story, about how I "hit the wall" in my ninth year of practice as a mental health clinician. I never saw it coming.

A Life-Changing Client Loss

You may imagine that my work life was like the TV image of the smug therapist sipping tea, nodding now and then, jotting notes and listening with indifference, then collecting the big bucks when the cuckoo clock sounds the hour's end. Think again. I was a trench worker that 9-1-1Pros would affectionately call a "shit magnet", like my friend, Jan! (Chapter 7.) This title in no way devalues the people I served. To the emergency responders, it just meant that my workload involved an inordinate number of really difficult cases that were highly stressful. While my colleagues in private practice also had tough cases, many of my clients suffered with complex PTSD and or severe marital problems, and many struggled with serious suicide risk.

Once I was trained in EMDR (see Chapter 9), clients experienced healing of their flashbacks and hypervigilance, so they told others in need. It was an enormous honor, and very rewarding, to provide this care to people during the worst seasons of their life. Yet, the cumulative stress of doing so much intensive therapy for so long had impacted me far more than I realized. One fall day, that stress reached its boiling point.

The day before, I'd seen a man and woman in my office for their sixth couples' session. Though my caseload was already too full, I'd agreed to see them as a favor to their close friend, my practice partner.

"C'mon, Jim…" he'd pleaded. "They just need some help with their marriage, and you're the relationship guy! Please?"

My gut said *no,* but my mouth said, "Okay." (Have you ever had a hard time saying "no" when you need to? Earlier in my career, I did.) Since their first session, this couple's marriage had improved, and we were close to finishing up. At the end of this particular session, the man's affect seemed strange and my gut stirred. This time I listened. For some reason I felt compelled to ask him the bottom-line question, "Do you have any thoughts of killing yourself?"

He assured me, "No. I've had thoughts in the past, but no. And if I did, Jim, I'd let you know. But would you be willing to pray for us before we go?"

I gladly did so, and he seemed more peaceful when they left my office.

Twenty-four hours later, in the middle of a therapy session, my office manager knocked on my door. She motioned me out in the hallway, closed the door behind us, and whispered, "The man you saw at three o'clock yesterday killed himself early this morning. His wife is waiting for you at her house."

I was numb. As I drove to their home I was flooded with sorrow, panic, guilt, and a tangle of racing thoughts: *what if I could of…I should have…he lied to me…what will this do to his family?* 9-1-1Pros who have handled calls when people completed suicide, and family members who have lost loved ones this way, can surely relate to this flurry of thoughts, emotions, and sensations that follow realization of the death.

As I came through the door, she said, "Oh, Jim: I'm so glad you're here. Sit down. Read this." It was his suicide note. In it, he apologized for lying and admitted he had known for years he would do this. Then he said, "…but wasn't' Jim's prayer yesterday wonderful?" I felt sick.

The Fallout

Upon return to my office, I immediately requested that two peers conduct a complete extensive review of my clinical documentation of this case to identify anything I could have done different to help save this man's life. Their review showed that my care had been without error. I didn't believe it and wasn't consoled. I couldn't shake the guilt or the sense of failure. An enormous exhaustion set in.

In every session during the next many weeks, I was hypervigilant about missing even a single clinical detail for fear that others might die. Yet my motivation and passion for work had vanished along with my energy. As the country song says, my "give-a-damn" was busted! I questioned if I was really qualified to be a therapist…

As I told this part of my story in class, I noticed Greg staring straight into me. He seemed to be absorbing every word. I continued…

Have you heard about the "frog in the kettle" experiment? Imagine you're the slightly demented scientist in charge; you fill the kettle half-full of water and place it on the stove. You add a lily pad for that homey touch, a tiny floating tiki bar, and a mini-screen TV. Then you set Mr. Frog inside and crank up the heat. Here's the question: Is there a point, as the water temperature gradually increases, and before it begins to boil, that our frog-friend will try to jump out? The answer is no. Frogs are amphibians, and one of their talents is to adapt radically to climate changes. But in this un-natural instance, Mr. Frog's natural tendency works against him. So he becomes an appetizer—if you're from the southern United States, you dip him in sauce and eat him. If you're from the north, you probably just cringed. But, no matter where you're from, if you don't know the signs of Compassion Fatigue, you're far more apt to end up cooked!

At this point, Greg wasn't smirking at my frog story, like the rest of his classmates. His head was hung low, and he was bouncing his knee. Something was definitely going on with that man…

I asked my students to write down the phrase, *Burn-out*, under the right handle of their umbrella drawings. Then I listed some of its features: fatigue, exhaustion, irritability, hopelessness, increasing cynicism, and more.

Then I continued my story…

The Frog in the Kettle

Folks, after my client's suicide, I realized that I had become the frog in the kettle. His death wasn't the cause of my compassion fatigue. It was the tipping point. The cause was the cumulative effect of excessive demand and traumatic events to which I was exposed (Secondary Traumatic Stress) over nine years.

How many times, before his death, had I been alongside others, feeling their despair, straining to help stop their flashbacks, listening to their painful histories, and trying to help them choose life as they teetered on the edge of death? At that point in my career, after being alongside people for about 12,000 hours of therapy, the heaviness of this trench-work had finally caught up to me. In retrospect, I could see that some of my symptoms of compassion fatigue had been slowly appearing and subtly intensifying for a couple years. But they hadn't seemed to really affect me; until this death. I had a great support system—my wife Linda, my faith, my family and friends. At this point though, even they weren't enough.

Although I could still function at work, I became over-worried about suicide, even in clients with little or no risk. That's called hypervigilance. The prospect of doing another 20 years of PTSD treatment with folks seemed impossible. I felt dread and exhaustion. And that's when I knew it was time for EMDR—not to administer it, but to seek it for myself. Fortunately, a few sessions of this therapy, which I call "The Whacky Eye-movement Treatment," provided me with immediate relief from the excessive guilt and hypervigilance that was plaguing me. It helped me regain my "mojo" and my passion for doing the work of therapy. Yet, there was more I needed to do.

As we discussed in Chapter 3, mild to moderate acute stressors knock you out of balance for a few minutes. But repeated exposures to Secondary Traumatic Stress, especially when very severe, and when combined with Burn-out, can throw you out of balance *permanently*. So, in addition to EMDR, I also needed to build a personal plan to regain my balance between life demands that drained me, and experiences that recharged me. I needed to strategically design and protect time for family life and self-care: time to rest (intentionally do "nothing"), exercise, eat real meals, and more play time. These are essential ingredients in the recipe for healing Compassion Fatigue. This became so clear to me the day I struggled to play *Candy Land*™.

Candy Land™

I remember coming home one day, a few weeks after my client's suicide, to find Linda and my eight-year-old daughter, Ami, sitting on the family room carpet with a board game between them. Ami shouted happily, "Daddy! We're playin' Candy Land™. C'mon, you can go next!" I sat down with them, as she placed a green playing piece on the Start space.

"That's yours, daddy. You can take your turn now." I reached for a card, like I had countless times before, and turned it over. It had two yellow squares on it, indicating that I should move my piece to the second yellow space on the board. I picked up Ami's red piece and moved it to the second blue square on the board. She looked at me in amazement, took my piece, and moved it to its proper place. Then she promptly rebuked me, "Daddy, what's wrong with you silly goooooose: this game is for children, six and older!"

You see, my hand was in the family room, but my head was at the office. I was replaying what the client had said, what I said in return, weighing risk factors and the likelihood they'd survive, while I was playing *Candy Land!*

Later that evening, Linda noticed how tense I was and pulled me aside, "Marshall, when's the last time you got yourself into a trout stream?"

The fact is, I'd assigned plenty of clients to get back out into nature during the past couple years, but I'd personally seen more trout on the wallpaper border in my office than in a stream.

"Go! Get outta here!" she said.

Finding the Stream Again

When my wife orders me to go fishing, my compliance rate is 100 percent! She knew whenever I went fishing I always came home recharged and in a better frame of mind. Linda's support reconnected me with this vital part of myself that I'd grown so out of touch with amidst caring for my family, my clients, and serving at church. Sometimes, too much of a good thing isn't a good thing. It was time to set some fresh boundaries in my life, like I taught my clients. But right now, it was time to *go fishing*. Within a few minutes, I had gathered and dusted off my gear in the garage, loaded it into my car and was on the road for the Maple River, north of Pellston, MI.

In a half an hour I was at the stream. The sun was just then melting into the tree line; the perfect time to fish for brook trout. I eagerly put on my full waders, rushed to assemble my fly rod, clumsily tied a fly to the line, and stomped down into the Maple River. My energy wasn't just driven by excitement; it was also driven by the hypervigilant inner voice: *Don't slow down, don't let down; if you do, something bad will happen.*

I could hear myself saying out loud, "I'm here to fish, so we've got to catch fish! Now, where will they be hiding?"

I scanned the water looking upstream, then, "There! Right there in that deep swirl of water under that low hanging tree, up river!" So, I began my cast, dialing my wrist back and forth, sending the rod back and forth over my head as I stripped off more line with each backward pull of the rod. As a long loop of line now trailed behind me, I took aim at that deep swirl, pointed my rod tip at the destination under that tree, snapped my wrist, and waited for the line to land softly on the water's surface. But the line never re-appeared in front of me. My hook had embedded high up in a tree behind me. Furious, I tugged hard to free the hook from the bark. *This can't be happening!* Gritting my teeth, I wrapped the fishing line around my hand and pulled backward slowly until the line, stretched to its limit, finally snapped and fell limp into the brush. The fly remained, half-buried in the bark, in full sight, irretrievable. Fuming, mumbling and snorting, I regathered the line and tied on a fresh hook, "I'm not givin' up! I'm here to fish. That's the hole where the fish are, and dammit, I'm gonna kill some fish today!"

Realizing

That had never been my attitude before. In fact, unless fishing for dinner, I preferred to remove the hook from the fish's mouth, hold them in the water, admire the colorful markings on their skin for a few seconds as they regained their strength, then release them gently back into the stream. But not today! It was time to kill fish; to win! Not be defeated; not feel *helpless* like I did after my client's suicide, or when so many times I couldn't free other clients of their suffering.

Resolute, I began my second cast. Back and forth went the rod, the line elongating over the water until it landed…smack dab in the limbs of that damned tree above my ideal fishin' hole! I was beside myself, furious again at being defeated. I twisted my upper body and jerked my arms away from the embedded hook to snap my line free. Then I just stood there sagging in my waders, with the remains of my line dangling in the water in front of me. That's when I suddenly realized how ridiculous this scene must have looked and what a hilarious YouTube video this would make. We could title it, *"Psychologist Finds Peace on Northern Michigan Trout Stream."* I'd been so jacked up on cortisol and hypervigilance for so long, my brain and body didn't feel safe letting down…until that moment of realization. Then I slowly tucked my rod under one arm, and just stood there, finally still and silent.

That's when I heard the river, for the first time in a very long time.

Being Where You Are

I looked down *into* the amber-colored water. On the river bottom were long ripples of blond sand, partially covered by smooth, rounded stones of all colors. Have you ever seen bright, effervescent green river grass dancing in the current? Two strands rose up from the river bed near the surface, swaying back and forth in unison. The sight was almost hypnotizing. How could I have been standing in this water all this time and not seen this? I looked up in astonishment; I was surrounded by beauty.

The leaves of Sugar Maple trees formed an almost iridescent golden, orange, yellow canopy above me and stretched with the river for as far as I could see. Spaces between the branches allowed beams of the evening light to shimmer on the water's surface. Standing there, in silence, I took a slow, deep breath.

Feelings of sadness and grief welled up as I realized what my wife already knew: I'd been away from this river, from refreshment that fed my soul and balanced me, and from myself, for too long.

I heard a single bird calling down river. Had she been there singing all along? Finally, I felt the river's powerful current rushing, and pressing against my waders. When I had first pushed my way into the stream, I'd been so tense, so driven that I couldn't even feel the river. How could this be? How could I be standing waist deep in a trout stream for half an hour and not even feel, see, or hear all that was around me? Then it hit me: *if I missed experiencing all this beauty, standing right here in the middle of this sacred place, what other sacred things in my life have I been missing the past couple years?*

How many times had I been in that family room physically, but not present mentally when my little girls were dancing for me, playing with me, or when… when a part of me was far away, worrying about a client at risk. Now the grief was enormous. It rushed from my heart and flooded my eyes. It was safe out here in the Maple, and I let my tears fall freely into the river for a while… until the peace of that place surrounded me, absorbed the pain, and fresh hope stirred. The bad news had been realizing what I had lost in those many months when the Compassion Fatigue had taken me over. The good news was that it wasn't too late to set a new course, to heal, grow, and take my life back. It was time to work on that plan to regain balance.

I'll finish my story soon enough, but what about Greg?

Greg's Chance for Realization

That day when class was finished, Greg's exit was very different than his entrance. He walked out like he was dragging a pile of bricks behind him, staring at the linoleum. Indeed, there was something going on inside this young man, and he needed support. But my gut said to give him space, for the time being.

The next morning it was chilly there at the State Public Safety Training and Standards compound in Salem, Oregon. This massive compound sat in the foothills surrounded by a tall, spiked, black wrought iron fence. The day began with a single bugle blasting Reveille; then cadets flew the colors and marched their drills. I made my way across the breezeway between the cinder block dormitory and the cafeteria amidst a flood of police and dispatch trainees and their instructors; all hustled to get in line for breakfast. Just before I entered the cafeteria door, I heard, "Mr. Marshall!" It was Greg. As I neared him, he rotated away from me and the flowing crowd so no one could see him.

"What's happening, Greg?"

It was his turn for tears. He brushed them off his face as he explained, "When I left home to come here, my wife told me I'd better figure out what's wrong with me; she said I'd become an asshole, and she wasn't sure she wanted to be married to me anymore. I thought it was just her; that she was just being a bitch. But then you laid out your story about Compassion Fatigue yesterday, and I realized: that's me! I've got every sign. I don't know what to do and I'm scared I'm going to lose my wife and my family. What do I do?"

Greg seemed ready, so I cut to the chase, "Are you willing to go to marriage therapy if your wife is willing?"

"Yes, I would."

"How about individual therapy? You're going to need professional help to assess what's really going on inside. If you don't get expert help to overcome the stress impacts from your work, your marriage probably won't work."

"Yes, I'm willing to work on my own stuff too."

"Okay, what would happen if you called your wife right now, told her everything you've realized and what you're willing to do to save your marriage? Would she hang up on you?"

"Well, I don't know if she'd hang-up on me, but I don't think she'd believe me. I've really become quite an asshole."

"Well, it can happen to any of us in the trenches for too long. The important thing is what we do when we realize it! Forget the beginning of class. Go for a hike out on that trail and call your wife. When you get done, then come to class."

Turning the Corner on Compassion Fatigue

About a half-hour later, Greg quietly reappeared in the classroom, and with stealth, took his chair in the back. He opened his workbook, found his place, and began taking notes. There was a big grin on his face. At the next break, he rushed to the front of the classroom, eager to report the results of his call. "She didn't hang up. She didn't promise to stay either, but she said as long as I'm willing to do the individual and marital therapy, she'll stick around long enough to see what happens."

Once all the other students had cleared out at the end of the day, we identified a qualified EMDR therapist for Greg, shook hands and he left. Now he was fully invested, and when he left he promised to update me.

About three months later I got an email from him. He and his wife were in marital therapy, still together, and improving. With help from the EMDR, he started to feel more like himself. Six months after the training, he sent me another update; his marriage was doing better than ever, and he was enjoying life and his family more.

The next year, I returned to Oregon to teach *Survive and Thrive*. While wrestling with my baggage in the parking lot, Greg showed up, all smiles, and helped me haul my stuff to the dorms. This time I was meeting the real Greg: a very warm-hearted, kind-spirited man, free of his own heavy load, free to be himself again. He seemed rested, energized, and more balanced. Since then, he has become a 9-1-1 leader and my friend. We've enjoyed sharing emails through the years and, Lord willing, we'll sit together again to support each other as two men who will always be imperfect but growing.

The Horns of the Bull Revisited

Beware the horns of the bull.
If you're tempted to judge a peer who behaves like Greg initially did, remember: *in ignorance, good people judge and do harm; but with new insight we can wonder compassionately and do great good.* My hope is that the stories and the information in this chapter will help you see what might be driving your own struggles. Then, rather than judging yourself and gutting it out longer, you'll follow the few steps I'm offering you below to overcome Compassion Fatigue. First though, since 9-1-1Pros seldom get closure, let me finish my own story. After all, we who do intensive caregiving are more alike than different. We can get lost in service to our own detriment, no matter what our credentials!

I thank God for my wife, family, friends—including Greg, my colleagues, and the river. That day on the Maple was the turning point for me. When I finally pulled myself out of the water, I was resolved to do all I could to restore personal balance. I began by taking a personal inventory: which of my responsibilities (volunteer and at work) could I reduce or let go of completely? Who could I ask for support—to cheer me on and hold me accountable in honoring my self-care plan? (I chose my brother-in-law, Tom. His encouragement and periodic kick in the pants was invaluable. And it turned out he needed the support just as much as I did.)

As imperfect as my own recovery efforts were, they helped me to enjoy doing full-time therapy for many more years after my client's suicide. The loving support I received, along with clinical help, and defining a plan to restore my balance, all combined to save my career and protect my health. In fact, that healing journey paved my pathway to the 9-1-1 Family. When my sister eventually asked me to create *Survive & Thrive* for telecommunicators, it was not only because of my clinical qualifications. She believed dispatchers would relate deeply to, and benefit from, my own journey through struggles as a fellow Extraordinary Care Giver.

Conclusion: Bringing it Home

Can you relate to my story or Greg's? If you can, you're in good company! As a 9-1-1Pro, you've probably experienced more disturbing, sad, and ugly stuff on the job than most humans ever will. So, (depending on other personal factors too) you may be a bit more at-risk to get Compassion Fatigue. You deserve whatever help you might need to overcome it. Remember this: it's not a character flaw. It's the natural fallout of exposure to excessive psychological demands over a long period. We can't control all the tough stuff we experience at work, but we can choose what we'll do to take care of ourselves so that we can enjoy all that matters most to us in this life. You've given so much to so many. Maybe now it's your turn to invest with the same intensity in your own wellbeing.

Don't try to diagnose yourself. If you're gut says you're struggling, please just use the *Additional Resources* below and you'll be on your way to reclaiming your well-being. First, take a few minutes to explore the three key chapter review questions. One more thing: remember that you don't need to go it alone. In the 9-1-1 Family, we're truly all in this together. Ask for the help you need to succeed.

ಬ೩೮ು

Questions for Reflection

To get the most from this chapter, you are encouraged to write your reflections here (in both the Kindle and paperback versions of this book).

- What was your main take-away from reading this chapter?

- What specifically made it valuable to you?

- How can you apply this take-away concretely to improve some aspect of your personal life and or efforts to support the wellbeing of 9-1-1Pros?

Additional Resources

Visit **https://www.9-1-1training.net/help-for-compassion-fatigue**. You'll find two attached resources: 1) the world's most trustworthy screening tool for Compassion Fatigue, called the *ProQOL (Professional Quality of Life Screening)*.
It's a quick and easy-to-use tool you can use to determine if you *may* struggle with Secondary Traumatic Stress, Burn-out or both aspects of Compassion Fatigue. Take the ProQOL, then score it according to the included instructions. It's actually fun to take. Then just read what your scores may mean using the provided explanations. If your scores are high on Secondary Traumatic Stress and or Burn-out, follow the recommendations, and take a couple minutes to build a self-care plan to overcome the struggle using 2) the 9-1-1TI resource just beneath the ProQOL, entitled *The CF Self-Care Planner*.

* Screening tools are not designed to diagnose mental health problems, nor are they able to do so reliably. Their purpose is to gain insight that can lead to more trustworthy definition of your struggle with clinical help, then to the treatment you may need. The ProQOL is an evidence-supported screening tool use world-wide. Please use it as directed.

Work Cited

Stamm, B. Hudnall. "Professional Quality of Life: Compassion Satisfaction and Fatigue Version 5 (ProQOL)." *ProQOL*, 2009-2012. **www.proqol.org**.

CHAPTER 11
9-1-1Pros: Sleep for the Health of It! Here's what you Need to Know

Craig Boss

Editor's Note

Everywhere I've traveled to train 9-1-1 telecommunicators to "Survive and Thrive," I ask the same question, "How many hours of sleep per every twenty-four hours do you think 9-1-1Pros get on average, including their days off?" In almost perfect unison, they shout the same alarming lyric, "Four to five or six hours." Yes, there is sometimes one "odd-ball" who impulsively blurts out, "Eight hours". They are fortunate to survive the day with their limbs intact! 9-1-1Pros covet the sleep they don't get. In this chapter, sleep expert, Dr. Craig Boss, will meet you right in the middle of your sleep struggles. He'll help you discover the benefits and inner workings of sleep, explore the factors that impair it, and he defines the health impacts of chronic sleep problems. But be encouraged, "Doc Boss" wraps up with great nitty-gritty strategies you can use to improve your sleep. Trust me: it'll be worth staying awake to read every word!

JM

CB

Whether you're a 9-1-1Pro or another type of emergency responder, it is often a badge of honor to be able to say that you've worked for twelve-sixteen hours, slept for four hours, and gotten every to-do list item completed outside of work. When working night shifts, swing shifts, and mandatory overtime, it can be dreadful going to bed; struggles getting to sleep and staying asleep can be so frustrating. Just a few hours later, the merry-go-round starts over again. My goal is to supply you with some core strategies and insights that can help empower you to be well by sleeping well!

Now please don't doze off as I lead you into a couple paragraphs of really important science. If you're going to succeed at improving your sleep, I really want you to understand some of the basics of what happens when you sleep. So, hang in there while I review some of the core concepts and science of your sleep.

Sleep is defined as the perceptual disengagement from the environment that (thankfully) is reversible. Yet, incredibly, and contrary to common belief, even during sleep your brain is very active. Sleep is broken down into two broad types: Rapid Eye Movement (REM) sleep, commonly known as "dream sleep", and Non-REM sleep. Non-REM includes Stages N1, N2, and N3. During N1, you sleep very lightly as you transition between wakefulness and the other stages of sleep. The majority of sleep occurs in N2. While in this stage, the brain and the body are being prepared to enter into deeper sleep. During N3, very slow, high amplitude, brain waves occur. As a result, we often refer to this stage as slow wave sleep. During this slow wave sleep, nerve connections are improved, and several restorative functions occur within the body. REM sleep typically cycles every 70-120 minutes after you initially fall asleep, and it is when dreams occur. It has been associated with positive benefits in memory and attention. In addition, your body is relatively paralyzed during the REM stage. As a result, we don't act out dreams. (Good thing, right?) So, if you were to pay cold, hard cash for specific stages of sleep, you'd want to invest it in REM and slow wave sleep!

Overall, the recommended amount of sleep for an adult should range from seven-nine hours each day, although there can be individual differences. With this said, sleeping less than six hours per day on a consistent basis over time actually increases health risks. I'll give you a few insights about this later.

Just as all of us thrive on routine, so does your brain. Consistent routine drives consistent circadian rhythms. Circadian rhythms refer to the "pre-wired" timing of your brain that regulates sleep and wake cycles. This is a key concept to understand, especially in a world of irregular sleep schedules. Now think of your days, nights, and your sleep as you consider the next few science facts.

Your Brain and Sleep

The instant you open your eyes and light strikes them, a message is sent to your brain signaling you are awake. When this message is sent, a whole cascade of chemical and neurotransmitter responses occurs, marking the start of your twenty-four-hour circadian rhythm. Signals are sent to minimize the gradual increase of sleepiness experienced by the brain. Everyone's circadian rhythms are unique. They are based on genetics and long-term routines of wakefulness and sleep. Classically, the circadian wakefulness signal starts between 5-7 a.m. This alerting signal continues to climb until the early afternoon. At that point, there is a normal, and predictable, leveling out.

Often, we experience drowsiness after eating lunch and believe food is the cause. Sure, if we just had a big Thanksgiving dinner that's a possibility; but the main reason is that the normal circadian alerting signal levels out for a brief period. This occurs in everyone's brain, and cannot be controlled. Then, typically two to three hours later, the brain increases this alerting signal, and we experience a "second wind." A relative "wakefulness maintenance zone" occurs, until the light in the environment around us starts to dim. Due to less light being detected by the brain via the retina, a message is sent to a small area in the brain called the pineal gland, which then releases melatonin. Melatonin then down-regulates the circadian alerting center, to prepare the brain for sleep. If we've remained awake since the time we got up for the day, our brain experiences more "sleep pressure" or sleepiness. As we maintain longer periods of wakefulness, the relative sleepiness of the brain is much higher.

After falling asleep, the brain is replenished, and sleep pressure slowly decreases. In essence, the sleep you are obtaining is filling your tank, preparing for the next day. To counteract the decreasing level of sleepiness, circadian rhythms decrease even more during the night to help maintain sleep in the brain. Ultimately, circadian rhythms reach their bottom. To continue to maintain sleep, the body's temperature drops to its lowest point between 3-4 a.m. This keeps the brain asleep until circadian rhythms begin to rise again at 5-7 a.m. So, if you start getting sleepy during this time while you are working, understand this is a natural brain response. This cycle then repeats itself during each twenty-four-hour period. Again, you have no control over this normal cycling, it is pre-programmed by your brain and can vary somewhat between individuals.

At this point, you may be asking yourself, "Why is this doctor going on about all this stuff? I just want to sleep!" The answer is, if you understand the basics, you can actually understand why you may have difficulty sleeping, as well as how to make your sleep even better. More on this in a bit.

Facts about Sleep

The study of sleep, and the impact it has on our lives, has become an important component of preventive medicine.

We have all experienced what it feels like to get inadequate sleep. We may not only feel sleepier during the day, but we find that we have difficulty focusing and concentrating. Numerous studies have evaluated the neurocognitive impact of inadequate sleep. These studies reveal that reaction times are prolonged and academic success declines. In addition, stroke and cardiovascular risk increases. A recent study of approximately 5000 patients revealed a correlation of increased stroke risk in those who sleep less than six hours/night on a consistent basis. Diabetes and prediabetes risk increases. Depression and anxiety risks worsen. Not good news, right? But knowledge is power, so, please, read on!

Motor vehicle accident risk increases by approximately six times with inadequate sleep. The potential of obesity increases based on the impact that inadequate and/or fragmented sleep has on appetite hormone levels. Headaches (migraine, tension, and cluster) may increase. Restorative effects, in regard to healing, are diminished. Cardiovascular risks increase including abnormal heart rhythms, elevated blood pressure, palpitations, and potential coronary artery disease. As you can see, sleep is a must when trying to minimize risk.

A Day in the Life of a Sleepy/Fatigued Person

A multitude of factors contribute to poor sleep, excessive sleepiness, and fatigue. These may include work stress, mood, medical conditions, shift work, financial stress, over use of stimulants, poor sleeping environments, and more. Let's review an example of a patient who is having difficulty sleeping.

John is a forty-year-old telecommunicator on the night shift. He has worked the night shift for the last several years. His work hours are between 7 p.m. and 7 a.m. He generally tries to sleep between 8:30 a.m. and 2-3 p.m. To relax before falling asleep, he enjoys watching TV in bed for thirty to forty-five minutes. Without the TV on, he feels that he cannot sleep well. He can fall asleep right away, but has difficulty staying asleep. Ole Yeller, John's Labrador, sleeps in his bedroom, often in his bed. This pet usually wakes him one time during his sleep, to go outside. Often, after sleeping for three to four hours, he feels like he catnaps for the rest of his time in bed.

John has tried over the counter medications for sleep with minimal success. He does not have a bed partner due to his shift work.

His last caffeine for his day is at 3 a.m., during a lunch break at work. This is either in the form of coffee or soda. He often feels that around 4 a.m. he has the most difficulty staying focused on his job and being productive. At that point, even with coffee, he begins to feel sleepy. Before his shift, he will, at times, take a nap or a brief rest for one hour at around 5 p.m. When he leaves his workplace, the sun is generally quite bright as he drives home. Once he is out of bed for the day, his biggest complaint is fatigue, not sleepiness.

This patient's history is not uncommon, especially for a night shift worker. Demographics also show that a night shift worker sleeps, on average, one to four hours less during a twenty-four-hour period as compared to a worker scheduled during a day shift. In this particular case, multiple issues are present that may undermine John's ability to initiate, and maintain, sleep. We'll walk through each component of his day, and his sleep, which may impact his sleep success.

Initially when John leaves his workplace, he is greeted with bright sunlight. Day workers might think that this would be a welcomed sight, but it isn't. The bright light activates the wakefulness center in the brain. When John and other night shift workers leave work in the morning time, they should put on their sunglasses before they step into the light of day. This strategy helps decrease the wakefulness signal to the brain.

As you'll recall from our discussion of sleep physiology, between 3-5 a.m., circadian rhythms hit their lowest point increasing the risk of sleepiness. John notes that he has more difficulty completing his tasks after 3 a.m. In addition, he has consumed caffeine at 3 a.m. Caffeine can affect sleep quality for hours after its use. Even when people can fall asleep readily after drinking caffeine, it will lead to increased sleep fragmentation, unknown to the person. Generally, in my practice, I ask all patients with difficulty initiating and maintaining sleep to avoid caffeine eight to ten hours before bedtime. This is tough advice to swallow, but research shows that when we drink caffeine even six hours before bedtime, it impacts our sleep quality. Even though it may seem like an impossible task to minimize your stimulants at first, your sleep will be maximized. This will then make your next day better, helping you to continue to decrease use of stimulants. You get the idea. When you make hard but important changes like this, you're developing *success cycles* that improve your health and performance.

Once at home, John climbs into bed with his loyal dog and turns the TV on to relax. At first, this might seem very comfortable to most people. Unfortunately, it's a setup for dysfunction. The act of lying in bed awake while watching TV promotes a conditioned response of wakefulness in bed-not to mention the terrible things that are often on television such as, news, and anxiety producing shows. Your brain then associates your bed with being awake, and you associate your bed with the ultimate frustration of not being able to sleep well; a destructive cycle begins. If you wake after falling asleep, your brain may have more difficulty reinitiating sleep due to the same association. You then begin fostering "bed dread."

The impact of watching TV in bed doesn't stop there. The light emitted from a TV can also encourage heightened wakefulness in your brain, similar to being exposed to sunlight in the morning. Alternatives to television may include a box fan, white noise machines, or readily available apps on smart phones that allow you to choose "sleep sounds" that are comforting. A very dark environment while you sleep is critical. You may want to consider black out shades and other accommodations.

Pets in bed can have equally detrimental effects on sleep. It may seem cozy, but often pets lead to increased wakefulness due to movement, proximity to our bodies, or demands while you sleep, such as needing to go outdoors. When you wake due to your pet, it may be more difficult to get back to sleep. Your pet will fall back to sleep without a problem. They quickly learn how to influence us for what they want. Often, loyal pet owners, like John, believe their pet won't sleep well if not in bed with them. Let me reassure you, your pet will sleep just fine outside of your bed, and they will always be happy to see you when you wake up.

After sleeping for approximately 3-4 hours, John wakes and has difficulty falling back to sleep. This may occur due to the factors above, but it can also be impacted by our underlying circadian rhythms. Remember what I discussed earlier-at approximately 11 a.m., the wakefulness signal produced by our brain is intrinsically higher. Even though a person may work third shift, this internal cycle may still affect your sleep quality. So, it is critical to minimize any potential factors that may increase wakefulness. This is also a reason that sleep medications often do not work well (in conjunction with the other factors noted) in people who work third shift.

A daytime nap can be a helpful way to improve alertness, especially if sleep hours are inadequate, or fragmented in some way. People often refer to "power naps" as the strategic use of sleep during the day, to combat sleepiness as well as fatigue. Indeed, naps can be very helpful, but just like any medication, they should be used at the right time to help optimize their effect. Taking a nap too late, or for too long can impact our ability to initiate and maintain sleep. Generally, it's best to take naps more than seven hours before bedtime, and not lasting longer than thirty minutes. For John, and for many people who work third shift, this kind of power nap minimizes sleepiness and fatigue during the work shift.

Yet it is also important to remember the impact naps can have on sleep later. Per our circadian rhythms, and how our brains are pre-wired for sleep cycles during a twenty-four-hour period, working night shifts flies directly against what our brain is innately programmed to do. Our brains are physiologically programmed for first shift work, except for a small minority of the population that have a true night owl programming. If too much sleep occurs late in the day, it will be harder to initiate and maintain it during our designated sleep time.

Once up for his day, John says he feels more fatigued than sleepy. Contrary to what most people believe, a person who does not sleep well may not feel sleepy but complain of fatigue. This may also be translated as tiredness, a lack of motivation, or feeling "blah." Others may feel depressed. It is always interesting to talk to folks who don't sleep well. At first, they will say they feel fine. On further questioning, they will often agree that they feel fatigued. Even more interesting, is to speak to a person after he or she has begun to sleep well. They will often reflect back and see how fatigued they actually were. Our perception of reality is truly based on our frame of reference.

Drugs and Sleep

The United States population is bombarded by many drugs that promote improved sleep. These include over the counter preparations, as well as prescription drugs. Interestingly, even more products are promoted to improve wakefulness and energy. Ironically, a vicious cycle begins with the use of stimulants to maintain wakefulness, and the subsequent use of sleeping aids to facilitate sleep. In addition, other medications used for various other disease states can affect sleep quality or increase sleepiness during the day. I'll cover a few of the prescribed and over-the-counter drugs that are available, but this is not a recommendation to use them.

Over the Counter Sleep Aids

Benadryl (Diphenhydramine): Diphenhydramine is probably the most prevalent active ingredient in over the counter products to help promote sleep. It is often combined with pain relievers (Acetaminophen, Ibuprofen, and Naproxen) as well. Diphenhydramine is a first-generation antihistamine. Histamines, as a general group, are alerting neurotransmitters. Being an "antihistamine," this class of drugs subsequently results in sleepiness. Often, over time, the effect of sleepiness decreases as tolerance to the drug increases. The normal dose of diphenhydramine recommended by manufacturers may often lead to next day fatigue and sleepiness. This may certainly impact safety while driving or affect concentration and cognitive function. Also, use of diphenhydramine may worsen urinary frequency and prostate symptoms for men with significant prostate enlargement. Occasionally, diphenhydramine may cause increased activation and alertness. It may also worsen restless legs symptoms in those who experience this problem.

Melatonin: As noted in the discussion above, melatonin is a naturally occurring hormone produced by the brain that inhibits the production of alerting signals that promote wakefulness. Melatonin is sold over the counter in a variety of dosages and in immediate and extended release formulations. Typically, melatonin helps us initiate sleep more than maintain sleep. Common doses are one to five mg taken one to three hours before bedtime. Don't be fooled; increased doses may possibly improve sleep, but at the potential cost of next-day side effects of fatigue and sleepiness.

Valerian: Valerian is an herb used to promote sleep and minimize anxiety. It is often referred to as "nature's valium." As with many herbal remedies, the exact mechanism of action of valerian is unknown. Studies regarding the effectiveness of this herb have been inconclusive.

Tryptophan: Tryptophan is an essential amino acid that is acquired via our diet. It is the precursor to serotonin and melatonin. Tryptophan is readily available in numerous foods that we consume including milk, oats, eggs, and meats (not just turkey). In the body, tryptophan is converted to 5-HTP which is then converted to serotonin. 5-HTP is available over the counter and is also used to promote sleep. Serotonin is an important neurotransmitter which can help with depression and anxiety. Serotonin itself is an activating neurotransmitter, but may, in some people, increase drowsiness (see selective serotonin reuptake inhibitor discussion below). So, when grandma talked about drinking warm milk to fall asleep, she was taking advantage of the potential impact of tryptophan!

Chamomile: Chamomile has been used for centuries for numerous medicinal purposes, including sleep. Today, one of the most common sources of chamomile is in herbal tea. Results of chamomile use, like most herbal supplements, often vary from one person to the next. Even if there is not a robust improvement in sleep, chamomile tea is a very pleasant way to end the day.

Prescription Medications that may be Used to Help Initiate/Maintain Sleep

In this section, my goal is to make you aware of the numerous medications most frequently prescribed to those who struggle with sleep. I rarely prescribe medications to patients for sleep. Frankly, my favorite medication to facilitate sleep is *none*! More than anything else, my desire for you is to be aware of these medications if they are suggested to you, or if you encounter them being described in the line of duty.

Ambien (Zolpidem), Lunesta (eszopiclone), and Sonata (zaleplon): These drugs act in many ways like the older benzodiazepine class of medications (that is, similar to Valium). But they are associated with a more limited function. For that reason, they are categorized in the "benzodiazepine-like receptor agonist" class. Depending on the formulation, they may help with sleep initiation, as well as sleep maintenance. The half-life of these drugs, depending on formulation, ranges between one and a half to five and a half hours. In general, these medications, and all prescription sleeping medications, are best used only for limited periods of time. Each of these medications, to varying degrees, may be associated with dependence.

Desyrel (Trazodone): This drug was originally developed to help treat depression but is now rarely used solely for this indication. Currently, it is most commonly used for insomnia, even though it does not have this indication. It has a sedating effect due to its effects on serotonin, and its anti-histamine properties.

Belsomra (Suvorexant): This is a much newer class of medication that targets the posterior hypothalamus of the brain. In this area of the brain, orexin which is an alerting neurotransmitter, is produced. Belsomra inhibits orexin which therefore causes sleepiness.

Rozarem (Ramelteon): Rozarem is a medication that targets melatonin receptors to help facilitate sleep onset but may not be as effective to maintain sleep. It does not produce dependence and may in some cases be more effective than melatonin alone.

Klonopin (Clonazepam), Ativan (Lorazepam), Valium (Diazepam) and others: These medications are benzodiazepines. They are typically used for the treatment of anxiety but in some cases are used to facilitate sleep, especially those with significant anxiety. Similar to the benzodiazepine-like receptor agonists, these medications typically are used for short periods of time. They may be prescribed for longer time durations in patients who have very significant anxiety. Benzodiazepines carry the potential risk of dependence.

Medications Used for Other Purposes that may Affect Sleep

Selective Serotonin Reuptake Inhibitors (i.e.: Prozac, Zoloft, Effexor, Celexa, Lexapro, and others):
This class of medication is widely prescribed for the treatment of depression and anxiety. They are an outstanding choice in this setting but may have significant impact on sleep and wakefulness. As the name implies, these medications increase serotonin, which is an activating neurotransmitter. As such, it is more favorable to take this class of medications when you wake up. This will decrease difficulty falling asleep at bedtime and staying sleep. Occasionally, people may sense increased fatigue or sleepiness when first starting this class of medication. Generally, with time, this side effect improves. However, if these symptoms persist during waking hours, moving the dose to later in the day will result in improvement, and minimize impact on the ability to initiate and, potentially, maintain sleep.

Beta Blockers (Atenolol, Metoprolol, Carvedilol, and others):
This class of medication is generally used for the treatment of high blood pressure and to slow the heart rate. So sleep may occur as a side effect. If you experience significant fatigue after initiating this class of medication, it is preferable to use them in the early evening (or suppertime). Most of these medications are offered with alternatives that can be used once a day and therefore are easier to dose in the evening.

Second and Third Generation Antihistamines: Cetirizine (Zyrtec), Loratadine (Claritin), Fexofenadine (Allegra):
These medications are used to combat seasonal allergies. In theory, they should not lead to significant sleepiness or alerting activity, but they may in some cases. Cetirizine is the most likely to cause sleepiness, so it is generally best to take it close to bedtime, to minimize the risk of sleepiness while awake.

Other Factors that may Affect the Ability to Initiate and Maintain Sleep

In addition to understanding our circadian rhythms, and how we can implement changes to improve our sleep, it is also important to realize that some people struggle with actual sleep disorders, and they may not even know it! There are over 100 classified sleep disorders. We will touch on one of the major disorders seen in sleep medicine.

Sleep Disordered Breathing

Sleep Disordered Breathing is a global term used to describe any changes in the upper airway, or in the physiology of breathing, that lead to significant sleep fragmentation. The majority of the U.S. population thinks of *obstructive sleep apnea* when a person is snoring and intermittently stops breathing. It is important to realize the significant impact obstructive sleep apnea can have on sleep and health, even during episodes when a person does not appear to stop breathing.

When sleep-disordered breathing exists, the airway is being compromised recurrently during sleep. This occurs primarily in the back of the throat, at the junction of the base of the tongue and the soft palate. As we fall asleep, the muscle tone in the airway decreases which, in susceptible individuals, leads to increased risk of the airway narrowing. As the airway narrows, oxygen levels may drop. The brain recognizes this is occurring and will subsequently arouse, to increase tone in the airway for normal breathing to resume. When this happens repeatedly, sleep is fragmented significantly. Of course, your sleep may also be interrupted when your significant other jabs you in the side with an elbow to make you stop snoring! Even Kevlar doesn't help.

As a result, even when people think that they are sleeping well, substantial sleepiness and fatigue can occur during waking hours due to the recurrent brief arousals that are happening throughout their sleep to maintain an open airway. It is a misconception that sleep-disordered breathing just affects those who may be overweight. This can occur in all people, especially in those with genetic predisposition, regardless of weight. In addition to breaking up sleep, sleep-disordered breathing can impede falling asleep. As a result, people may perceive they have insomnia when, in actuality, a collapsing airway is inhibiting them from falling asleep.

So, what does someone do if they suspect they have sleep disordered breathing? This condition can be diagnosed with a sleep study, which can be done at home with portable sleep monitors, or in sleep centers. Sleep studies done at home monitor the airway, effort of breathing, and oxygen levels. They are used solely to facilitate the diagnosis of obstructive sleep apnea and are not used to diagnose other subtler forms of sleep-disordered breathing or sleep disorders. When sleep medicine physicians have multiple concerns regarding possible reasons for sleep fragmentation, overnight sleep studies in accredited sleep centers, are recommended. These studies evaluate multiple variables that may be impacting the ability to initiate and maintain sleep and are much more sensitive in evaluating subtle forms of sleep-disordered breathing.

Untreated sleep-disordered breathing can lead to numerous health risks already discussed, along with broken sleep leading to significant levels of fatigue and sleepiness during the day. So, diagnosis and treatment are really important. The most well-known treatment for sleep-disordered breathing is Continuous Positive Airway Pressure (CPAP). This involves using a CPAP unit which generates air pressure in combination with a small mask that goes either over/into the nose or a mask that covers both the nose and the mouth. The air pressure helps maintain airway patency, which decreases brain arousals and drops in oxygen levels during the initiation and maintenance of sleep. Often, people envision Darth Vader or a fighter pilot when they think of using CPAP therapy. In reality, up-to-date masks have become much more comfortable, and easy to use.

Other options for treatment are also available, including custom oral devices that help move the lower jaw forward, which leads to opening of the airway. These devices are best made by dentists who have expertise in making and adjusting them appropriately. They are best suited in the treatment of uncomplicated mild to moderate sleep-disordered breathing when no other significant medical history is present.

Weight loss may also have a significant impact on sleep-disordered breathing. A ten to fifteen percent weight loss can lead to improvement. Weight loss decreases the amount of fatty tissue in the airway, which leads to less restriction during sleep. In addition, it allows for more ease of breathing at the level of the diaphragm. As previously noted though, even very significant weight loss may not fully treat sleep-disordered breathing.

In some individuals, sleep-disordered breathing may be positional, occurring almost solely when they sleep on their back. If this is identified during a sleep study, and minimal other medical issues are present, positional therapy may be recommended. This helps facilitate a person to maintain a lateral position during sleep.

Surgical intervention of the posterior airway may be considered, but this is generally best used only in mild to moderate sleep-disordered breathing. Unfortunately, even in this setting, the risk of recurrence is high. Because of this fact, surgery of this type is not commonly used as treatment.

If you have concerns of sleep-disordered breathing, or other sleep disorders, talk to your doctor. When sleep disorders are diagnosed, and properly treated, your sleep can improve tremendously, while at the same time decreasing risk to your body in the future.

Hot Tips to Sleep Tight

Sleep hygiene is the term used when discussing the various measures, you can implement on a daily basis to optimize your sleep. I have highlighted some of these points already in the context of John's challenges, but here's a summary of the important steps you can take to make your sleep the best it can be no matter what shift you work. I realize that your 9-1-1 work demands, and the hours you work pose a real challenge to getting good sleep. The following points are things to consider to optimize any component of your sleep/wake routine that can lead to improvements in your sleep.

1. Adequate and consistent hours of sleep, similar to diet and exercise, are essential to healthy living. Your body and brain thrive on consistency when it comes to sleep. Having an erratic bedtime and wake time leads to erratic sleep. This is especially true even when you might have a day off. Don't allow yourself to stay up and wake up excessively late on your days off. This leads to disruption of your circadian rhythms going into days that you work. As a result, your ability to initiate and maintain sleep may be affected adversely.

2. From his informal survey of several thousand dispatchers, Jim Marshall reports that most 9-1-1 Pros get an average of between four and six hours of sleep per every twenty-four hours. So, I know that you really struggle finding a way to get more sleep time. As hard as it may seem, try to make a commitment to maximize the number of your hours of sleep per twenty-four. I understand the demands of irregular schedules and night shift. Yet, when you commit to consistency in sleep to the fullest extent your schedule will allow, the inconsistencies in your life can improve!

3. Avoid substances that can impact your ability to initiate and maintain sleep.

4. Caffeine: Every effort should be made to minimize drinking caffeine eight hours before your bedtime. Caffeine can affect your ability to get to sleep and stay asleep. Those who say they can go to sleep after consuming caffeine probably are extremely sleep-deprived and/or have developed a significant tolerance to caffeine. Even if this is the case, sleep can still be disrupted, and you don't even know it. Making changes in caffeine use can be done gradually. Start with discontinuing caffeine one hour earlier per day every third day until you hit the goal of 8 hours before your bedtime time. As this is completed and other hot tips are instituted, your sleep, as well as your ability to function the next day, can improve!

Alcohol also leads to significant disruption of sleep. Initially, it may help people get to sleep but as it is metabolized, wakefulness may result. If you have difficulty initiating/maintaining sleep, use of alcohol before bedtime should be avoided and if you do, never in excess. Try to keep at least four to six hours between your last alcohol and bedtime.

5. Discontinue TV, computer, cellphone and any other handheld screen device use an hour before bedtime, and do not use screen devices in the bedroom. Technology is a great thing, but it leads to increased wakefulness signals in your brain. Remember that being awake in bed conditions your brain that this is normal. Instead, read something relaxing outside of your bedroom with some soft backlighting. This will help you wind down. If you believe the world may end if you miss your favorite program, record it and watch it at a more convenient earlier time.

6. Don't allow yourself to watch a clock during the night. If you wake and have difficulty falling back to sleep, a clock next to your bed can lead to an increased level of frustration about being awake. When it comes to alarm clocks, set it for your wake time and cover it. Don't lull yourself into believing, "I don't need an alarm because I wake naturally." By setting an alarm, your brain is eased of the burden of ensuring that you wake on time, and you'll get more sleep.

7. Try to develop strategies to leave some of your stress and frustrations outside of your bedroom. Yeah, I know, telling a dispatcher to avoid stress is like telling the ocean to avoid salt! Your brain is so full of "stuff" when you get home. For 9-1-1Pros and others with the most stressful jobs, it can really help to list your concerns and worries about the day a couple of hours before your bedtime. I refer to this as the "Worry List of Life." Do this outside of your bedroom. Jot down your concerns and a plan to deal with them (or at least one step toward that goal). Do not keep a pad next to your bed to write things down. This will only cause you to focus on the stressors. In addition, avoid negative TV shows and, God forbid, national news, or any other stressful media. Consider doing something that is relaxing, such as meditating or stretching (especially after a long shift of sitting).

8. If your brain is racing when you lay down in bed, consider using relaxation breathing which can help you stop the negative cycle of thoughts. I frequently recommend the "4/7/8" breathing sequence. This strategy distracts you from ruminating over concerns you've already worked to let go of for the night. First, breathe in and out through your nose deeply and slowly, for a total of four breaths. Once you breathe in all the way on the fourth breath, hold your breath for a count of seven. Then breathe out over a count of eight. Repeat this sequence. At the

same time, picture a person, place, quotation, or phrase that brings you comfort or peace. Repeat this as needed until you fall asleep. There's no single right way to do this breathing strategy. You may find that more deep breaths and less time holding your breath, or breathing out, is best for you. The key is not to try to force yourself to relax or fall asleep. Just tune in to how you feel as you do these relaxation steps.

9. If, while trying to do the breathing exercise, you find that you're focusing on noise in your environment, consider using a fan near your bed or "sleep sounds" readily available on smart phone devices/apps.

10. Exercise and a regular daily routine can lead to improvements in sleep. When exercising, try to avoid workouts too close to bedtime. Increased core body temperature near bedtime can delay your ability to fall asleep.

11. Keep your bedroom cool, dark, and quiet. A cool bedroom will help facilitate better sleep. Remember how the body temperature drops during the night.

12. Avoid big meals before bed. Try to keep at least 3 hours between your last meal and bedtime. If hunger strikes then, consider a small, higher protein snack such as cottage cheese, yogurt, or a small handful of almonds.

13. Avoid late day napping. Minimize any napping to seven to eight hours before bed. If you do take a nap, keep it to twenty to thirty minutes. It will refresh you, but not affect your sleep quality at bedtime.

Hot Tips Around the Clock

I know that when first looking at the recommendations above, many of us who have worked or are currently working third or rotating shifts are simply ready to throw in the towel. Before you do, remember that even taking small steps of implementing change is the first move in being able to make leaps of improvement in your sleep. After reviewing the Hot Tips, think seriously about how you can develop consistency and process change in your life. Again, the goal is to first optimize the time that you have to sleep and then to build out. I want you to be empowered by being able to take some control. After doing so, you can develop your own success cycle when it comes to sleep! Here are the points I want to emphasize when it comes to sleeping better in a world driven by first shift:

1. Dim down the light hitting your eyes when leaving work. If it is sunny outside, get your sunglasses on even before you leave your workplace

building. Minimize the natural alerting signal of light.

2. Set yourself up for success with an environment conducive to sleep at your home: black out shades on windows, cool room, white noise (fan, sleep sounds, classical music), eye shades in addition to black out shades on the windows, ear plugs. Have it all ready even when you leave for work.

3. Consistency breeds consistency. Routine builds routine. Your brain loves both when it comes to sleep. Even if your schedule is changing each week, take charge with consistency. Your first two days or so of sleep may not be optimal, but it will improve compared to not having a routine.

4. Take a pause when you get home. Give yourself time to wind down with some of the thoughts noted earlier. Don't undermine your success. Be deliberate as you get ready for bed.
5. Track your success and encourage your coworkers. Within the context of the information that you've learned, and as you implement change, help your friends who you might see are having problems with sleep.

A Word to Our Sponsors

For all of you who develop shift schedules, I know that it is a crazy world especially when needing to cover a stressful twenty-four hours. With this said, I would encourage you to think about ways that you can take some of the information presented to help optimize how scheduling can be constructed. If your employees obtain better sleep, they will in turn produce better work and be a happier group.

1. Consider creating shifts that last longer than a week so that routine and timing can improve when it comes to sleep. Rotating schedules cause significant disruption in sleep. If possible, create a four-week cycle of staying on one shift.

2. Depending on the demands of your center, consider twelve hour shifts to build consistency in routine and sleep timing. Maintain a schedule for four weeks at a time.

3. Find the night owls. Some of your employees are simply (and often genetically) third shifters. Ask your group if some would rather work third shift all the time. If so, consider letting them maintain their third shift all the time. By doing so, this decreases in some measure the number of third shifts that need to be covered by those who would prefer days or afternoon shifts.

The demands of 9-1-1 work are numerous. By optimizing your sleep, you will be able to approach your work knowing that you are ready to handle the mental and physical requirements of your job with more confidence. Remember that sleep, just like your specialty training, is an important component of doing your job well, minimizing burn out, and decreasing the risk of other medical conditions for the future. I'm hopeful that when you understand and implement the principles I've introduced, you will be able to realize your full potential, not only in your sleep, but your personal and professional life as well. Sleep for the Health of It!

Questions for Reflection

To get the most from this chapter, you are encouraged to write your reflections here (in both the Kindle and paperback versions of this book).

- What was your main take-away from reading this chapter?

- What specifically made it valuable to you?

- How can you apply this take-away concretely to improve some aspect of your personal life and or efforts to support the wellbeing of 9-1-1Pros?

Additional Resources

- *Consider reading the now classic, and quite entertaining sleep book, Power Sleep, by Dr. James Maas; and also his more recent Sleep for Success: Everything You Must Know About Sleep but are Too Tired to Ask, co-authored by Rebecca S. Robins*

- Stay tuned for the upcoming class, *9-1-1Pros: Sleep for the Health of It!*

9-1-1 Pros: Sleep for the Health of It!

by Dr. Boss and Jim Marshall. Direct all inquiries to Info@911training.net.

CHAPTER 12
Enough Fat Jokes Already! Seven Steps toward Winning the 9-1-1 Obesity Challenge

Jim Marshall

Introduction

Eating is a Very Personal Issue

Few topics are more sensitive and personal than eating and struggles with obesity. As readers battling food issues read articles or books on this subject, they may feel a familiar flood of thoughts and emotions. Hopefulness may tangle with skepticism about yet another promise of fast and permanent weight loss that seems too good to be true. Thoughts of past failure may stir feelings of discouragement mixed with self-judgments and shame. And if they are a 9-1-1Pro, they may also feel a big dose of cynicism anticipating that they'll take yet another stab at losing weight, only to fail again. I can assure you; this Chapter offers no false promises of quick and sustained weight loss. It does offer real hope through exploration of several factors that, in combination, make weight gain more likely for 9-1-1Pros *and* steps they and their leaders can take to improve these factors.

Respecting the Complexity of the Challenge

Have you ever said, "You have no idea how hard I've tried to lose weight!" You are probably not alone! I can't prove this, but I'd bet my home equity that most people who struggle with obesity have said far more disparaging things to themselves at different stages of the struggle than others have said to them. And that's really something, given the things that well-intended humans can say! It's extremely discouraging, even clinically depressing, when a person has toiled hard for years with small victories of weight loss, only to be followed by weight gain. The weight goes down twenty pounds, it goes up twenty, on and on for years; ending up at the same weight (and health risks) as when they started. Self-criticism and lowering self-esteem may take over in the form of negative self-talk that fuels even more depression—and weight gain.

- *I would succeed if I just practice more self-control.*
- *I'm just not trying hard enough.*
- *I have no will power.*
- *Maybe I just don't have what it takes.*

What an excruciating cycle; especially when you're successful at most everything else in your life! But there's also good reason for hope...

Good Cause for Hope

Telecommunicators are bright, courageous, tenacious, persevering, and often even sacrificial. They often muster the grit and determination to withstand twelve, sometimes even sixteen hour shifts for days on end. If grit were the only criterion for permanent success in weight management, this chapter wouldn't be necessary. Hope will not be found in pushing yourself to practice *more* self-control, try even *harder*, and rally *more* will power. Yes, grit is an essential ingredient for change, but the real hope for lasting improvement is through understanding the variety of factors that drive the food struggle in the 9-1-1 family. By identifying those factors and defining steps to manage them more effectively, we may achieve better health than we've ever had before. *That's* the goal of this chapter.

Seven Steps toward Winning the 9-1-1 Obesity Challenge

The Importance of Setting Realistic Expectations

As a trauma therapist, I learned long ago that offering simplistic solutions to people struggling with serious long-term problems was worse than doing nothing at all. There are *no cookie cutter solutions* to complex problems. But that doesn't mean there aren't solutions or that change isn't possible! But the possibility of change will depend on seeing the full picture. The steps I offer here, related to each factor suspected to drive 9-1-1 obesity, will not, in themselves, fully address the challenge. But the more steps we take, the further down the road to improvement we're apt to travel.

Headway in decreasing obesity in the 9-1-1 center is a shared responsibility. Dispatchers can go a good distance in improving their own health if they are empowered with the information they need. Yet leaders, too, must work to improve work conditions shown to increase weight gain and provide the resources their employees need to increase the probability of success.

Here are the seven steps for decreasing obesity we'll explore:

1. Get empowered through increased awareness of health risks of obesity
2. Improve 9-1-1 Work Design to increase opportunity for physical activity
3. Increase knowledge about the role of cortisol production in eating
4. Boost training in stress resilience to activate skillsets as needed in real-time
5. Break free from the Suck-it-Up/Eat-it-Up Emotional Code
6. Practice Self-Compassion to reduce self-criticism
7. Wonder Compassionately and Heal Trauma (Note: if you have endured life-long struggles with obesity, you may want to read this section first.)

Let's get started.

Step 1: Get Empowered through Increased Awareness of Health Risks of Obesity

What You Need to Know

Researchers Lilly and Allen found that 54.7% of eight hundred and eight 9-1-1Pros were either obese or morbidly obese (Lilly & Allen 262). This rate is significantly higher than the national adult rate of 36.5% during the same period (Ogden 1). This is an alarming statistic, and should certainly prompt our industry to jump into action to help reverse the problem. Yet, the more common a problem is within a community or a group, the more *normal* it seems. Since being overweight or obese has long been common in our 9-1-1 centers, and throughout the industry, we, as a 9-1-1 culture, may have become so accustomed to it that we no longer see it as a problem; it's just the norm. We don't think about risks connected to what is just normal. To put it simply, we become desensitized.

And, on the personal level, if I'm already deeply discouraged about a problem and I'm convinced there is nothing I can do to change it, then why dwell on it? This makes good sense. So, as a 9-1-1 culture, and as individual members, our vision of the problem and the risks associated with it fades from view. Both factors work together. So, life goes on in the comm center and the risks associated with obesity remain a distant thought.

Fortunately, there is cause for hope for 9-1-1Pros as we explore the next six steps and pursue change related to them. And, with reason for hope, it becomes more tolerable to recognize the risks and work strategically to reduce them.

So, let's first define what we know about the risks of obesity; not as a scare tactic to motivate change, but to affirm the importance of not giving up the good fight.

I have always believed that it was possible to be obese yet still be in pretty good health without being at big risk of early death or disease. Most Americans also believe this to be true. As it turns out, this is false. I know, that is sobering, but it's important to know. Obesity produces a combination of factors, known collectively as *metabolic syndrome,* which significantly increases health risks. This syndrome is defined as, "elevated waist circumference and triglycerides, low HDL cholesterol, hypertension, and glucose intolerance" (Violanti 194). Complications of this syndrome include higher risk of heart disease and Type 2 diabetes.

Because of the risks associated with metabolic syndrome, the American Medical Association officially designated obesity a disease in 2013. They believed increased awareness was the first step in empowering folks to succeed in their battle with obesity.

A major new study, completed in 2017, supports the wisdom of the AMA's effort. This study found that "people with obesity considered to be healthy were 49% more likely to develop coronary heart disease, as well as were 96% more likely to have heart failure" (Sandoiu). For this reason, the authors of this study came to a powerful realization:

> The idea of being healthily obese is a myth. Our work shows that so-called 'metabolically healthy' obese individuals are still at higher risk of coronary heart disease, cerebrovascular disease, and heart failure than normal weight metabolically healthy individuals. The priority of health professionals regarding these patients should be to promote and facilitate weight loss, as it is with any other obese patient (Sandoui).

These findings prove that many members of our 9-1-1 family are at greater risk of living shorter, less fulfilling lives, unless they are taking active steps to lower these risks. Yet, they are less apt to do that if they don't realize those risks and they've come to see obesity as just normal in the comm center. So, they would be less apt to seek and discover new information and steps that they can take to protect themselves.

What You Can Do

- Just by reading the medical facts above you've already, hopefully, gained more awareness of the risks related to obesity. Now you can build your knowledge base. While we tend to look to our doctors to tell us if there's a medical risk, they often don't share hard facts, like those above, with their patients. 9-1-1Pros deserve to know the risks they face so that they can decide how to rally an adequate defense. Your first step in planning to help reduce obesity in your 9-1-1 center is to embrace this knowledge as inspiration to pursue good solutions.

Step 2: Improve 9-1-1 Work Design to Increase Opportunity for Physical Activity

What You Need to Know

There's really no way to overestimate the role that 9-1-1 work design plays in obesity. Let's consider the design of 9-1-1 work at the console for a minute. *Traditionally* it includes:

- The requirement to remain within a small space (the console area) which confines physical movement, especially when understaffed
- Long hours
- Typically, few, and in many 9-1-1 centers, no breaks during which greater movement would be possible
- Work is performed predominantly while sitting

One of the greatest contributors to weight gain and chronic diseases is sedentary behavior. The fact is, traditional 9-1-1 work design significantly increases obesity struggles, because it places major limitations on the dispatcher's physical activity. Fortunately, in recent years, the 9-1-1 industry has made some progress in trying to improve work design at the console. Industry associations have encouraged conference presentations and published articles on the topic. Corporate partners have developed hydraulic consoles that rise, to enable work performance while standing up. Also, companies offer treadmills designed for use during active dispatch work. Increasingly, dispatchers who are given these opportunities are taking advantage of them. Those who don't, may be less aware of the dangerous health risks of remaining sedentary through their careers. And excessive work hours, extended night shift work and rotating shifts can impair sleep promoting increased struggles with obesity (see Chapter 11).

What You Can Do

- Leaders should aggressively seek funding and support for purchase of treadmills. Far from being work frills, they can: improve health, foster weight loss, and boost performance, morale and retention of employees.
- Leaders should strive to make it possible for dispatchers to take regular breaks throughout the day.
- Dispatchers with elevating consoles can stand up intermittingly through their shifts; all 9-1-1Pros can do body stretches and other in-place exercises as much as the demands of a given shift allow.
- Dispatchers can consider buddying up with a peer to start and maintain a team regimen, walking for 30 minutes before or after work.
- See the Additional Resource section below for more information about sedentary behavior.
- If you are a leader, consider forming a PSAP committee to evaluate how much opportunity for physical activity is currently available (at the console and in the PSAP) and how it could be increased. Also, if you are a leader, consider volunteering to serve on the committee.
- Evaluate how scheduling is impacting employee sleep patterns since sleep deficits and impairment can increase obesity.

Step 3: Increase Knowledge about the Role of Cortisol in Eating

What You Need to Know

Let's look to the smart folks from Harvard for a couple gems of insight about the stress response and eating that ought to set your head spinning with some new thoughts in support of Step 2.

> In the short term, stress can shut down appetite. A structure in the brain called the hypothalamus produces a corticotropin-releasing hormone, which suppresses appetite. The brain also sends messages to the adrenal glands atop the kidneys to pump out the hormone epinephrine (also known as adrenaline). Epinephrine helps trigger the body's fight-or flight response, a revved-up physiological state that temporarily puts eating on hold (1).

Wait! Let's pause for a moment. I know the fight-or-flight response isn't news to most of you. But let's be sure we didn't miss the first of two gems from these Harvard folks: your appetite is not just based on *when you ate last*. Even if you hadn't eaten for hours, and were ravenous before that awful 9-1-1 call, your appetite probably vanished in a split second when all hell broke loose. Have you ever gone without eating when you're stressed out? It isn't just because you're 'busy." It's because your hormones are running the show here. And not just governing appetite suppression. Let's read on…

> But if stress persists it's a different story. The adrenal glands release another hormone called cortisol, and cortisol increases appetite and may also ramp up motivation in general, including the motivation to eat. Once a stressful episode is over, cortisol levels should fall, but if the stress doesn't go away—or if a person's stress response gets stuck in "the on" position—cortisol may stay elevated (1).

This is a huge point: you're actually motivated by a sustained stress response to eat, and to keep eating! My next question may be the most rhetorical one I've ever asked: are 9-1-1Pros more apt to trigger a stress response that gets "stuck" in the "on" position than other workers? Just take another look at 9-1-1's Nine Big Risk Factors we unpacked back in Chapter 3:

#1: No Warning Before Potentially Traumatic Calls
#2: The Big "C" of 9-1-1—Lack of Closure
#3: Telecommunicators are Psychologically On-scene but Physically Unable to Reach It
#4: 9-1-1Pros "Send Their Own" into Harm's Way
#5: Limited Sensory Engagement with Those on Scene
#6: High Call Volume and Frequency
#7: The Crazy-Tasking Demand
#8: Little to No Downtime to De-stress: for cortisol to cease production we need to feel secure that no new threat is imminent
#9: Lack of Appreciation and Professional Respect

These 9-1-1 stressors in any combination will almost certainly and significantly increase the chance that you will be in a sustained fight-or-flight response throughout your shift. So you'll be motivated to eat too much. But if that's the case, what happens over a longer period? 9-1-1Pros are more apt to experience Chronic Stress. This term does not mean that you are constantly producing cortisol. It means you activate the stress response excessively over months and years with too little down time between activations. You may either produce cortisol, or experience the left overs, which flow almost constantly within your blood supply. Therefore, you're more apt to remain in a vigilant state, on edge; especially since, as a telecommunicator, you don't know exactly when that next hot call is coming.

What You Can Do

- Respect that your eating patterns at work are not just due to "lack of motivation or will power."
- Recognize that 9-1-1Pros are apt to over-eat unless they learn to manage cortisol-production.
- Build the skills needed to succeed at optimal management of cortisol production. That leads us to Step 4!

Step 4: Boost Training in Stress Resilience to Activate Skillsets as Needed in Real-Time

What You Need to Know

Throughout the United States, only a small portion of our 9-1-1 telecommunicators have been trained to utilize empirically supported stress management and resilience skills that can help them manage their stress responses. As we will discuss in Chapter 15 there is an official industry standard that states, "Public Safety Answering Points shall establish Comprehensive Stress Management Programs" (NENA 22). This mandate has helped increase awareness and pursuit of stress help for many centers. However, PSAPs have yet to learn that this standard exists, and many of our leaders (whether they are familiar with the NENA standard or not) simply do not have the funds to purchase this training.

What You Can Do

- In Chapter 6, I shared some of the powerful skills that my students learn in *Survive and Thrive*, including the ChoicePoints™ strategy. So, if you are struggling with 9-1-1 stress and eating, a first helpful move forward might actually be reaching back to that chapter for a few moments. Review how you can use the ChoicePoints and resilience skills to manage stress through your work day. By optimizing your stress responses one event at a time, you may reduce cortisol-driven craving. Yet, there's more you can do...We can also use the ChoicePoints strategy specifically in response to the *craving* for food at the console. Fortunately, we often receive clear cues when cortisol is activated. These are cues you can use to do something smart for self-care.

  Stress cues come from three different inner sources: your *automatic* thoughts, emotions and body sensations. You can use your attunement to these cues as prompts to actively manage your eating patterns in the comm center.

- To master your eating choices, learn the cues which signal your cravings. Here are some examples of what those cues look like:
    - **Automatic Thought**: "I just want to eat something, I don't care what it is, but if it's in sight I'll eat it… (This may explain one of the most frequent and hated 9-1-1 refrigerator violations: eating food from containers with someone else's name on it.) Or perhaps the thought is: "Oh man, they brought us pizza again. I shouldn't, but it looks so good! I just need some good comfort food right now…"
    - **Automatic Emotion**: tension, nervousness, anxiety, or sorrow that you're trying to fend off from a bad call, headache
    - **Automatic Body**: hunger pangs, even though you've already eaten

You've probably just edited this list and replaced my examples with your own. So, that means if they occurred at work, you could probably *notice* them. *Noticing* those cues is a core skill in the ChoicePoints strategy, because once you notice them you can activate the skills to regulate your stress response and hopefully decrease the craving. Now consider these points:

- Visit Chapter 6, to review and practice Heart Focused Breathing, CAD Breathing and the Prep Technique when you notice the cues as craving first kicks in.

- Keep this in mind: the goal is not to use your in-the-moment attunement to your craving to become your own self-critical food-cop. It is to practice non-judgmental awareness of cues for self-care; to help you distinguish true hunger from cortisol-driven craving (which may pass quickly with skill-use and helpful distractions).
- Remind yourself that when you practice these skills as a choice for your own self-care, you will feel less like you are depriving yourself of food when you don't obey the craving.

Step 5: Break Free from the *Suck-it-Up/Eat-it-Up* Emotional Code

What You Need to Know

For years, as I've spent time with 9-1-1Pros at their comm centers or in my classes, I've heard an oft-repeated message, "We battle with our weight, because we're emotional eaters." Emotional eating is defined as, "The use of food to modify negative mood states" (Levitan 783). But not everyone who works in a 9-1-1 center is an emotional eater. (That doesn't make them better, just different, as we'll see in a minute.) So, what inclines one person to do more emotional eating than someone else? First, the intense demands with callers in distress naturally incline dispatchers to shelf their feelings to stay objective on the call. Yet, I believe the bent toward emotional eating depends in part on your Emotional Code.

In Chapter 5, we defined our Emotional Code as, "the mindset that governs what we do with our emotions." When a loved one dies, do we feel sorrow, sadness, cry when needed, and seek support (which reflects a healthy emotional mindset)? Or, do we push on, work even harder, and distance ourselves from the pain, never looking back? This is an example of what I call the Suck-it-Up code. Whether our Emotional Code is healthy or not, we gain nothing by judging it. We can gain much, though, by figuring out if it is working for or against us.

In Chapter 5, we also established that the Suck-it-Up Emotional code dominates the 9-1-1 culture, and the larger emergency responder culture. Some suck up their emotions with distractions like excessive gaming, drinking, and work. Some do a combination of all of these. Many 9-1-1Pros find food as the ideal way to keep painful emotions at bay, since it works quite well. And, let's face it, a handful of Oreos is gonna win my vote over a stalk of celery most days of the week. Newsflash #2: sweet, fatty food tastes good! They're also the most popular pick (over salty-savory foods) among emotional eaters. But there is, of course, the depressing downside (apart from higher risk for Type II diabetes):

> Emotional eating increases an individual's tendency to consume more food than physiologically needed. Increased intake leads to increases in body mass index (BMI) scores and the probability of having a clinical diagnosis of being overweight or obese (Fox 194).

So, a cycle ensues: emotion-driven, over-eating = obesity = increased risk for chronic disease. With zero judgment intended, I call this the Suck-it-Up/Eat-it-Up Emotional Code. Now let's look at what you can do to pull out of it.

What You Can Do

- Begin by respecting why the 9-1-1Pro is so inclined to adopt the Suck-it-Up/Eat-it-Up Emotional Code. An enormous amount of distressing emotion floods in from callers daily!
- Revisit Chapter 5 to evaluate and rewrite your emotional code, and to practice seeking and sharing emotional support with your peers (and loved ones).
- Use the ChoicePoints strategy to notice when you're inclined to stuff distress that will lead to emotional eating and activate a stress resilience skill. Review Chapter 6 as needed to practice the skills.

Step 6: Practice Self-Compassion to Reduce Self-Criticism

What You Need to Know

In my class, *The Power of Peer Support,* I playfully bait my students with the following, seemingly naïve, question, "Why do you 9-1-1Pros think you have to be so perfect all the time? I mean, nobody's perfect. You guys are harder on yourself than any group of professionals I know!" Their answers usually lead us right to what drives intense self-criticism in dispatchers:

- "All our calls are recorded."
- "Our calls are graded as part of Quality Assurance, there's almost no room for error."
- "Our field responders will complain if we make the slightest mistakes."

Then somebody blurts out the biggest, most powerful reason why most (not all) dedicated 9-1-1Pros dread even making small mistakes and may beat themselves up relentlessly when they do:

- "When we make mistakes, people can die."

Oh, okay then. There is *that* to consider, too. When 9-1-1Pros say this, they are thinking about two groups of people. Yes, the public; whether they are guiding a mother in performing CPR on an infant; sending firefighters to an address when screaming or language barriers make it hard to confirm that address; or countless other life and death scenarios where humans can make mistakes. But also, if you ask any group of dispatchers, "what matters most at the end of the day for you as a 9-1-1Pro" (as I have countless times), you'll always hear the same response, "Everyone goes home safe." Of course, they are speaking of their field responders. If you're a telecommunicator, you're probably nodding your head in agreement right now.

As dispatchers, you feel an enormous sense of responsibility for the safety of the field responders you send on calls for service. And every time you know there will be risk involved, the pressure to do everything right returns tenfold. Ironically, even if you are 100% dedicated to bringing "everyone home safe," you also know this is the one thing over which you have no control. To which I always get the response, "Well then, by damn, at least I can do everything humanly possible to improve the odds for the better."

This makes total sense. And my goal isn't to change the work ethic it represents. The problem that must be addressed is how you, as a 9-1-1Pro, are impacted psychologically when people do die, or are seriously injured on your watch. And that depends on how well you can accept your human limits when you face them; how able you are to practice self-compassion and kindness. This is not the same as "letting yourself off the hook" and avoiding acceptance of responsibility when we fail. With self-compassion, we will recognize the failure, feel appropriate sorrow, and pledge to improve if needed. Yet, we will also affirm that mistakes are inevitable since we are human. If we are consumed with a sense of failure, intolerable guilt follows, and an ever-increasing self-critical mindset to prevent the next mistake.

Very understandably, 9-1-1Pros are especially at risk of this extreme mindset because so much may be at stake when you fail at the console. And this brings us to my point about how to reduce over-eating.

Psychologist Kristen Neff, a pioneer in the study of self-compassion, has helped prove that we achieve more success with self-compassion versus criticism. It turns out that in pursuits like weight loss, the harder we are on ourselves by habit, the harder it will be to change the habits we most want to change.

> In areas where it is hard to fool ourselves—when comparing our weight to those of magazine models, for instance…we cause ourselves incredible amounts of emotional pain. We lose faith in ourselves, start doubting our potential, and become hopeless. Of course, this sorry state just yields more self-condemnation for being such a do-nothing loser, and down, down we go…Even if we do manage to get our act together, the goalposts for what counts as "good enough" seem always to remain frustratingly out of reach (Neff 5-6).

See if you can relate to this example: after years of terrible eating, you've spent weeks studying diets and plans for healthy eating. You finally find one you think will work and get started. You pull it off without a hitch for a couple weeks, but then, amidst more stressors at home and work, you drop the ball two days in a row. Discouragement sets in and you begin to silently berate yourself. Dr. Neff's message: your conditioned harsh response to this slip-up will almost certainly be what dooms your effort, not the slip-up itself.

What You Can Do

- Actively practice self-compassion. The ChoicePoints strategy can also help you here. Take a few minutes to prepare and practice this strategy to reduce self-criticism and boost self-compassion:
    o Identify and write down some of the harsh or critical statements you tend you say (or think) to yourself.
    o For each criticism, write a kinder replacement statement.
    o Imagine one of the situations that typically would trigger the self-criticism. As you visualize that situation, take deep breaths in and out of your heart and focus on the affirming statement instead. By doing this you may be able to put a new mental template in place that will make this shift from self-criticism to self-compassion easier to do.

- If you know that you're inclined to berate yourself, buy Kristin Neff's book! I urge you to do this, not because I earn a percentage of Dr. Neff's book sale (which I don't), but because I know your investment in fully understanding self-compassion will require more than the brief introduction this chapter affords. No cookie-cutter solutions, remember?
- Go to the *Additional Resources* section below for information on her book and her website which include other resources you can use to boost self-compassion.
- If you know that the berating will likely not improve by using the ChoicePoints strategy I proposed above, consider Step #7 below, respecting and dealing compassionately with underlying trauma.

Step 7: Wonder Compassionately & Heal Trauma

Recently I was in the classroom with the 9-1-1 family leading the *Survive and Thrive* resilience experience. This was a group of telecommunicators selected by their leaders to pursue training to become *Certified 9-1-1 Peer Supporters* (Chapter 16). I emphasized that together we would make the room a safe place for members to share, as they chose, never under pressure to do so. As we traveled through those two days, the group became extraordinarily bonded. Many students took risks to relate personally to our topics, and they were rewarded with strong support and encouragement from their peers. Then I shared Lilly and Allen's findings about high obesity rates in the 9-1-1 industry (discussed earlier in this chapter). I expressed my concern that *self-shaming about eating drives deeper discouragement* and depression, fueling worsening food struggles. This really resonated with the class members. One 9-1-1Pro courageously took the lead by acknowledging that her failure to break this lifelong cycle of uncontrolled eating was breaking *her*.

Let me emphasize that the discussion that followed, as described here, is never one I would pull a class into. I carefully govern and guide our discussions. This time, the person who shared felt confident that this was a smart risk for her, and I supported her choice. This woman was one of the most senior and highly respected dispatchers in the room. She placed her hands-on top of her stomach and said to the full class, "I've struggled with obesity my whole life." Then she looked at me and said, "Jim, I've tried to lose this weight so many times. I lose some, but I always go back to how I ate before. It's hard *not* to hate myself." She described how shame, disgust, and a sense of failure would always follow the over-eating. "So, what do I do?"

Getting to the Kinder More Powerful Truth by Wondering Compassionately

I could see the deep disappointment in her eyes, the weariness from years of fighting with herself unsuccessfully, yet still a longing to successfully manage her weight and be healthy. Knowing that she and I had already connected as 9-1-1 family through our time together in class, I reflected, and then offered to lead her in a brief exercise *wondering compassionately*. We could do this either in the moment during the class or privately during a one-on-one time together while on break. She elected to go ahead, with her classmates present. So we began. I said: "I'm going to just start a sentence as if I am you speaking, then I want you to just do your best to finish the sentence. Don't respond at all if you don't want to. There will be no right answer. Just say whatever seems true." She affirmed her willingness, so I started the statement:

"A part of me says, 'I should be able to keep myself from grabbing those cookies and putting them in my mouth. What's wrong with me? I am an adult. This is my choice!' Yet to be honest, as bad as it sounds, as embarrassing as it may be to admit, there's another part of me that says…" She finished the sentence quickly; "I want it. It tastes good. It feels like a blanket to me. But I shouldn't…"

I jumped in because she had just slipped back into judging herself, even as she was able to identify the huge need that food met for her on a core level: "Wait, back up. I'm going to continue where you left off: 'Sure, maybe I shouldn't feel this way, but the truth is, I want to eat this. It feels like a blanket, like comfort to me!' Is that right?"

She affirmed this was how she felt. I quickly assured her that she did not have to continue this exercise amidst her peers, and that we could do this together during a break. Yet, she wanted their support and encouraged me to continue the exercise.

I said: "…Listen, you said earlier that you've struggled with eating your whole life. Let's wonder compassionately together. Can you recall feeling that food was like that blanket for you when you were a girl?"

"Yes, it was."

"Okay. We don't have to go into any details, but would it be accurate that there was some pretty sad, hard stuff happening back then?"

"Yes", she said.

"You don't have to answer. But if you choose, I'm going to start another sentence for you, and then you finish it." I began the next sentence with a hesitant yet angry tone as I suspected she might have felt years ago.

"There's a part of me that says I shouldn't eat this pastry. I'm disgusted with myself. What's wrong with me?' Yet, to be really honest, the other part of me feels like 'you know, screw you, I will eat this if I want to, because…

She added: "… it is comfort to me, and I want to!"

"How much comfort did you get from others back then, to help soothe your pain about what was happening to you?"

"Not much. None, really."

"Were you getting criticized for over-eating? Was somebody trying to make you stop eating the sweets?"

"Yes."

"You've done a great job. Is this okay, or should we stop?"

"No, I'm good. It's okay"

"Okay, then. Let's go one step further, just wondering compassionately. I can't know this, but is it like a part of you says, 'I'm gonna eat this because it comforts me, and also maybe because, you know what? Screw you! I'm gonna eat it because it's one thing I do have control over, and it comforts me, and you can't stop me!' Can you relate to this?"

"Um, yeah. Yes."

"So, look; your whole life you've been beating up on yourself, angry that you can't control what and how much you eat. You acknowledged that you've been really mean to yourself for years about this struggle. I want you to consider something. Just for a moment, can you look back in time and see that young girl who was sneaking food, and finding comfort in it?"

"Yeah, I can" she said.

"I think there are plenty of people in this room right now who know you are a loving person. Could you possibly imagine going to that young girl, your younger self, with some of that love, to offer her your kindness, your understanding, to begin helping her heal?"
She said, "I think so".

This was not a therapy session. It was an exercise. But if it had been a session, I may have offered to guide this woman in connecting more deeply with, and learning to actively love on, that younger part of herself; to exchange self-loathing, for self-compassion, then to seek healing of the traumatic experiences that fueled her early need for comfort. This brave 9-1-1Pro received a great deal of support and affection from her classmates that day as I carefully transitioned our class discussion beyond her. Our group then shared a third day together on the topic of peer support. Her transparency about this struggle with food turned out to be a core part of the shared experience that brought everyone together. It reinforced their shared realization that even the strongest 9-1-1Pros need help and are courageous to seek it, from professionals and from their peers. I'm confident that this woman will pursue therapy to heal the self-condemnation that had, for a lifetime, blocked her best chances for success. Wondering compassionately had served as a key to her future.

She hadn't known what else to fill her sadness and aloneness with as a girl, other than by eating the most comforting foods she could find. It just so happened they were also the foods that would threaten her health over a lifetime. Since she had no other real options for comfort, and since kids are usually limited in their ability to self-soothe, she locked into compulsive eating. Of course, she would also become psychologically dependent on the *experience*: the flavors, the full feeling, the comfort, and the sense of control it brought her. But that didn't make her stupid or pathetic or bent on self-destruction. She was trying to solve a problem.

Without realizing it, she had been beating up on that little girl for years, after each episode of overeating. Perhaps you can relate personally to her story. You too may have learned to whisper mean things to yourself again and again, in disgust. And each time, that young part of you may have felt even more shame, more alone and—here's the catch-- more hunger for comfort! Rather than being motivated to eat less, it is possible that the more shame you felt as a child, the more desperate you became for soothing to fill yourself with the one thing you discovered would bring comfort—*more sugary, fatty food.* This is not something to be judged. It is something to consider with kindness.

I'm not trying to make excuses here. The goal of this exploration isn't to blame parents for childhood struggles to avoid responsibility for adult behaviors. We are just trying to wonder compassionately, because sometimes we cannot succeed in taking full responsibility unless we reach the truth about what motivates our most self-defeating behaviors; and more often than not, it is kindness that leads the way to truth. Kindness is a light shining into places where healing happens. Without wondering compassionately, we become locked into a futile pattern of attempting to "take responsibility" by bludgeoning ourselves after each failure, with the same ruthless accusations. We may become convinced we're just losers, through and through. Such condemnation never leads to powerful behavior change, because it is ignorant of what drives our struggles.

What You Can Do

- Reflect on this exchange between our 9-1-1Pro above and me. Jot down some notes. How and how much can you relate to her and to what she recognized? If you are strongly resonating with this discussion, or if you sense that it fits but feels threatening, please consider seeking some good therapy help from a trauma therapist who is certified in EMDR (see Chapter 9).
- Unless advised by your physician, practice wondering compassionately about eating struggles, with the support of a qualified therapist, before pursuit of restrictive diets. Extreme weight loss attempts can be set-ups for failure (if not carefully guided by medical experts) and can set off a cascade of strong self-criticism, discouragement and increasing likelihood of failure. Compassionately accounting first for the psychological struggles in your relationship to your body, before you seek weight loss, is a foundation for success in improving your health.

Conclusion and Additional Recommendations

At the Personal Level…

If you've been fighting the good fight with weight and eating for a long time, don't give up. Always begin with the guidance of your physician and other expert assistance they may recommend. And rather than making this self-care effort something you feel you must do alone, consider a peer that you could trust to walk alongside you, offering support. In my own work to improve my physical health, I had stalemated for a long time; until I asked my brother to team up with me. That made a big difference. You *can* do this.

At the PSAP and 9-1-1 Industry Levels

9-1-1 is an industry; but it is also a family. Let's address this struggle together, strategically. All of us who have been a part of the family for years know that there has been widespread concern about this problem for a long time. Our professional associations (NENA and APCO International) have welcomed an increasing number of conference presentations and articles dedicated to the issues of healthy life style and nutrition. More must be done. A formal, unified and strategic initiative in the industry on obesity is called for, given the serious health risks cited earlier. Yet, this is a hard issue to face on personal, agency and industry levels.

Perhaps there has been an unspoken fear that openly addressing the problem of obesity in the 9-1-1 family is akin to telling your brother he is ugly. If we truly care about someone, we don't intentionally hurt their feelings. Yet caring takes different forms when the risks are as great as those facing our 9-1-1 Pros in conjunction with obesity.

I urge industry leaders to advocate for federal funds to support further research, such as Lilly's, in which they sought to identify the impacts of 9-1-1 work on obesity. Researchers can only go beyond preliminary studies like this through funding. I also encourage formation of a blue-ribbon task force composed of all 9-1-1 stakeholder groups, joined by scientists, who can help to fully define the problem and create resources and guidelines for 9-1-1 centers and their employees.

ଔଓ

Questions for Reflection

To get the most from this chapter, you are encouraged to write your reflections here (in both the Kindle and paperback versions of this book).

- What was your main take-away from reading this chapter?

- What specifically made it valuable to you?

- How can you apply this take-away concretely to improve some aspect of your personal life and or efforts to support the wellbeing of 9-1-1Pros?

Additional Resources

- For an in-depth understanding of Self-Compassion and help growing more compassionate with yourself, purchase Dr. Neff's book, *Self-Compassion: the Proven Power of being Kind to Yourself* (2015).
- Visit Kristin Neff's website for free resources to measure your level of self-compassion and to practice self-compassion meditations. **http://self-compassion.org/**
- If you have grown deeply discouraged about your obesity consider seeking professional counseling, and exploring the group support of Overeaters Anonymous: https://oa.org/
- Consider reading the article: *Sedentary Behaviour: A Threat to Global Health,* by Jessica Brichta, World Obesity: https://www.worldobesity.org/news/wo-blog/november-2015/sedentary-behaviour-threat-global-health/

Works Cited

Fox, Susan and Egan, J. "Emotional Eating: Feeding and Fearing Feelings- What Psychologists Need to Know." *The Irish Psychologist*, vol.43 issue 8, June 2017, pp. 194-200, www.researchgate.net/publication/318402381_Fox_S_Egan_J_201 _Emotional_Eating_Feeding_and_Fearing_Feelings What_Psychologists_Need_to_Know Irish_Psychologist_43_194 200

Harvard Health Publishing. "Why Stress Causes People to Overeat." *Harvard Health,* February 2012, **www.health.harvard.edu/newsletter_article/why-stress-causes** people-to-overeat.

"Integrated Chronic Disease Prevention and Control." *WHO*, World Health

Organization, www.who.int/chp/about/integrated_cd/en/.

Levitan, Robert D., and Caroline Davis. "Emotions and Eating Behaviour: Implications for the Current Obesity Epidemic." *University of Toronto Quarterly*, 8 August 2010, muse.jhu.edu/article/390250/pdf.

Lilly, Michelle and C. Allen, C.E. "Psychological Inflexibility and Psychopathology in 9-1-1 Telecommunicators." *Journal of Traumatic Stress*, vol. 28 no 3, 11 May 2015, pp 262-66. doi: 10.1002/jts.22004

Neff, Kristin. *Self-Compassion: the Proven Power of Being Kind to Yourself.* William Morrow Paperback, 2015.

NENA. "NENA Standard on 9-1-1 Acute/Traumatic and Chronic Stress Management." *The National Emergency Numbers Association (NENA)*, 5 August 2013, p 22, c.ymcdn.com/sites/www.nena.org/resource/resmgr/Standards/NNA-STA-002.1-2013_9-1-1_Ac.pdf

Ogden, Cynthia et al. "Prevalence of Obesity Among Adults and Youth: United States, 2011–2014." *cdc.gov*, no. 219, November 2015, pp 1-8. **www.cdc.gov/nchs/data/databriefs/db219.pdf**

Sandoui, Ana. "Can You Be Healthy and Have Obesity? Not Really, Says Major Study." *Medical News Today*, 21 May 2017, **www.medicalnewstoday.com/articles/317546.php**.

Violanti John, et al. "Atypical Work Hours and Metabolic Syndrome Among Police Officers." *Archives of Environmental & Occupational Health*, vol. 64 no. 3, 2009, pp. 194-201.

CHAPTER 13
"I'm just Sick and Tired of Being Sick and Tired. Help me."
An EMS Doc's Personal Battle Through Self-Medication and Addiction

S. Marshal Isaacs

Reader Caution: this chapter contains a story involving struggle with suicide. There are no gruesome details and there's great cause for hope in this story. Still, if you've been personally touched by suicide, have yet to heal, and know you're easily triggered by such stories, this could be very tough reading. We advise you to pass over this chapter; or at the very least, "buddy up" with a peer to read it, stay attuned to how you're impacted, and seek professional support as needed. Whether you read this chapter or not, be sure to read Chapter 9: *Does Your Console Need a Reboot?" EMDR Therapy for Healing Traumatic Stress & Self-Care.* If you are considering killing yourself, please just set down the book and give a call to the National Suicide Prevention Life Line, a fully confidential 24/7/365 help line. Their number is 800-4273-8255. Or text HOME to the Crisis Text Line at 741741 in the United States.

Editor's Introduction

I met Marshal Isaacs at the 2016 Pinnacle EMS Conference in San Antonio, Texas where we were both speakers. His Saks Fifth Avenue wardrobe and confident demeanor exuded class and evidenced his Manhattan upbringing. This was one highly privileged and educated man at the top of his career! I assumed that he was qualified and motivated to speak on the topic of addiction in the EMS profession because he was an emergency physician. Marshal cleverly built his session on a false pretense: he successfully led his audience to assume that we saw Marshal Isaacs. After all, we were looking right at him, standing right in front of us. But, in the middle of his fairly predictable PowerPoint-driven presentation, he pitched us a curve ball. He pointed to the huge projection screen. There, looking down on us, appeared this dirty bedraggled man whose face had no more life than a corpse and his eyes cast a thousand-mile stare.

"That is the real Marshal Isaacs," he said.

A few folks couldn't hold back an audible gasp. People looked around at each other, stunned. The contrast between the man on the screen and the man at

the podium was breathtaking. We really had not seen Marshal. Not how he knew we needed to see him, to understand his journey to the lowest point in his life, nearly to death, through recovery, and to the lectern that day.
In this room, full of a few hundred people, there was a near-sacred silence. Personally, I was overcome with emotion thinking of the courage this prominent physician had rallied to bare himself publicly. Yet, it was precisely his telling of this personal story that moved me and many others, to wonder compassionately about our co-workers suffering with addiction, and to act to help save them. That's why I asked Marshal to share his story with you in this book; so that we will have the eyes to *see* our 9-1-1 family members—and perhaps ourselves-- at risk, and summon the courage to offer, or ask for, help. In the first part of this chapter Marshal shares his story with you. The second portion is an interview in two parts that I conducted with him to learn more about his personal experience with addiction, and how we can apply his lessons and insights to the 9-1-1 family.

A final note: as the reader, beware of falling into the predictable error of assuming this chapter doesn't apply to you since it seems to be about just alcohol and drugs. There are many ways we can self-medicate, and many things to which we can become addicted: high-adrenaline work, sex and pornography, toxic relationships, compulsive gambling, spending, and, yes, eating. I say yes, because the need to medicate 9-1-1 stress may be a factor in the industry-wide struggle with morbid obesity, and that can be deadly. Overweight 9-1-1Pros need to avoid judging themselves and get empowered by compassionately striving to gain more insight about what is driving their eating patterns. Addiction may or may not be a factor. Many factors contribute to weight gain, especially in 9-1-1. Still, if you are one of those discouraged by your weight gain, you may be able to relate to and be greatly encouraged by Marshal's message here.

For now, it is important for all of us to keep one thing in mind as we face any addiction: simplistic solutions, and self-condemnation driven by ignorance and shame never lead to healing. But, with new insight, we can wonder compassionately and do great good for ourselves, and our 9-1-1 family members who struggle. We hope this chapter will help you do precisely this kind of compassionate wondering, to gain new insight, and heal, or help your peers heal.

JM

PART 1: Marshal's Story

I had my first beer when I was 14 years old. I was a social drinker (just one or two drinks—not intending to get drunk) for all of 5 minutes. After that I *never* drank socially again. I only drank to get drunk. And not a little bit drunk, but shit-faced drunk. I cannot tell you why that was. I *do* know alcohol did for me what nothing else up until that point had done: it gave me confidence. It helped me feel like I "fit in." But most importantly, it helped quiet the noise in my head, or if it didn't quiet it, alcohol helped me to not care about it. This became "reinforcing."

I learned when I drank (and later, when I found drugs) that I believed they made me feel better. Over time, they stopped making me feel better and instead they made me feel *much* worse. In retrospect, alcohol and drugs made me feel nearly nothing at all, and I only thought that was better than what I felt when sober.

I want to be clear about this next point: I had a good childhood. I have great parents and a sister I love very much. The only trauma I experienced in childhood was self-inflicted. It was "all in my head." Through the counseling I underwent in recovery I learned many of my earliest thoughts were "dark." They included subjects and things most young children do not think about or if they do, they ask adults about them and then they move on. But, I could not move on. I obsessed over these thoughts until it made me physically ill. I could not talk about them. They were too disturbing for me put into words, and even if I tried, the responses or explanations I received were not adequate for my troubled mind. As I got older, I came to believe my thinking was not only substantially different from most others but sharing my thoughts was disturbing to others. And so, I kept them inside where they festered. When I used alcohol and drugs, my thoughts were either quieted (numbed), or my response to them felt less troublesome for me.

By age fifteen I was drinking hard liquor, and by sixteen I was smoking pot. I started college when I was seventeen and before my eighteenth birthday, I had tried nearly every recreational drug there is.

It should come as no surprise that within six months of entering college I was dismissed from the accelerated six-year medical school track I was in, and I was cut from the college swim team. To say I wasn't really fully present for college would be an understatement. To be frank, I'm not even sure how I was accepted into medical school.
Once in medical school, I knew it was important for me to buckle down and pay attention. But I was drinking and using regularly, so during my first year, I

was as mentally absent from medical school classes as I'd been in my undergraduate years. That didn't work out so well for me. At the end of my first year, the Dean invited me into his office and said, "Marshal, you appear to have had a really good time during your first semester. So, we'd like to invite you back to do it again." My performance had ranked me number one hundred in a class of one hundred. That was a bit of a wake-up call, and my dad, who was paying my tuition, was more than a little bit frustrated with me. He sat me down and essentially said, "Stop wasting my damn money! Do you want to do this or not?" The fact is, I *did* want to do it. I felt I was meant to become a physician, particularly an EMS physician. After all, as a young boy and teenager, I chased ambulances, fire engines and police cars on my bike after school. Becoming a 9-1-1 physician was what I felt I needed to be.

Somehow, I was able to buckle down, and I even graduated at the top of my class. I didn't stop drinking or using drugs, but I was able to keep it "in check." I undertook emergency medicine residency training in Pittsburgh, and completed fellowship training in EMS at Stanford, still drinking and still partying—but only when I was "off duty."

After fellowship, while still fairly young and most definitely immature, I was fortunate to be appointed to serve as both the Medical Director for the San Francisco Department of Public Health's Paramedic Division as well as the San Francisco Fire Department. That's when the wheels started coming off. Initially, I was "just" partying on a Saturday night, along with an occasional extra day thrown in there. Then the slope steepened. I progressed to using on Fridays *and* Saturdays, and before I knew it I also needed a "hump day." So, I was using on Wednesday, Friday and Saturday. But of course, Sunday is also part of the weekend and, come to think of it, Thursday was almost part of the weekend too. That left only Monday and Tuesday as my days off from drinking and drugging each week—and even they disappeared, eventually.

Ultimately, I could contrive any excuse to drink or use, *I can party because it's been a really good day* or *I'm going to use because it's been a really bad day*. In the end, the only excuse I needed to drink, or use was it was a day ending with the letter "Y"—like MondaY, TuesdaY. I'd justify using simply because "I'm breathing," although I was beginning to suspect I might not be for much longer.

I knew I was in trouble long before I crashed and burned. But, I didn't know there was a way out. Even if you told me there was a way out, I wouldn't have believed you. To be honest, in the dark recesses of my mind, I did not want a way out.

I also rationalized that the reason I needed a release was because of all the death, suffering and abuse I saw in the course of performing my jobs; it was a way of coping with the stressors in my life. I *deserved* the escape that drinking, and drugging gave me. This is where the whole cumulative impact of Post-Traumatic Stress Disorder (PTSD) and anxiety disorders needs to be recognized as a factor for people struggling with addiction. This is not an excuse, but a recognition that escaping from traumatic experiences was one of the mental drivers. I kind of knew I was self-medicating and that it was just making my life worse, but my disease convinced me that it *was* working. Until it didn't any longer.

About a year before I came to Dallas, I was offered the opportunity to apply to be Medical Director for the New York City Fire Department (FDNY). At that point I wanted to return home. My mom was starting to fade away due to early Alzheimer's Disease and I wanted to be there for her and my father. I also believed I needed to get out of San Francisco. I was pretty sure I was going to die if I didn't. I applied and went through a six-month search process for the NYC job, but that fell through at the last minute due to politics. Then, when Dallas heard I might be "available" they picked me up like a free agent. I had already made the emotional separation from San Francisco, and Dallas was still closer to New York than San Francisco. I didn't know it at the time, but I was also looking for a *"geographic cure."*[1]

I thought maybe if I got out of San Francisco, I could either moderate my drinking and using, or stop altogether. I didn't realize I would be taking my disease with me to Dallas, but, that's exactly what I did. When I got there, I may have slowed down for a few weeks, but that did not last very long.

Soon, I began calling in sick, missing appointments and commitments, and that pattern just spiraled over the next two years. I remember sitting at a stoplight in early June 2009. I had gone to work late because I had stayed up late the night before. Once at work, I did the bare minimum of what I could get away with, and then I rushed out around 3 p.m., so I could get home to start drinking and using again. That June day, I sat at that stoplight and experienced "a moment of clarity." I said to myself,

> *Is this it? Is this what I've become? I just do the bare minimum at work if I can even make it to work and then I rush through it because all I can think about is my next drink and my next drug. I have lost nearly everything that means anything to me, except my job and even that is at risk now. My friends don't want to be with me, and don't trust me. My family has no idea what's going on in my life, and I have not been there for them. My work colleagues are rapidly losing confidence*

in me. In fact, I know they suspect something is wrong with me. I am completely alone and hopeless. Is this "it"?

The traffic light turned green. The answer came to me, and it was crystal clear. *Yes. This is it. I'm done.*

I had arrived at what some refer to as the "jumping off place." This is the place where an alcoholic accepts he or she can no longer live with alcohol and drugs but cannot imagine a life without alcohol and drugs. We must then either jump off from that place to a new life in recovery, *or*, for far too many, the jumping off place has a much more tragic meaning and ending. I was heading toward tragedy.

I was regularly considering suicide, having developed a plan and even my own funeral (still trying to control the un-controllable!) I went home that day and arranged for a colleague to take my on-call duties for the weekend.

That was a Thursday night and I didn't have to be at work again until Monday morning. I thought I should go out the only way I felt was fitting; ingesting so many drugs and so much alcohol I would just slip into a coma or have a seizure, a stroke, a heart attack, or whatever. I just did not want to wake up. That was the plan. But I fucked that up, too, (which, in hindsight, was a very good thing). I knew I had done enough alcohol and drugs to kill an elephant, yet, when 5 a.m. Monday rolled around, I was still here. I remember, in that stuporous state, thinking, *how is this possible? How am I not dead?* I considered shooting myself, but I didn't have a gun; and I just couldn't bring myself to jump off my balcony, nineteen floors up.

I was due to take charge of a portion of the Parkland emergency department at 7 a.m. I had already been warned that if I showed up late again or didn't show up at all, I would be fired and reported to the state medical board. Somehow that was worse than the thought of trying to fake it through the shift. So that's what I did: I showered and drove really slowly to work. Of course, that didn't work. I don't remember very much after that, but I was later told I was found passed out in an empty resuscitation room.

I was promptly relieved of duty, escorted to the administrative offices and told I was going to be drug tested. I had already considered stealing a patient's urine sample, but I realized a urine sample from a random ER patient might have more drugs and alcohol in their bloodstream than I did! … and I'd probably turn up pregnant! So, I didn't go with that plan.

My "airplane" was literally out of fuel and out of airspeed and I was out of ideas. With nothing left to hide, and nowhere else to go, I watched my slow-motion crash and burn. I said to the staff, "I'm just tired. I think I have a problem. Please help me." Four hours later, I was on a plane to inpatient rehab in Mississippi, where I stayed for three months.

Rehab was the worst thing I have ever been through, and *the best thing that ever happened to me*. I believe my life, and career, was saved by God, by staff at Parkland and UT Southwestern, the City of Dallas/Dallas Fire-Rescue, and that shithole rehab facility in Mississippi. I could not be more grateful, as that is when my second chance at life and career began. It was June 8, 2009.

ଓଃଔ

Part 2: Marshal Isaacs' Interview with Jim Marshall

When Marshal finished sharing this story, and before the interview formally began, I felt compelled to say, "This might seem trite, but I'm also grateful you survived. We both know people who didn't. Because you survived, you're living life as a gift now, for others. I don't want to add a burden to you, but your life is a gift to our emergency response family."

Marshal replied, "Thank you for saying that. It doesn't sound trite at all. I've been told I am a walking miracle. And I believe that to be true."

Then Marshal revealed why he was willing to take time with me to share his story, "I really have only one purpose now. While I love being the Medical Director for Dallas Fire-Rescue and the UTSW/Parkland BioTel EMS System and a Professor and emergency department doctor, those are my roles. They are not my purpose. My purpose today is this: don't drink, don't drug, tell the truth, and be of service to others. That's it. It's easy. Don't get me wrong. I work really hard in my recovery program, but it is not that hard to say, 'today I am not going to drink alcohol. Today I am not going to get fucked up on drugs. Today, I will tell the truth and be of service to others.'

I began recovery almost 9 years ago, but it took some time before I recognized the gift I'd been given. After all, how many people are given a second chance in life and career? So now, I need to give back…"

From there, our interview commenced with a cascade of questions opening up the rest of Marshal's story, and his thinking about self-medicating, recovery, and life. I think you'll find his answers are far from dry lecturing; they're free of cheap advice, and full of down-to-earth, powerful insights bound to be immediately helpful. Each section begins with a heading that captures the focus of that part of the interview.

❧

1: The Problem

Addiction and Lying

Jim: What's the biggest line of BS you would tell yourself, so you could use again?

Marshal: That I could handle this. That I was still in control. That I was not in danger. That I was *not* an alcoholic or a drug addict.

There were so many more lies I told myself:
- *This is not a problem for me, I can handle this.*
- *I work really, really hard and do good things for people so I deserve to party hard.*
- *If you saw the shit I saw in my job you would drink and drug too!*
- *I'm not hurting anyone but myself.*

To be a really good addict you need to be a really good liar. If you're not a good liar, you can't justify using and you'll be found out very quickly. I was a very skilled liar and manipulator. I was also very good at lying by omission about my substance use and many other things. If you didn't ask me a question precisely I figured I didn't need to answer you precisely. To me that wasn't lying, that was surviving. I spent so much time and so much emotional and spiritual energy lying and covering up and manipulating. It was exhausting. I couldn't keep track of who I told what. I don't do that dance anymore. That alone is such an amazing gift. If you ask me something now, I'm going to answer you with the truth as I know it. And if you don't like my answer, that's your shit. It's not my shit.

Addiction, Shame and Guilt

Jim: So, was part of that emotional and spiritual drain due to carrying the weight of the shame you felt about lying and manipulating?

Marshal: *Yes!* The shame and guilt were there on so many levels. I have great parents who brought me and my sister up really well. And they instilled good values in us. One of those values is *don't lie*. Yet, I did. I lied to stay alive, to continue drinking and drugging without being found out. That was so discordant with what I was taught and what I believed was right. I also felt shame and guilt for not showing up for work, showing up late, and for not being available when I was paged [messaged] by my staff who needed my assistance. When I was drunk and high I did things I wasn't proud of. That led to shame, and guilt too. I dealt with all that shame and guilt the way most alcoholics and addicts probably do: they drink and drug more.

Facing Addiction in the First Responder Culture

Jim: What is your first thought about how your story relates to 9-1-1 telecommunicators and other first responders?

Marshal: Many 9-1-1Pros can probably relate personally to my story—whether they struggle with their own demons, or the struggles of a loved one, or a work peer. I want them to understand how I began recovery and that I have at least some vision for how the journey of recovery can lead to a much better life.

9-1-1 telecommunicators, firefighters, paramedics and EMTs work within a "Good ole boy network," within which there's a longstanding stigma about addiction. So, when these professionals struggle with abuse, often they are shunned. As an industry, our leaders must commit to addressing that stigma, so our agencies can invest in building support programs. So telecommunicators and other responders will actually feel safe using these programs to get help for alcohol and drug abuse, and the PTSD, anxiety and depression that often drives addiction.

I recently presented my story at an EMS conference. The participants' response was overwhelming. They said "It's about time! We want more, and we want to help." One gentleman came to me afterward, he was crying and said, "Thank you, I wish this support program had been in place a year ago, because my brother, who is a firefighter, recently killed himself."

The Slippery Slope and the Power of Stigma Among 9-1-1 and Other First Responders

Jim: This is the crux of the matter. 9-1-1Pros I've deeply cared for, have lost their lives, their officers, and their loved ones, in the same way. Living on that slippery slope of unhealed traumatic stress, self-medicating and addiction can be deadly for 9-1-1Pros, or other responders, especially when they are battling it all alone. And they end up alone when they are too ashamed to ask for help, *and* when they believe they ought to be able to "suck it up" and handle it themselves.

Can you speak to how the shame makes the struggle with addiction even more of a slippery slope for first responders?

Marshal: Yes. Let me read you a quote. And don't be put off by how formal it sounds. This is a kickass statement that powerfully answers your question. It's about physicians but certainly relates to 9-1-1Pros too.

> Although physicians' elevated social status brings many tangible and intangible rewards, it also has an isolating effect when they are confronted with a disease such as addiction, which has a social stigma. This *isolation* can lead to disastrous consequences both in delaying the recognition of and intervening in the disease process--as well as in the attendant risk of death by inadvertent overdose or suicide (Berge).

A challenge for 9-1-1 telecommunicators struggling to accept the reality of their addiction is that they may feel they've become "one of those derelict" members of society—those they deal with routinely on 9-1-1 calls—the same folks for whom they have some fairly nasty names. That self-judgment is part of the stigma that emergency responders face. They believe they are supposed to be different than those they serve. So, if they struggle, they are apt to believe they are somehow less worthy than their peers. They may see it as a moral lapse in character.

Traditionally, the fire service, EMS and medical professions adopt a culture that tends to be fairly "testosterone driven"—and the women employed in these professions have become part of this culture! We live in a very macho, *no-fear* mentality. We are taught to "suck it up" when faced with difficult emotional situations whether loss, grief, or tremendous trauma (with exposure to dead bodies, child abuse, etc.). We were *not* taught to manage our feelings or talk about these stressful things.

In fact, in the fire service, EMS, law enforcement and emergency medicine fields, we are taught the response to a bad shift is "let's go have a liquid dinner (or breakfast)." So, alcohol use, and by extension drug use, was and still is, encouraged--without reckoning with the even greater risk this poses to our peers, who may be genetically predisposed to addiction and mental illness.

Jim: You've just said a hugely important mouthful, Marshal. Telecommunicators live and operate within this first responder culture you've described. That 9-1-1 workforce is still predominantly female, so you'd think they'd be more apt to share feelings and seek support for emotional struggles. But 9-1-1Pros, whether male or female, naturally have a need to be accepted, and respected, as equals by the bigger first responder culture. So, most 9-1-1 personnel have believed they must live by the "suck it up" emotional code (see Chapter 5).

That makes it more likely they'll try coping with stress by stuffing distress, and self-medicating, which can put them on that slippery slope towards abuse and addiction.

So, as a recovering person, how do you define self-medicating? And again, by using this term, I'm not judging somebody for struggling with it, just seeking clarity about what's healthy and what's not.

Marshal: It's any activity we engage in to take our minds off that which is causing us emotional or spiritual distress—And which kicks you in the ass, somehow, sooner or later.

So, self-medication is anything that helps a person escape from things that feel too uncomfortable but may be toxic in the long run. It could be alcohol, drugs, food, gambling, porn or sex taken to excess. It could be self-deception, or any other thing in a long list of stuff, that ultimately is self-defeating. A lot of alcoholic addicts like me found that alcohol or drugs were a "shortcut." We found the thing that did it the fastest or best, and we were like "that's it!" For people like me, that's that. It doesn't matter if it was the first time you ever smoked pot, drank wine, took a pill, put a needle in yourself, or kissed an elf. Whatever. You're done (until you get help). For us, self-medication immediately became an addiction. But what we were looking for was *relief.*

By contrast, healthy coping strategies could be talking it out with a friend, meditation, yoga, prayer, exercise, quality time with family or friends, hobbies—anything you engage in that most reasonable people would consider to be healthy alternatives to self-medicating or to just plain suffering in silence.

Jim: So, you're saying self-medicating takes our minds off our distress. Do you think most folks who end up addicted were trying to find a way to escape pain?

Marshal: I think the word pain is too broad. It may not always be pain. It may be anxiety or a feeling of anxiousness. But certainly, pain is the most extreme on that scale. Let's say you take someone like me who feels socially inept or somewhat shy and you tell them they're going to need to be in a social situation. I wouldn't say being in a social setting would produce "pain," discomfort, yes, but not pain. So, if you gave me a drink or a drug before that event it would be easier for me to engage.

Jim: I know you're not an Addictionologist, but what is addiction as you see it?

Marshal: Many people in recovery believe addiction is a physical, emotional and spiritual malady. Depending on the substance you're addicted to, there are biochemical changes in your brain that contribute to making, and keeping, you addicted. Then there's the mental obsession that accompanies this biochemical change—the feeling that one has to have more of the substance, and the compulsive behavior that is so hard to control. There are also spiritual issues connected with addiction. I've yet to meet an alcoholic or drug addict, who, at their core, didn't have spiritual struggles contributing to their troubles that didn't need some level of resolution.

Grappling with the term "Addiction"

Jim: The term "addiction" is an intense term, and it can be threatening. Using alcohol as an example, what's the difference between just enjoying it and being addicted, in your view as a recovering person?

Marshal: You're the mental health professional, but in my opinion, it has to do with consequences. Some people can use alcohol or drugs without negative consequences. Most alcoholics or addicts have tremendous consequences as a result of their drinking and using. Some have the ultimate consequence of death. Yet another group of people clearly *abuse* substances without becoming addicted. Some of these people also have big consequences. The best example is the young person who misjudges their ability to stay sober during a night of drinking. Then, because they lack maturity and good judgment, they choose to get behind the wheel when they're intoxicated.
They may kill someone, themselves, or both. That person is not an alcoholic. They had a lapse in judgment that resulted in a horrific consequence.

By contrast, people who are addicted continue to engage in patterns of use with continued and increasingly bad consequences. They cannot stop, despite often significant efforts on their parts to do so.

Jim: I think you've done an excellent job capturing the major components of addiction. This definition fits very well with what I've taught clients and students. The definition offered by The National Center on Addictions not only supports your definition, but also the keys to recovery. They state that addiction is:

> …a complex disease, often chronic in nature, which affects the functioning of the brain and body. It also causes serious damage to families, relationships, schools, workplaces and neighborhoods. The most common symptoms of addiction are severe loss of control, continued use despite serious consequences, preoccupation with using, failed attempts to quit, tolerance and withdrawal. Addiction can be effectively prevented, treated and managed by healthcare professionals in combination with family or peer support (Defining Addiction…).

Marshal: To understand how my mind operated when it was controlled by addiction, imagine you offered me this proposition, "Marshal, I have this one beer for you (or this one glass of wine, this one toke, one pill or one line). You *will not* be able to get more. Maybe tomorrow night, but not until then. Would you like to have just one and then nothing until the next day?"

Do you know what my answer would be? I would say, "No, I don't want one drink, because it's not enough." Why? Because it would actually cause me more pain to start drinking or using without the ability to continue than it would be to not start at all. For years that realization is what kept me from partying on nights when I knew there was something really important for which I had to wake up at 5 a.m.

In recovery we talk about our "drug of choice." For some, it is alcohol, for some it is opiates or cocaine. My drug of choice was *more*. More of anything that would make me feel different than how I felt at baseline.

The Definition of Insanity

Jim: So, what was your internal dialogue driving this quest for more?

Marshal: It was this: *Marshal, if you're gonna start using drugs or alcohol at 3 p.m., you know you'll still be awake abusing the next morning at sunrise—you've proven that over and over again. You said this will not happen and yet it happens again and again. Every time. You know it before you drink that first drink or take that first drug. You know you must be up at 5 a.m. to be in the ER before 7 a.m. So, don't start.*

But my addiction would respond, *"No. This time will be different."* But, it never was.

Jim, *so* many times I've said to myself, "This time I will go to sleep and it will be fine." I will drink like a "normal person." It became a pathetic running joke with myself. Friends would ask, "Are you partying tonight?" I would say, "Yeah I think so. I'll party a bit and then I'll go to sleep at midnight." I'd then laugh at myself, because I knew that I wouldn't stop. I was the living definition of insanity—doing the same thing over and over again expecting a different result.

Jim: There will be some of our readers who read this description and will say "Oh, well he was a full-blown addict. I can drink five or ten beers a night, still get up in the morning and function fine. I'm a heavy drinker, but I'm not an alcoholic. So, leave me the hell alone!" So, what would you say to that reader?

Marshal: I'd say put your affairs in order, because there is a good chance you're going to die. This is a progressive disease, and the first symptom is denial. I said that same thing for many years, "Look, I can party like a beast and still get up in morning to go to work." I could do that until I couldn't do it any longer. Some people *can* do it for years, and some people will go from being a regular person to losing everything in a matter of weeks or months.

How Addiction Progresses

Marshal: Some people can drink heavily or do drugs for years without disaster. They appear to be what we'd call *functional alcoholics* or *functional drug addicts*. It can take many, many years before they start to have more serious problems and ultimately fail. Other people can get drunk every day and somehow, by the grace of God, reach eighty or ninety years of age, and still be okay. But they are, by far, the exception. We all know people who appeared to be fine. They'd been a social drinker, or perhaps they had never even tried drugs. Then, one day, something happens in their lives that leads them to using. Within weeks, or months, they are living under a bridge, or, worse, they end up dead.

The progression is that fast sometimes. Once it gets you, it is a spiral that is hard to pull out of and you're in trouble. Some have a spiral that starts wide and slow and for others the spiral is very fast and very steep.

Jim: At this point some of our readers might think you're saying that anyone who drinks alcohol will end up in trouble sooner or later. I know that isn't your point. Moderate drinking is defined as up to one drink per day for women and two for men. And many folks can maintain this use without ever increasing their general use beyond that level, and without ever developing any pattern of bad consequences (in relationships, health, legally, or at work). Yet there are plenty of good folks out there who may not develop a full-blown addiction leading to a death spiral but they do abuse alcohol or substances to self-medicate feelings related to anxiety, unresolved trauma or depression. For them, the fall-out can include worsening depression, less impulse control, more impaired judgment, and more risk of suicide. So self-medicating is full of risk even if someone never becomes addicted. Life gets really complicated and, as you said, for some it happens quickly, for others, over time. Your thoughts?

Marshal: You're raising the issue of "comorbidity"—when people struggle with two or more disorders occurring at the same time. This brings us to the proverbial question: *which came first: the chicken or the egg?* Do people drink because they are depressed, or are they depressed because they are chronically abusing? It can go either way. For me there was no question. I have had some underlying emotional struggles in the past, but there is no question. I absolutely experienced depression, hopelessness, and, eventually, thoughts of suicide as a direct result of my alcohol and drug use. I know this because once I was treated, I was no longer suicidal.

Jim: Right. As you said, it can go both ways. Some folks struggle first with a mental health problem, like clinical depression, and then find alcohol as a self-medicator, which becomes an addiction. Others first become addicted to a substance, which then sets them up for greater risk of depression, and symptoms of other mental illnesses. In either case, the evidence now supports treating both conditions at the same time by doing our best, as clinicians, to understand how they are connected, then working to lessen the substance abuse and the distressing symptoms (Integrated Treatment…). I can tell you it's not always easy to identify the "co-occurring" addiction! Folks struggling with an underlying addiction are often incredibly talented in convincing themselves and others they aren't addicted. No judgment intended here. Can you relate?

Marshal: Absolutely. I used to pride myself in saying I never drank or used when I went to work. That was true. For years I prided myself on saying, "I may be an alcoholic, but I'm not like those scumbags who get fucked up at work."

You know what? That was complete and utter deceit, because I sometimes went to work with either no sleep, little sleep, or still under-the-influence from partying the night before, the day before, the week before, and from the cumulative weeks, months, and years of using. The truth is I was impaired or recovering from using. That was evidence of extremely poor judgment and as with most alcoholics/addicts, I had little if no insight into my problem.

∽∽

2: The Recovery

Faith and Purpose to Live and Be Sober

Jim: What helps you the most to stay sober?

Marshal: Fear of going back to that shithole of a rehab facility in Mississippi! Just kidding. What *really* keeps me sober? I want to say God, working a program, working with others. I do not want to squander the second chance I've been given in life and career. I do not want to go back to being *that* person. I was miserable and I never want to experience that kind of pain ever again.

Jim: Can you explain what you mean? Everybody's in such a different place with the whole idea of God and the role of spirituality and 12 Step Groups in recovery from addictions. Does spirituality or God have a part in your recovery?

Marshal: I have to believe it is the biggest part. I don't have a choice. I've tried it without believing, and for me it works better *with it*. So, while I have, and will continue to entertain the possibility that I am deluding myself, I choose to believe there is a higher power, which I choose to call God, that wants me to stay sober. And, even without that, I truly believe I have been given this gift which compels me to try to be of service to others.

One of the deepest fears, among the addicts I've come to know during the past eight and a half years is *there really isn't any point to life*. Alcohol and drugs take away or diminish that fear. We rationalize that if there is no point, *why not be drunk or high?*

Today, I know there is a point. I don't claim to know what the point is... (he laughs) ...But I do know that I'll probably never stop trying to figure it out. For me, for today, there is enough of a point if I can do something to help relieve someone else's suffering, pain, or anxiety, just a little. That may just have to be enough.

How to Know if you're Addicted

Jim: How can a person know when they're addicted?

Marshal: There is a very easy exercise to determine if you're having a problem with alcohol and/or drugs. Try to control the amount and frequency that you drink or use. If you cannot control that, then you may have a problem. If you continue drinking and using despite the negative fallout in your life, you may have a problem. If you came to me and asked, "Can you help me figure out if I'm an alcoholic or drug addict?" I'd say no one can truly decide that for you. Clinicians can reliably diagnose substance use disorders, yet the person must be able to accept that diagnosis. If you continue drinking or using you may eventually figure it out on your own, but that could entail some very serious consequences including, loss of employment, jail, or even death. If your drinking or using is progressing and you're experiencing consequences related to your drinking or using, then you have a problem. It's that simple.

It's like saying, "I'm not sure if I have an allergy to peanuts, but every time I eat peanuts, I get a skin rash, and I'm worried I could end up in full blown anaphylactic shock." If you cannot eat peanuts without getting a rash, and if your rash and symptoms are getting worse the more peanuts you eat, then it's insane (NUTS!) to think you aren't allergic to peanuts.

D-E-N-I-A-L means that I *Don't Even Know I Am Lying* (to myself).

Rallying to Seek Support from Family and Friends

Jim: Many responders have been taught that folks who need mental health help are too weak to handle their issues alone. Here's the ironic thing about that. It takes a lot of courage for firefighters to run in the direction of the fire when everyone else is running out of the blazing building. Likewise, it takes a lot of hutzpah for the telecommunicator to lean into the 9-1-1 call from the mother who is screaming that her baby's not breathing. Well, as responders, it also takes a hell of a lot of courage, on the personal level, to face our deepest pain and fears, and ask someone to walk through the healing process with us. In my view, asking for therapy help, or peer support, is the farthest thing from weakness. Your thoughts?

Marshal: I completely agree, Jim. No one goes to treatment or begins a recovery program because things are going great in their lives. So, seeking help means you must be honest enough with yourself to admit something has gone wrong. That takes courage.

Jim: Yes. I believe it also takes peer support. 9-1-1 centers in the U.S. are now establishing peer support programs so a struggling 9-1-1Pro can confidentially seek support from a peer who: has also been to hell and back, who can listen, tell their own story, and set an example of healing through brokenness. A Peer Supporter can also be the one who'll say, "I'm not going to give up on you…And I'll go with you to that counseling appointment!" (See Chapter 16: *The Power of 9-1-1 Peer Support: The First Line of Care and Prevention for the Frontline of Dispatch.*)

Marshal, when we are considering fully admitting we have a problem, we need the support of friends, family, and often a licensed counselor. How do we break through the shame to reveal we have a problem, maybe an addiction, and we need help?

Marshal: That is one of most difficult things. Until you can admit your struggle to yourself, then you're probably not going to get help unless you are "found out" and compelled to seek treatment. For some people, it is easier to first turn to someone else and say they are having this problem and ask, "Can you help me find help?" Sometimes it just takes that one person who knows what the next step can be. It's so hard to admit when we have a problem with alcohol, other substances, PTSD, depression or anxiety disorders and we need professional help. Each person has to decide how open they will be about their struggle, and who they will open up to. It's so personal.

When I got home from treatment in Mississippi, I felt the right path for me was full disclosure. Some people thought I was crazy to be so open about my alcoholism/drug addiction. My dad was *very* concerned, not because he was ashamed of me…He was worried being open about it, especially in the first few months of my recovery, would cause problems for me.
But I'm grateful I made that decision early on in my recovery. It has helped me, and hopefully now I can help others.

Giving Support to a Struggling Peer or Loved One

Jim: If somebody is reading this chapter and realizes a coworker or a loved-one needs immediate help with a problem that has reached a crisis stage, what would you advise them to do?

Marshal: Seek help themselves from a professional for advice on how to proceed in helping their colleague, friend or loved one. And don't try rescuing the peer by yourself. A wrong approach or confrontation can be detrimental. Find someone either through a clinician, a local 12-step program, or church. All you have to say is, "I need help because I don't know how to proceed here." There *is* help if you seek it out.

Jim: Thank you, Marshal, for this encouragement and for helping the 9-1-1 Family reflect together on how to face the challenge of addictions and self-medicating. If readers have questions for you, can they email you?

Marshal: Of course. My email address is: **marshalisaacs@gmail.com**

Conclusion

In this chapter, Marshal has taken the risk of being incredibly vulnerable and transparent. He did this for you, knowing that sometimes we need more than information; we need a human being to serve as a bridge to the help we need. To add to Marshal's efforts here, I'll also take a risk and get personal to emphasize a few resources that can make an enormous difference for you (or those you're concerned about).

My father, an incredible human being, struggled with alcoholism for many years. At age fifty-seven, he began his recovery. Words can't express what that meant to me and for the rest of our family's life. In addition to our support, three resources were really important:

1) Dad, like Marshal, entered an extensive inpatient recovery program to get a strong start. This isn't necessary for everyone, but it was for him, and he knew it.
2) When Dad left the inpatient program, he sought the help of a licensed mental health professional specializing in addictions. Though he was an educator, he'd been trained early in his career as a psychotherapist—he knew the benefit of having a professional who understood his struggle, could help him build a solid plan for a sober life, and coach him through the initial wobbly stages of recovery. And,
3) He courageously overcame his shame and walked into an Alcoholics Anonymous (AA) meeting. As a highly educated, professional man, he

could have rationalized that he shouldn't need this help. But he knew that was a bunch of bull. He never became fanatical, but he was diligent, and continued attending meetings for most his life until his death at age eighty. (See the link to AA in Works Cited section at the end of this chapter.) In those meetings, dad shed decades of shame, let others challenge his early denial, and I'm certain he was a gift to lot of other folks in that room too. Think what you may about AA, but those anonymous people who walked the Twelve Step path alongside my dad helped save his life. So, AA was a gift to our whole family.

Three decades ago, Dad placed the special bronze AA coin he'd earned on the celebration of his first three years of sobriety in my hands. I'm holding it in my hand right now, as I reread these words. I'm so grateful my father finished strong and left a legacy to his children and grandchildren—not of perfection, but of acknowledging his need for help, and of triumph. We're each living out our legacy one day at a time. If you can personally relate to the struggles with self-medication and addiction we've described in this chapter, I hope you'll consider seeking the resources that Marshal and my father have used to win their battles, to fulfill your own legacy.

Now, before you head to the next chapter, be sure to take a few moments to reflect on the questions below and check out the Additional Resources.

Questions for Reflection

To get the most from this chapter, you are encouraged to write your reflections here (in both the Kindle and paperback versions of this book).

- What was your main take-away from reading this chapter?

- What specifically made it valuable to you?

- How can you apply this take-away concretely to improve some aspect of your personal life and or efforts to support the wellbeing of 9-1-1Pros?

Additional Resources

The resources offered below were selected by the volume editor, J. Marshall to provide help related to struggles including, yet extending beyond those addressed in this chapter:. You will find links to organizations offering help dealing with alcohol, drugs, food, gambling, and sexual activity. Keep in mind, without judging, that there can be a fine line between self-medicating and addiction. The objective is to seek help when it is needed.

- The official website of Alcoholics Anonymous: **https://www.aa.org/**. This site offers tremendous information to explore AA, including a meeting finder. (Yet, see also Addiction.com below, for additional help locating meetings.)
- Addiction.com. This website helps you locate a 12 Step meeting (related to a variety of struggles) in your local area.
- American Addiction Centers (AAC): This is a for-profit organization but they worked to create recovery programs for first responders suffering from addictions. Call: 877.620.8491. Visit their website: AmericanAddictionCenters.org.
https://www.addiction.com/meetingfinder/
- The official website of Gamblers Anonymous: http://www.gamblersanonymous.org/ga
- The official website of Overeaters Anonymous: **https://oa.org**
- SAMHSA's National Helpline, 1-800-662-HELP (4357). This is a "confidential, free, 24-hour-a-day, 365-day-a-year, information service…for individuals and family members facing mental and/or substance use disorders. This service provides referrals to local treatment facilities, support groups, and community-based organizations. Callers can also order free publications and other information.
https://www.samhsa.gov/find-help/national-helpline
- Addiction 101. An educational website that serves as a first place to land in learning about and seeking help for sexual addiction: https://www.addiction.com/addiction-a-to-z/sex-addiction/sex-addiction-101/

Work Cited

Berge, Keith H. et al. "Clinical Dependency and the Physician." Mayo Clinic Proceedings, Volume 84, Issue 7, July 2009, 625-631.
"Defining Addiction Changes Everything." *National Center on Addiction and Substance Abuse*, 14 April 2017,
www.centeronaddiction.org/addiction.

"Integrated Treatment for Co-Occurring Disorders: The Evidence." *Substance Abuse and Mental Health Services Administration,* 2009, store.samhsa.gov/shin/content/SMA08-4367/TheEvidence ITC.pdf.

End Notes

[1] For more information about the concept of "geographic cure", see: **(https://www.amethystrecovery.org/the-myth-of-the-geographical-cure/)**

CHAPTER 14
"Where was God in All This?" Recognizing and Traveling Through a Crisis of Faith to Rebuild Spiritual Resilience

Jim Marshall

In chapter 10, I shared interwoven stories of two people who traveled through Compassion Fatigue, a man I renamed "Greg," and me. In that chapter I described Compassion Fatigue as an umbrella with two handles. One handle represents the first component, "burnout" which impairs energy, attitude, mindset, relationships and potentially physical health too. The second handle is the "secondary traumatic stress," also known as vicarious traumatization. This is trauma you experience when exposed in the line of duty to other people's traumatic events, resulting in struggles with fear, difficulty sleeping, recurring images of the events, and or "…avoiding things that remind you of the event" (Stamm 5). However, in that chapter I did not address the very real possibility that, along with this psychological fallout of Compassion Fatigue, there can also be spiritual fall out—a Crisis of Faith.

It seems essential to explore Crises of Faith with you, as the 9-1-1 family, because you are Extraordinary Care Givers (ECG, Chapter 10). You're exposed to far more life-and-death trauma than most people. So, the risk of Compassion Fatigue and a Crisis of Faith is higher. This crisis, as I define it, involves the loss of confidence in what we believe about God and His interaction with us. This crisis includes damage to our faith, incurred through our suffering that makes it hard to know what to believe spiritually. A Crisis of Faith can lead to tremendous growth in the long run, but in the midst of it, the struggle is unwelcomed.

For sure, there are vast differences in the faith and spirituality among the ranks in our comm centers, just as there is in our country. While I identify myself as a Christian, some folks have deep spirituality that doesn't include faith in God. If you are happily agnostic or atheist, a lack of faith in God is, of course, not a crisis at all for you. So, this chapter may not apply to you *personally*. Yet, you may have loved-ones and co-workers whose faith includes belief in (and now struggles about) God. They may come to you, not because you share their beliefs, but because they know you care for them and are safe to talk to. Hopefully in that case, this chapter will provide you with more insight as you offer them a listening ear.

I know from my own experience as a trauma therapist (and a fellow ECG) how people can experience Crises in Faith. The unique combination of stressors experienced by telecommunicators that impact them emotionally, mentally, and physically can also affect them spiritually. For me, being vulnerable enough to tell my own story is worth it, if there's a chance it will help 9-1-1Pros in their own Crisis of Faith to find a pathway through it to vital spirituality again. In my view, the goal of working through this crisis is not to reassemble every element of our understanding of God so it is just as it was before. Instead, it is to grow a deeper, more mature spirituality that can stand strong, yet flex to encourage and energize us and others in the face of our uncertain futures. I call this type of faith spiritual resilience.

The Institute of Heart Math defines spiritual resilience to also include our "commitment to core values, intuitions, and tolerance of others' values and beliefs" (McCraty 49). It involves embracing a worldview built on compassion for others and for ourselves, openness to ideas beyond our own, and living in accordance with our values, which the Institute recognizes as part of integrity.

Along with these aspects of resilient spirituality, my own faith includes belief and confidence in the presence of a being that is both transcendent and fully present with us. One who has power and love to guide, strengthen and keep us secure through our lifetime here on earth. Spirituality that includes a belief in a higher power or God, for me and for many, also includes the belief that there is a heaven. My belief in Heaven is also a source of hope now and for a future, during and beyond our experience in this lifetime. Yet I also believe we are *south* of Heaven, where a lot of inexplicable and tough stuff happens. So, I seek connection with God through prayer and depend on support of loved ones and friends for strength to endure hardship. This is what I believed and how I experienced faith before my own crisis, and what I believe today. But during that Crisis of Faith, much of it was up for grabs.

I'm being open about this experience, so those who may be in the thick of their own seasons of doubt will not have to travel through them alone; and so that they realize that such seasons are *normal,* especially for Extraordinary Care Givers. With this realization, ECGs will hopefully feel like there is room, as a person of faith, to doubt that faith and to talk about those doubts. Hopefully they will feel enabled to ask the hardest questions and even vent anger at God with a friend alongside that gets it. This is the road *through*

Crises of Faith. It's rough, but as we traverse it with support, we can acquire a far deeper, more resilient spirituality.

My Story: "If God is All Loving...Where was He Then!"

In my story of Compassion Fatigue, I talked about "hitting the wall" after the loss of a client to suicide. This one event was actually the proverbial tip of my emotional iceberg. It slowly emerged to the surface; pushed into sight by an enormous group of traumatic experiences that had built up within my psyche during the first nine years of my clinical career. I had helped many people who seriously struggled with suicide risk; and they made it through their tough seasons to enjoy better years. However, in so many of those cases, while they were mid-stream in crisis, I could not know for sure, whether they would live or die.

Even though I was a trained therapist, I hadn't realized how those crises, combined with my daily responsibilities, had impacted me. (In those days, education about Compassion Fatigue was not part of our clinical training or even on the radar of most therapists.) I seemed to be functioning well in all areas of life through those years since graduate school, amidst big demands at work and at home. While it was hard to hear so many grizzly stories from folks in therapy, it was richly fulfilling work and most all of my clients improved and moved on. I didn't have huge anxiety, flashbacks, nightmares, or other symptoms of traumatic stress. Nor did I feel the cumulative impact of my exposure to trauma on my work life—until my client's death.

In addition to the struggles I described in Chapter 10, this death broke open a flood of religious questions and doubts. I found myself asking one of the most important, yet difficult existential questions, "If God is really *present*, always there for us—if God is really all-*powerful*, all-*knowing*, and all-*loving*—then where was he when this happened? …And when…?" My *Where was God* list was long. Since my late teens, I had enjoyed a faith in a God who I experienced as being present, reliable, caring and powerful; a source of comfort, security, guidance and hope. Now it seemed that He either did not possess those qualities or did not exist at all.

Myth: Doubt is the Opposite of Faith

For many, doubting is considered the opposite of faith. And so, it is something we should not do. In fact, doubting is a part of developing an *authentic* faith. It is rare for most people who have endured a great amount of tragedy to be free of doubts about God. To forbid ourselves from doubting is to imprison within us enormously potent discouragement, possibly even despair. Such pain can be released and replaced with hope when it can be shared with those who may have also traveled, or at least can empathize with this dark road.

You'll notice that this notion, "we shouldn't express our doubt", sounds a lot like practicing the old paramilitary "Suck-it-Up" Emotional Code (Chapter 5). Not a great idea for our mental health. And as it turns out, sucking up our distress is not a good idea for our spiritual health, either. It can be a freeing experience to admit doubt to ourselves, to give ourselves permission to openly express it and the painful emotions that accompany it. As we acknowledge thoughts and feelings about hardships that are tangled in doubt, we are actually entering a new portion of road which leads beyond that darkness—especially when we walk it with a supportive, nonjudgmental person.

Champions of Faith Freely Doubted

In the Scriptures, there is an ancient record of a king, David. In his childhood, he had extraordinary faith which made him fierce in the face of danger. As a young man he was a warrior beyond compare. As a king he was unsurpassed in his power, wealth, and the success of his reign in the province of Judah. David was also human—a very flawed human. He blew it in some very major ways. He also struggled at times with massive fears that were actually fully warranted. (It seems in those days there was always a sniper or two trying to kill him.) He openly expressed his fears to God in his prayers that still survive today.

At one point, David thought he saw the proverbial writing on the wall: his assassins were closing in and it looked as if there was no way out. Death felt very near. In despair, he didn't write another piece of poetic prayer proclaiming huge trust in God's faithfulness as he had many times before. This time he scrawled one of the most famous, seemingly faithless accusations of God recorded in the *Bible*, "My God, my God. Why have you forsaken me?" (Psalm 22:1). Forsaken means to utterly abandon someone and leave them to die.

How could David, this giant of faith, accuse God of just turning his back on him when he needed Him most? First, it was honestly how he felt, and he found it hard to contain himself. Second, he somehow knew it was okay to lay it all out there without worrying about getting struck with a lightning bolt for *lack of faith*. Perhaps he had come to know the character of God so well that, for him, this was as natural as a little child pounding on their father's leg at nap time, crying, "Why?" The Scriptures affirm this was the case, recording words believed to be spoken by God himself saying, "I have found David, son of Jesse, a man after my own heart…" (Acts 13:22).

If you'll allow me a little of liberty in paraphrasing this ancient statement, it sounds as if God is saying, "This man David, Wow! He pursues me, my love, and our relationship as if he wants me more than anything else in his life." David screamed in the face of the Deity, "My God, My God. Why have you forsaken me?" because somehow he knew there was room in the relationship for total authenticity. And for those afraid of the lightning bolt for doubting, consider this: when David was screaming at God, he was turning *toward* Him, not away from Him. In his active, honest doubting, he was actively relating to God. Rather than feel even more alone in the moment's desperation, he told God everything on his mind. He got it out, he released it. No sucking up anything.

For many devoutly religious people, this way of relating to God may seem sacrilegious and wrong. If you've traveled through your hardest times without struggling with doubt, I'm sincerely happy for you (perhaps even a little envious). But if we must keep silent with God when we're suffering most, our spiritual vitality will, along with our mental health, be apt to suffer in the long run. I'm not encouraging folks to live out a life of faith laced with perpetual doubt. There are seasons, though, where honestly expressing our doubts about God is the most authentic pursuit of our faith; no matter what it sounds like to others.

Let's look at just one more example where someone of great faith expressed doubt. In the Christian faith tradition, Jesus is considered to be fully human, yet also fully divine. I know, that concept is a real head bender, and we won't launch into theology trying to fathom this mystery. I bring up Jesus not to preach or proselytize. He just happens to be perhaps the greatest example of how doubting God is a part of loving Him. Even secular historians and leaders of non-Christian faith traditions elevate Jesus to the position of prophet and Holy Man.

Let me set the stage for the point about doubt that I want you to see. Jesus referred to himself as the "Son" of God, and referred to God as his "Father" (John 17:1). His teachings in Scripture reveal a deeply intimate relationship between this Father and Son. Jesus would not deny this relationship even when they threatened him with capital punishment. Yet, at the height of his suffering—he, the one with unparalleled faith—spoke words to God that were no more confident than King David's. In fact, while in tremendous pain after sustaining extreme torture, he quoted the very *same* words David had spoken a thousand years before him, "My God, My God. Why have you forsaken me?"

Did God really abandon Jesus? It sure seemed like it to him! And what he said to God fit that moment.

9-1-1Pros, you're pretty good at being blunt and to the point, right? Your "get down to business" mindset is essential in dispatching life-and-death scenarios. So, if King David and Jesus himself felt the freedom to be blunt with God when it really mattered, maybe you can too! This step is part of exchanging that old "Suck-it-Up" Emotional Code with a healthier one; perhaps it might sound something like, "In the worst moments of life, it's okay to turn to God and tell Him what I really feel, no matter what it is."

Fleshing Out a Game Plan for Surviving a Crisis of Faith

I hope you've gained a fresh perspective about how we can relate to God when our struggles fuel doubt—perhaps you've even gained a little more permission to be real with God when you travel through your hardest times. Yet, during those times, we're also in great need of support from human beings! We could say that sometimes we need that support more than God. I'd say, since God is unseen and we are flesh and blood, we sometimes need to experience more of God *through* people; people who can be physically present alongside us. In fact, this human experience was what pulled me through my own Crisis of Faith.

I had grown to care deeply for Don, my client who suicided. At the news of his death, I felt flooded with sorrow for his family.[1] There was a profound sadness tangled with guilt and helplessness. I knelt on the floor of my office, crying. I cried out to God for help. My pleading was followed by empty silence. Doubts rushed in to fill the vacuum, *what if we're really just alone down here. It's just us.* The vulnerability and aloneness in this moment was probably the most profound of my lifetime. The office was now closed and my secretary had gone for the day. She left the front door unlocked, since I was still "doing paper work" in my therapy room. Then I heard that door open, and I looked up.

Within a second, the handle of my inner door turned, squeaked, and two massive men burst in: Pastor Jim Larsen and Reverend David Behling. They were two of my closest friends in Petoskey. We served together on the elder board of our church. Jim was the brightest, most unorthodox pastor I'd ever known. That's what I loved about him the most—no matter what you said to that man, his love was guaranteed. He welcomed doubts and would give you room to vent them, free of any compulsion to set you straight. He knew about King David, and he certainly knew about Jesus!

David Behling, was our hospital chaplain and had come alongside more families in tragedy than any other clergy in our area. His heart and compassion are enormous. You need to understand that my client was also a pastor. As fellow clergy, Jim, David and Don had spent many years serving our small town. At some point, in the weeks I'd been seeing Don, he had apparently confided that I was his therapist. David, as hospital chaplain, had likely learned about Don's death upon its discovery, and rallied Jim to join him—ASAP. They both knew me well. And they expected I'd feel everything I was feeling the very moment they arrived.

The hour I spent that day with Jim and David, and their continued support in the months that followed, buffered my Crisis of Faith. Their love didn't vanquish it completely, but they stood together with me, on behalf of (and in much the same manner) as I believe God would, if He were flesh and blood. Sometimes when we can't muster faith, people of faith must lend us theirs. Jim and David did that. Not by sharing Scripture verses (though, carefully, they did) nor by trying to *convince* me God still existed. Rather, they simply showed up, listened, made room for doubt, and kept showing up. I knew their source of strength and in whose name they loved me. And somehow, as I look back now, I can see that they helped sustain my thread of faith until it could grow strong and resilient once again.

Before we wrap this chapter up, let me encourage you to consider a few concrete steps than can help you travel through a Crisis of Faith.

- Affirm that the crisis is normal, even healthy and transformative, though it doesn't feel good at the time.
- Take a moment to think about who you view as a person of mature faith. Are they someone you could trust to come alongside you when you're suffering? If so, consider calling them. Arrange a time to sit together to talk about faith, and maybe even share a copy of this chapter with them. (You have my permission.) Build that friendship, so it's there for you when you need it most.
- Seeking support from others doesn't have to be an either-or proposition. In addition to the friend you choose, consider who, among the ordained *clergy* in your area, would be most supportive of you during a Crisis of Faith. Try reaching out to them to talk, too.
- If your gut tells you that you're struggling with deep depression or other overwhelming feelings, seek a trustworthy recommendation for a good licensed mental health professional in your area. Practice a healthy emotional code by setting up an appointment to begin counseling. And by all means, if you need support, consider asking the friend or clergy you selected above, to come along with you for the drive to your first appointment.
- Most folks don't consider themselves writers. The idea of "journaling" usually conjures thoughts of flowery, poetic entries. But if you're thoughts

about God are tangled up, as mine were in the midst of my hardship, spiritual journaling can be extremely helpful. There's no formal process you need to follow. Just experiment with writing out your unedited, raw thoughts and feelings about your situation. As your thoughts begin to flow, decide if you're ready to write them as a letter directly to God. As you write, just notice what it feels like without judging your thoughts.

You can then decide if you want to share your journal entry with a friend, clergy member or therapist to help you release more of the distress. This may even lead to great conversation about God. My discussions with David and Jim did not offer tidy answers to my hardest questions about God. In fact, their acceptance of me without trying to force theological answers to those questions somehow helped me accept what I could not understand. And this helped to restore my peace with God and my ability to turn toward Him.

Conclusion

Doubt is part of faith. Ultimately there is no prescription, no "cookie-cutter solutions" to make our Crises of Faith easy to pass through. Hopefully, my story of struggle will empower you to walk authentically, and with support through yours. We're not meant to live this life alone, and fortunately we don't have to.

My prayer for you is to experience the freedom to be genuine with your heart and your faith, and to receive comfort on every step of the journey.

Questions for Reflection

To get the most from this chapter, you are encouraged to write your reflections here (in both the Kindle and paperback versions of this book).

- What was your main take-away from reading this chapter?

- What specifically made it valuable to you?

- How can you apply this take-away concretely to improve some aspect of your personal life and or efforts to support the wellbeing of 9-1-1Pros?

Additional Resources

- From a Christian Perspective: *The Question that Never Goes Away*. Philip Yancey (2014). This author originally pushed the limits in facing doubt about God in his first book, *Where is God When it Hurts*. This volume, brings Yancey's last thirty years of experience to take us even further.
- From a Jewish Perspective: consider Rabbi Harold Kushner's *When Bad Things Happen to Good People* (Original publication, 1981). Don't be deceived by publication dates. This book is timeless.
- All faiths: *The Wounded Healer*, Henri Nouwen, (1972). I still have my copy. This old book has become a classic, because it so powerfully makes the point that love in action speaks far louder than words. Nouwen also helps caregivers to recognize their own need for care. While he was a Catholic priest, his fame spread because of his relevance to all people, irrespective of faith tradition.

Works Cited

The Bible. King James Version, 2018, www.kingjamesbibleonline.org/.

McCraty, R., Atkinson, M. "Resilience Training Program Reduces Physiological and Psychological Stress in Police Officers." *Global Advances in Health and Medicine,* vol. 1 no. 5, 2012, 44-66.

Stamm, BH. "THE PROFESSIONAL QUALITY OF LIFE SCALE: Compassion Satisfaction, Burnout & Compassion Fatigue/Secondary Trauma Scales." *The ProQL Manual,* August 2005, **www.compassionfatigue.org/pages/ProQOLManualOct05.pdf**.

End Notes

[1] Many years have passed since Don's death on November 6, 1996. His widow had been grateful for the care I'd provided them, and we maintained some contact in the few years afterward... Just last year, as I prepared to write this chapter, I reestablished contact. She had moved to live near her adult children. She had worked hard and successfully to heal. When I told her of my desire to share the story of Don's death,

Ginger whole-heartedly agreed. She is convinced that talking about suicide, rather than denying its pain, is part of healing. For this cause, she even welcomed me in using their real names, as I have.

SECTION III

HOW TO SURVIVE & THRIVE TOGETHER: KEY ELEMENTS OF A RESILIENT 9-1-1 CENTER

CHAPTER 15

The NENA Stress Standard: The "Shall" Document with Eight Solutions that Can Save 9-1-1 Lives

Jim Marshall

Introduction

Reading about policy or standards can be as exciting as watching a sloth makes it way down from a tree. Virtually every organization in the world depends on good policy to succeed in their mission. Can you imagine a PSAP without policies? Of course not. However, if a leader in Oklahoma and a dispatcher in Maine both opened this book's Table of Contents, odds are close to zero that they'd choose to read a chapter about policy development before one about a dramatic personal story. That's why this chapter about policy comes after the many chapters filled with personal stories already shared in this book. But, don't skip it! If you've read the stories of 9-1-1Pros in the previous chapters, you hopefully recognize how critical it is to assure that all 9-1-1Pros have the resources they need so their stories can reach the happy endings our authors have achieved: healing, resilience and a great quality of life at work and at home.

9-1-1 Leaders Share Concern for Employee Well-being

Frontline dispatchers in some PSAPs have become deeply discouraged, believing that their leaders 'don't get it'—they don't understand 9-1-1 stress and the enormous toll it can take on 9-1-1Pros. In some cases, these frontliners may be right. Yet, after literally hundreds of hours of discussions with frontliners, 9-1-1 directors and industry leaders, one thing is clear to me: there is, generally, a very high level of concern and desire among our 9-1-1 leaders to protect and empower their dispatch personnel.

Many 9-1-1 leaders have worked to secure funds to get their dispatchers to stress training. Many are seeking their participation in critical incident debriefing sessions, starting morale committees and encouraging wellness programs. Yet, these initiatives and more resources must be provided to all 9-1-1 Professionals. The extraordinary stressors faced by our telecommunicators require strategic and comprehensive planning.

Leaders Face Real Obstacles

Two factors make it difficult for 9-1-1 leaders to translate their concern into comprehensive efforts to achieve that objective. These are not excuses for limited efforts to protect the resilience of 9-1-1Pros, but they are real factors and must be recognized and addressed so that good leaders can assure the resources their employees need to safeguard their well-being. *First,* whether running rural, suburban or big city comm centers, most of our directors are almost constantly *running on tilt.* They carry responsibility for their employees and the performance of their centers under heavy scrutiny from their governing boards, field response agencies, the media, and the public.

Systematic stress management efforts can seem unfeasible since a myriad of other immediate demands tug at leaders: getting the budget approved so the center can run, and people get paid, recruiting more employees to resolve understaffing, immediate personnel issues, equipment breakdowns, new towers, new radios, new CAD, getting NG9-1-1-ready. Every project requires more meetings, memos and policies. Governing bodies operating our PSAPs must evaluate our 9-1-1 directors' need for administrative support to accomplish all that is expected of them, including safeguarding the resilience of their personnel. Without adequate support, they will be more likely to focus on the immediate and urgent demands listed above and wellness initiatives may be left undone. Hopefully leaders and their governing bodies will see from the information provided in this book (see especially the case study in Chapter 20) that many of the metrics they seek to improve can be boosted by prioritizing resilience.

The second factor limiting 9-1-1 leaders' efforts to safeguard the resilience of their personnel is that many still lack awareness of the stress risks faced by their personnel; and they often do not know where and how to begin stress management initiatives. 9-1-1 leaders are experts in emergency response. They are not stress experts, psychologists or experts in organizational health. Therefore, they usually are not sure what to do *strategically* to help their people with 9-1-1 stress. But that's why we wrote the next two chapters (and the next two sections).

The Good News: You Can Start Somewhere. Here's How!

If you are a 9-1-1 leader, I hope you'll be encouraged, because this chapter, and those in the remainder of the book, are dedicated to equipping our leaders (and their governing bodies) with information they need in order to lead their PSAP in implementing comprehensive resilience solutions. As a leader, whether you are fortunate enough to be well funded or struggling just to keep the lights on, please just do all you can to put the following guidance offered in these pages into practice. Let's get started.

The NENA Stress Standard: Eight Solutions that Can Save Lives

The National Emergency Number Association (NENA) Standard on Acute/Traumatic and Chronic Stress Management is a national 9-1-1 standard. It is *the* policy that, if put into practice, can literally save the lives, mental health, performance and retention of our Very First Responders. The solutions to 9-1-1 stress risks provided in the Standard resulted from several years of work from 9-1-1 dispatchers, leaders and experts in mental health. This full document can be accessed and read by downloading it at the link provided in the Additional Resource section at the end of this chapter. Here, we select and address key sections of the Standard to make it easy to digest and put into practice.

The NENA Standard states that all "Public Safety Answering Points [PSAP] shall establish Comprehensive Stress Management Programs [CSMP]..." These CSMPs provide eight care elements to their personnel. They include:
1. Training in Stress Management
2. Onsite Educational Material
3. Critical Incident Stress Management
4. Identification and access to local trauma therapists
5. Employee Assistance Programs
6. PSAP Peer Support Programs
7. Ongoing certification training in high stress call types
8. Personal health incentivizing programs (option)

How We Will Approach the Eight Solutions

In this chapter, I will walk you through each of these eight solutions so you can more easily build your CSMP and put these solutions into action at your PSAP. We will list and describe each of these solutions (quoted verbatim from the NENA Stress Standard) and offer "Discussion" whenever helpful to support your efforts. Let's begin with Solution #1...

Solution #1: Stress Management Training

Throughout this book we have established the risks associated with 9-1-1 work. 9-1-1Pros certainly want to live a long life, perform well at their jobs and enjoy their families. And their leaders want the same thing. As a work culture, 9-1-1Professionals (including frontliners, supervisors and managers) are a highly responsible group; and they work very hard taking care of citizens, their field responders and their families. Here's the challenge: the more focused we are on taking care of everyone else, the less likely we are to prioritize self-care too. Yet, as 'Extraordinary Care Givers', 9-1-1Pros experience extraordinary stress. And that means they must be equipped with extraordinary skills to safeguard their mental and physical health. Of course, this is a shared responsibility. First, since their job exposes them to intense stress, their employing agencies fulfill their responsibility (in accord with the NENA Stress Standard) by providing them with stress management training. And dispatchers fulfill their responsibility by investing in the training and applying the insights and skills they gain from it.

In a moment, we'll look at the topics the NENA Standard states will be included in stress management training. Each one of these topics is important. Yet, there are a few additional ingredients of training that we need to point out. These 'intangibles' will make all the difference in protecting the mental health and resilience of our 9-1-1Pros. Many 9-1-1Pros will enter the class with serious depression, others with PTSD. This course may be their best opportunity to realize this need and to seek initial support. I will refer to my experiences with dispatchers in teaching my course, *Survive & Thrive*, as I discuss these 'intangibles':

- As the instructor, I must expect, and make possible, the chance that dispatchers will make decisions in the class that will be life-changing. This is not something I can orchestrate or force. It happens regularly, because all members of the class help create conditions in which 9-1-1Pros can recognize their most important needs within the discussions we create *together*.
- The classroom must become an emotionally safe space designed and guided to encourage (without manipulating) candid, heart-level discussion among all participants. In my class we discuss how safety will be created. Rule number 1 is strictly adhered to: honor complete confidentiality. Class is a judgement free zone, and no one will be allowed to dominate the discussion. As the instructor, I also emphasize that we can never know what a peer may be struggling with, how much they may need peer support during the class. We have lost members of our 9-1-1 family in the U.S. to suicide at an alarming rate in the past five years. A course in stress management may be an opportunity for a 9-1-1Pro in distress to feel deeply supported and shift directions toward help rather than ending their lives.

- One of the greatest privileges of my career has been sharing private one-on-one's (or two-on-ones when a dispatcher asks their peer to join us for support). During these times, 9-1-1Pros have often decided to accept help bridging to a local EMDR therapist we locate while still together. And peers agree to come alongside to help make follow-through easier.

- 'Top-down' lecturing and unloading of facts and information do not promote deeply internalized learning that leads to changes in self-care. In all my classes I make the same statement at the start, "If we don't co-teach today, we might as well go home right now. Each of us in this room has life experience that brings value to us all, whether you started in dispatch this week, or 25 years ago…." 9-1-1Pros cite this highly interactive, co-teaching classroom experience as an invaluable aspect of *Survive & Thrive*. They report that it helps them major life decisions to improve their self-care and seek professional assistance.

- The management of class discussion must foster maximum acceptance of personal responsibility for change. It is understandable that many 9-1-1Pros feel overwhelmed by conditions in their workplace. So, related complaints about PSAP leaders will inevitably come up as part of stress management training. While class discussion needs to allow for such venting and related peer support, it must be constructive. Here's my point: If dispatchers believe they cannot be happy until their leaders make work conditions in the center better, they may be sentencing themselves to a career of misery.

    Of course, PSAP leaders should do all they can to optimize work conditions. But a pivotal question in self-care for any of us is, "What do I do with what I can't control?" Hopefully, despite our circumstances, we are each striving to cope constructively, rather than being controlled by circumstances which we cannot change. This is the value of resilience skills and the ChoicePoints strategy: to heighten real-time attunement to our options to rally our resources, rather than drain them in the face of circumstances we cannot control.

With these important training 'intangibles' in mind, let's look at the specific *topics* related to stress management training called for in the NENA Standard.

The NENA Standard states:

"Public Safety Answering Points shall [provide]... Stress Management Training, minimum of 8 hours in length for all PSAP personnel, addressing the following topics:

- The nature of stress, stress disorders (acute/traumatic, chronic), mental and physical health impacts of unmanaged stress

    Discussion: for 9-1-1Pros to protect themselves from the serious mental and physical impacts of 9-1-1 stressors, dispatchers must understand basics about the "psychophysiology" of stress (the way in which the brain interacts with all systems of the human body when stress occurs--when demands exceed our personal resources). The information taught to telecommunicators should be from credible sources supported by science.

- Exposure to the above stress types specifically within the PSAP

    Discussion: self-care in the face of high risks of these stress conditions requires 9-1-1Pros to be fully knowledgeable about them. This education serves as primary education and, for some dispatchers already struggling, it can be life-saving. I have had countless private conversations with 9-1-1Pros at the tipping point who allowed me to bridge them to professional help. I don't believe they would have decided to receive help unless we had carefully discussed these psychological risks in class.

- Negative impacts of traditional military denial of traumatic stress on personal health and work performance/importance of supporting and personally embracing proactive stress management

    Discussion: Chapter 5 provides a complete discussion of this topic by exploring the powerful role of our Emotional Code: what we believe we should do with what we feel.

- Education on coping skills and strategies including Therapeutic Lifestyle Changes (TLC, See Terms and Definitions section in the NENA Standard)

- Utilization of specific skills activating the Relaxation Response (see Terms and Definitions section in the NENA Standard), including progressive muscle relaxation, diaphragmatic and coherence breathing, and imagery/visualization

Discussion: skills such as those listed here must be modified for real-time use by 9-1-1Pros due to the often-non-stop demand of call-taking. In the *Survive & Thrive* course, we carefully discuss the science of resilience and build the skills that protect it and optimize performance and health. A portion of that training is presented in Chapter 6. Training must also equip 9-1-1Pros to recognize when and how to activate these resilience skills to manage their stress response (see next item/training topic below).

- Principles and skills for management of emotion and thinking under duress

   Discussion: the ability of 9-1-1Pros to effectively manage their emotional distress is crucial for their performance at the console, especially with difficult and highly distressed callers. This ability is also a key to improved attitude, relationships and morale of employees working together in the PSAP. In Chapter 5, as in *Survive & Thrive*, I teach the *ChoicePoints Strategy*™, designed to create awareness of stress 'cues' so that resilience can be activated in real-time to increase management of the Stress Response, emotions and actions.

- Principles and skills for effective PSAP communication, conflict resolution

   Discussion: within the limits of an eight (even sixteen hour) course, it is difficult to fully equip 9-1-1Pros in conflict resolution skills. Yet, one of the primary keys to conflict management in employee relations is overall self-care protective of personal resilience. If our 'inner battery' (Chapter 6) is charged, we have more self-control, better judgment and impulse control. Here, too, mastery of the ChoicePoints strategy can prevent and help resolve conflicts that are often triggered when we 'obey' our emotions, rather than notice the stress 'cues' that a wiser option is available.

In addition to its value in decreasing negativity and improving customer service, stress management training can potentially help save lives and salvage quality of life, marriages, and families.[1]

Stress Solution #2: Onsite Educational Information

"Public Safety Answering Points shall [provide]…on-site PSAP educational materials and resources about stress related risks, information about available local and online resources to manage stress, including traumatic stress disorders, chronic stress and related health problems...the role of nutrition, exercise and sleep in prevention of stress disorders and stress-related diseases."

Discussion

These educational resources may be in the form of single page handouts, brochures, books or DVDs related to the variety of topics listed below. Throughout the United States 9-1-1 centers are using minimal square footage within quiet rooms or other dedicated spaces to install a bookshelf for resources like this. (See the Additional Resources section at the end of this chapter for free prepared materials addressing the topics above.) Other topics discussed in these education materials could include:

- Work related stress risks: this involves acknowledging that 9-1-1 work is stressful and that there is risk of stress related conditions related to performing this work. Contrary to the concern that this kind of acknowledgment can promote overuse of sick leave and FLMA, the greater likelihood is that employees will seek preventive help before problems become severe. Thus, a reduction rather than an increase in sick leave.
- Available resources to manage stress: this includes information educating telecommunicators about stress and how to improve resilience and manage stressors in daily life.
- Traumatic stress disorders: all 9-1-1 telecommunicators should be provided with information that explains traumatic stress disorders and other impacts of trauma. It can include a list of signs to look for and how to access local clinicians who are trained in evidence-based treatments to provide healing of trauma.
- Chronic stress: this is a condition resulting from the cumulative impact of overproduction of cortisol in the line of duty. Chronic stress can impact physical health. Fortunately, it is preventable and treatable if employees know the signs to look for and are encouraged to see their physician or healthcare provider.
- Related health problems: consider materials available from your local public health department on prevention and treatment of other stress-related conditions such as high blood pressure, diabetes, and obesity.
- The preventive roles of nutrition, exercise and sleep: while plenty of information on nutrition and wellness is available online, it is unlikely

an employee who spends much of their life sitting at a computer will take the steps to search for that information. They want to leave work and think about family, not possible problems.

The stigma about seeking mental health care runs so deep among emergency responders that even the presence of on-site educational materials, if explicitly supported by leadership, can be lifesaving. For leaders to provide and inform 9-1-1 employees about all these resources is more than just a gesture of support. It helps to actively create a culture of psychological support and care. When these materials are provided, and personnel are urged to become familiar with them and seek help as needed, a single brochure, with information about a local trauma therapist, could save the life of an employee who, unbeknownst to everyone else, has been struggling with flashbacks, depression and possible suicide risk.

9-1-1 Stress Solution #3: Critical Incident Stress Management

"Public Safety Answering Points shall [provide]… PSAP SOP [Standard Operating Procedure] establishing procedures assuring participation of PSAP personnel in Critical Incidence Stress Management [CISM] activities including debriefing sessions when involved in traumatic call events; and as needed in relation to such events. PSAP leaders are also strongly encouraged to promote CISM certification training by at least one PSAP employee to serve as the on-site CISM support person fostering effective use of CISM by PSAP employees. Printed materials and online information should also be provided informing employees about how to access CISM resources, and encouraging appropriate use (e.g., addressing the question: 'When should I ask for help?')."

Discussion

Critical Incident Stress Management is too often equated only with critical incident stress debriefing sessions. However, CISM is a comprehensive crisis intervention system of psychological first aid as developed by Dr. Jeffrey Mitchell of the International Critical Incident Stress Foundation.
It includes services that are provided to groups or individuals by a team including at least one mental health professional and trained laypeople. The services range from preventive educational support for those who may be involved in traumatic experiences, support in the acute crisis stage, and psychological first aid after traumatic events have occurred. The CISM model includes several components:

- Provision of educational information in both written and presented forms
- Defusing sessions which occur within hours of an event: this does not involve intensive processing of the experience. Rather, it is the equivalent of a supportive check-in, taking the pulse of those involved, inviting individual support, and assuring them of follow-up care in the days to come. That care, according to the CISM model can include both individual and group forms of...
- Critical incident stress debriefing: while this is most popularly administered as a group experience, CISM team members are also trained to provide the support on a one-on-one basis.
- Post-incident follow-up support to check-in on the status of participants and provide more care as needed

Group debriefing is typically provided throughout the United States to law enforcement officers and firefighters (and medics, depending on their agencies) after tragic events involving loss of life. However, most telecommunicators are still not included in these supportive events. Many still believe that because 9-1-1Pros are not physically on scene, they cannot be significantly psychologically impacted during an event. This belief is inaccurate and has been a source of disappointment and resentment among telecommunicators in the U.S. for many years.

Possible Benefits of 9-1-1 Participation in Group Debriefing

During the past thirteen years of training 9-1-1Pros, I have asked those who have participated in group debriefings how beneficial these experiences were. The majority have said that they were helpful and cite several reasons, offered here with my comments:

- They were grateful to be acknowledged and included among the other responders as a matter of respect
- The group process provided them the opportunity to hear other perspectives and achieve a level of closure they would not have otherwise experienced. This can produce tremendous relief and resolve errors in the thinking and images dispatchers created in real time. There is no strong evidence suggesting that these debriefings help to prevent PTSD, yet it stands to reason that increased closure and resolution of unfounded guilt could decrease a telecommunicator's unprocessed psychological distress. This certainly could decrease the likelihood of developing PTSD at least related to the specific incident.

It could also decrease the likelihood of self-medicating and other unhealthy coping strategies.
- 9-1-1Pros' participation in the sessions may have also helped to improve their relationships and shared performance with the field responders who participated in the debriefing.

Reliable results and positive experiences for participants in group debriefing require that groups are always led or assisted by a licensed mental health professional or a member of the clergy who has completed training in clinical pastoral education (CPE). Group leaders must be capable of exercising real-time clinical expertise and judgment to assure that all discussion of the critical incident is carefully managed to avoid increasing traumatization. They must also be able to maintain close attunement to all members of the group process identifying those who might be struggling most and assuring individual follow up care.

Other members of the clergy who are not trained in CPE may seek to lead these groups with the very best of intentions. They may be generally very competent in providing spiritual support to our emergency response groups and may be highly trusted by the leaders of these groups however without the essential clinical training, there is greater risk of doing harm in the attempt to do good. For that reason, the 911 training Institute urges leadership of group debriefings be only entrusted to those clinically trained, with the assistance of lay leaders. Non-CPE clergy could certainly serve in this supportive role.

Risk Factors of 9-1-1 Participation in Group Debriefing

I do believe that 9-1-1 Professionals can benefit from being involved in group debriefing experiences after tragic events in which they were involved. However, caution should be exercised. In addition to the risk that is introduced by underqualified leadership, there are several other factors that need to be considered carefully if 9-1-1 centers are to engage their people in group debriefings:
- Even when group debriefing sessions are properly led by qualified teams, there is inherent risk when engaging a group of responders and processing traumatic experiences together. Even when all participants appear to be stable throughout the discussion, appearance is not a reliable indicator of actual level of emotional disturbance. Debriefing sessions are often held at times that are inconvenient to participants because they must be conducted whenever possible amidst many people's schedule demands. Participants may be eager to leave at the end of the meeting and it is

difficult for two or a few leaders to keep track and check in with everyone before they leave. The inability to carefully assess the well-being and mental status of participants before they go is concerning.

For this reason, I believe group debriefing sessions should only be conducted with clear points of agreement between the session leaders and the agency leaders hosting the debriefing. These points would include:
- o emphasizing to all participants the desire of leaders to check in with them before leaving upon completion of the meeting
- o urging all participants to take personal responsibility for seeking support as needed
- o providing all participants with printed information about available qualified trauma therapists before they leave class
- o Plans will be made assuring meaningful individual follow-up with all participants within 72 hours of the meeting.

- Participation of 9-1-1Pros in debriefings must always be voluntary and never mandated. I have always been grateful when 9-1-1 leaders make a special effort to be sure their personnel are invited to debriefings because of the benefits they can receive, but also because of the powerfully supportive message this sends to their employees. However, telecommunicators have reported being mandated to these group sessions and with few exceptions stated that this was an experience that negatively affected them. Debriefing sessions should never be mandatory since we can't know how individuals will be impacted by their participation. If an employee is already overwhelmed by work or home crises (sometimes both) or their mental health is suffering significantly, their immersion in a highly intense debriefing could have damaging effects on their well-being.

In contrast to psychological debriefings as we are discussing here, leaders certainly maintain the right and the responsibility to mandate all involved staff to participate in tactical debriefings to evaluate and improve performance. But in their own thinking, they must be clear about the distinction between these two types of debriefing, to avoid the error of making them both mandatory.

- Invitations issued by leaders for their personnel to participate in debriefings should make clear when they are exclusively for psychological support in contrast to tactical debriefings. When those leading debriefing sessions are not properly trained, there is more likelihood that psychological debriefings will degrade into tactical debriefings, where fingers are pointed and blame is assigned. This is obviously a very detrimental experience for participants. In *Survive and Thrive*, I advise dispatchers to respectfully step out of such meetings. If the meeting was led by properly trained leaders, they will likely recognize when such a slip into tactical debriefing occurs. So, if a dispatcher leaves the room to safeguard their own well-being, one of these leaders can be expected to follow them out and offer needed support.

- The third risk factor is not about the way in which debriefings might be conducted but about what comes *after* the debriefing. There's also risk when emergency response leaders believe that they are providing all the psychological care that their personnel need by sending them only to debriefings without other additional professional support services or resilience training. There is greater risk of personal mental health crisis when responders believe that psychological first aid (such as debriefing sessions) is or is expected to be accepted as adequate support following tragic events. Responders are then less apt to seek those additional services they may need, especially when they adhere to the old Suck it-Up emotional code discussed in Chapter 5.

In summary, I do believe leaders should advocate for participation of their 9-1-1 personnel in group debriefings when they were involved in tragic incidents. However, when they extend this invitation to personnel, they should also inform them of the risks discussed, and refrain from making participation mandatory. Such an invitation provides telecommunicators with the option to use this resource. Yet, my general recommendation to them and to their leaders is to pursue individual support after critical incidents, when such support is possible. Unfortunately, only very few 9-1-1 centers in the country have developed peer support programs. Over the years, leaders and frontliners have requested that the 911 Training Institute create such a resource. Finally, in 2017, in response to these requests and the obvious and growing need, I developed the Certified Peer Supporter Program. It is designed specifically to address the unique stressors faced by telecommunicators through individual support on a 24/7/365 basis, with the support of a licensed mental health professional. We will explore that Peer Support Program in the next chapter.

9-1-1 Stress Solution #4: Evidence Based Treatment (EBT)

"Public Safety Answering Points shall... Identify local therapists specializing in treatment of stress and traumatic stress disorders who utilize evidence-based therapies recognized by the Department of Defense and the Veterans Administration to be effective in the treatment of PTSD. These therapies include...[Cognitive Exposure Therapy, EMDR, and/or Prolonged Exposure (PE). Note: this list is revised from language in the Standard.] Encourage proactive use of therapy by PSAP personnel."

Discussion

In the Introduction to this book, I told the story about the beginning of my clinical career in the late 1980s. At the time, we lacked effective treatment for Post-Traumatic Stress Disorder. This was dismal for those suffering from PTSD (now also called Posttraumatic Stress Injury, PTSI) and it wasn't much better for those of us striving to help them find relief. Fortunately, in 1990, I was trained in a new, ground-breaking treatment called EMDR. This treatment was probably responsible for saving a number of my client's lives. It probably also saved my career. I shifted from feeling a difficult combination of empathy and helplessness for my clients before using EMDR to feeling a sense of hope, optimism and fulfillment after I began utilizing this treatment. The world of clinical and research psychologists had believed (as many erroneously still do today) that PTSD was incurable. It turns out, fortunately, that we were all wrong!

In 2011, the U.S. Department of Defense and the Veteran's Administration concluded a massive review of all existing treatments of PTSD for which there was any evidence base. They sought to determine which, of all these therapy approaches, was truly effective in resolving PTSD symptoms. Their results: only three cut the mustard and made their list of recommended treatments, and EMDR was one of those three (VA/DoD). Since 2005, I have strongly recommended that EMDR be considered the treatment of choice for all 9-1-1 telecommunicators for PTSD/PTSI.

In Chapter 9 of *The Resilient 9-1-1 Professional,* Sara Gilman and Reannon Kerwood provide an extensive and fascinating look into their successful treatment of 9-1-1 Professionals using EMDR. They help you learn what an EMDR session looks like and about the liberating outcomes 9-1-1Pros have experienced as a result. In their chapter's Additional Resources section, Gilman and Kerwood also point you to free resources we've developed and provide on the 911 Training Institute website to help you learn more about EMDR, and how to locate and select a qualified therapist in your area. If you, your personnel, or your loved ones suffer with PTSD and other emotional struggle for which you or they have yet to find effective help, this is a must read. It's also essential so you're prepared to assist your PSAP peers or employees to find help in the future. With the resources provide here, it'll be much easier for you to put a check in the 'completed' box as you work to finish the planning of your PSAP's Comprehensive Stress Management Program.

9-1-1 Stress Solution #5: Employee Assistance Programs (EAP)

"Public Safety Answering Points shall... Establish (if not currently provided), educate and encourage employee use of Employee Assistance Programs that provide confidential counseling for all PSAP personnel, with funding of initial session(s) to encourage employee use. PSAPs are urged to seek EAP contracts with clinicians familiar with 9-1-1 and who specialize in treatment of traumatic stress disorders (see Stress Solution #4).

Discussion

Employee Assistance Programs can be an invaluable resource in preventing escalation of impacts from 9-1-1 stress and personal issues in the life of all 9-1-1 Professionals (at all levels of the organization). However, EAPs can be unhelpful if they lack knowledge of the unique 9-1-1 stressors (Chapter 3) and the emergency responder culture, and if they lack clinical skills to treat traumatic stress.

In *The Resilient 9-1-1 Professional,* we thoroughly discuss the EAP solution. In Chapter 17 you'll find a full interview with EAP expert Randy Kratz who defines the elements of a best practice employee assistance program in service to the 9-1-1 centers in Dane County, Wisconsin. In addition, I provide you with a guidance document, *Assuring Best Practice in 9-1-1 Employee Assistance Programs* (Chapter 17 Appendix). This document can be used by 9-1-1 directors and their agency's Human Resource departments in discussion with current or potential EAP providers, to assure best practice care of 9-1-1 personnel. Members of 9-1-1 governing bodies are also urged to read Chapter 17 and this appendix so they are prepared to support optimal selection of an EAP for the PSAP.

9-1-1 Stress Solution #6: Peer Support

"Public Safety Answering Points shall... Establish PSAP Peer Support Programs. These programs utilize call center staff who are trained to provide confidential emotional support upon request of a PSAP employee without administering advice or solutions. Peer support is not a substitute for professional counseling but serves to defuse stress and staff conflicts while encouraging people to move toward responsible solutions and professional therapy assistance as needed."

Discussion

Each the solutions called for by the NENA Stress Standard provide an essential ingredient in fortifying 9-1-1 Professionals against stress risks. Yet, Peer Support plays a uniquely crucial role. No one can understand, empathize and come alongside a 9-1-1Pro like a 9-1-1Pro! Well-trained peers are the first-line of defense against stress risks for the Very First Responder. Because of the crucial role of Peer Support (when combined with a foundation of self-care through Stress Management Training), Chapter 16 is dedicated entirely to explaining this solution of the Stress Standard.

9-1-1 Stress Solution #7: Call Mastery Training

The authors of the NENA Stress Standard recognized that dispatchers who are properly trained in all aspects of their work will be more confident and therefore better able to cope in the face of enormously stressful call taking and dispatching. How do you define 'call mastery'—successful management of a 9-1-1 call? Since 9-1-1Pros cannot control what happens on scene or the choices that other people make in their lives, call mastery can't be defined by the outcomes of the call or the dispatch. Given these very real limitations, 9-1-1 call mastery must be defined as managing the call—in accord with the highest available level of training and resources—irrespective of the outcomes.

As described in Chapter 6, the brain and body work to produce a healthier hormonal cocktail when we are confident rather than feeling helpless in the face of a stressful experience. Specifically, when we are dominated by fear we activate only cortisol and other stress hormones. However, when we are confident we also produce dehydroepiandrosterone (DHEA), also known as the Vitality Hormone. This combination enables us to peak performance while preventing stress related illnesses and increasing our sense of reward at very difficult tasks.

These science facts support the need for basic dispatch training for all telecommunicators. A growing number of states in the U.S. have established training standards and created funding mechanisms assuring training to their Very First Responders. Yet, the majority of our states still lack 9-1-1 training standards, so many 9-1-1Pros significantly lack in training. Fortunately, with assistance and a forum provided by Coordinator of the National 9-1-1 program, Laurie Flaherty, a group of 9-1-1 stakeholders has established the United States' first *Recommended Minimum Training Guidelines for the Telecommunicator*.[2] (For a copy of this document, see the Additional Resources section at the end of this chapter.) So, the industry is heading in the right direction. And, fortunately, the NENA Standard already defines the national requirement for training related to managing calls involving mental illness and suicide risk. This training is especially critical. Here's why…

9-1-1-Training in Calls involving Mental Illness and Suicide

In Roberta Troxell's 2008 study, dispatchers reported that calls involving huge emotional distress and suicide are also apt to activate intense fear, helplessness and horror. This combination of emotions is evidence of being psychologically exposed to a traumatic event. Two factors call for prioritizing training for all 9-1-1Pros in managing calls involving mental illness and suicide: these calls are more complex than most all other medical dispatch calls, since presentation of symptoms is less uniform and caller cooperation is often far more compromised by their mental status; and the risk of violent death during the call. Consider my earlier statement, how high confidence modifies and optimizes cortisol production. The psychological and physiological health of the telecommunicator *and* their best performance on the call are both protected by being properly trained in this call type. In other words, such training is ethically essential for the good of both caller and calltaker.

Many dispatchers the United States still have not had training in management of calls involving suicide and serious mental illness. With the alarming number of incidents across the country of suicide-by-cop, 9-1-1 leaders are reaching for help to acquire this training, amidst serious funding restraints. Online training represents one solution to increase the access to such training.

Proposing a Best Practice Standard: Protecting the Caller and the 9-1-1Pro

Should non-physicians, including 9-1-1 Professionals, conduct and train their peers to conduct emergency *medical* interventions to callers? That depends. We would all agree they should not *if* they are creating those interventions themselves. Our 9-1-1Pros will readily acknowledge that they (like me) are not trained or qualified to assume primary responsibility for developing medical evaluation and treatment models. However, 9-1-1Pros *can* conduct and train peers to conduct medical interventions if they are trained to use protocols developed by physicians specializing in emergency medical science designed (with invaluable input from 9-1-1Pros). These experts can assure that the initial design and implementation of the interventions is based on best current science.

In the same way, training on management of suicide calls requires that the curriculum be developed by mental health professionals with special knowledge of suicidology, mental illness, diagnostic evaluation and intervention. So, in accord with our reasoning above, we can ask: should a non-mental health professional assume primary responsibility for development of such training curriculum for 9-1-1 telecommunicators? No. However, 9-1-1Pros can be trained to conduct powerful evaluation and interventions with callers at risk of suicide if they are equipped with training and tools designed by mental health experts. Yet, I do not consider it advisable for non-mental health professionals to train 9-1-1Pros in suicide call management. We must also recognize that among telecommunicator's in our classrooms, are those who may be actively struggling with suicide and at risk of being more greatly distressed if material is not presented and discussion managed with great sensitivity to this risk.

In response to requests from frontline telecommunicators and their directors, I have developed a certification course, *Certified Emergency Mental Health Dispatcher* (CEMHD) to equip telecommunicators related to the course objectives cited above within a more comprehensive curriculum. I have integrated telecommunicator self-care and real-time use of resilience strategies into this course, so that 9-1-1Pros can buffer the stress involved in managing suicide calls while managing their emotional distress in real time for optimal performance.

The curriculum for these courses must be developed from sources directly produced by experts in the field of psychology and suicidology. Information from journalists or laypeople should not be used as primary sources for key information in these courses. Throughout the years dispatchers in my courses have recognized errors in previous education, for example about how to talk to a person at risk of suicide. Those errors were due to instructor ignorance and may have decreased the ability of telecommunicators to work effectively with such callers at risk. My goal here is not to judge but to help set a standard for design and delivery of 9-1-1 courses on topics involving mental health, so that 9-1-1Pros are prepared for excellence. This is, of course, critical for optimal service delivery to the public at risk, but also in providing the telecommunicator with the ability for genuine call mastery and well-founded confidence.

While I won't define the full curriculum from my courses on these topics, I will highlight just a few that are essential to be covered in training.
- Destigmatizing mental illnesses to boost empathy in call-management
- Preparing dispatchers with a mindset to withstand real-time psychological distress for optimal performance and self-care
- Identification of factors driving suicide behavior
- Exploring the empirically defined components of suicide: desire, capability, intent, and buffers
- Effectively building an alliance with the caller
- Gaining skill in assessment of suicide risk and in intervention to prevent suicide

In my course, *Certified Emergency Mental Health Dispatching*™, dispatchers are introduced to *LifeBridges FlexProtocol*™, a tool designed to equip 9-1-1Pros for effective assessment of suicide risk by identifying the empirically established components of suicide cited above. (911 Training Institute is currently working to create a CAD-based software version of this LifeBridges protocol as a comprehensive stand-alone protocol with capacity for integration with other protocol programs.)[3]

9-1-1 Stress Solution #8: Health Incentivizing Programs

Increasingly, throughout the United States, government agencies are creating health incentivizing programs for employees to encourage improved self-care in both physical and mental health. These programs generally involve providing resources to educate employees about all aspects of health and fitness and provide opportunities for self-improvement with some kind of incentives attached. I would encourage you to review Ivan Whitaker's chapter (23) for a successful example in which a 9-1-1 leader has implemented such a program with the help of his morale committee. One aspect of his approach is especially noteworthy: since the financial reward of reduced sick leave use was so small per person he decided along with the morale committee to pool the earned funds for use in financing enjoyable evenings with food provided. This is a wise approach since there is a real question about the effects of health and fitness competitions for employees.

Such competitions may actually lead to demoralization and longer-term failure in advancing physical health when goals are not reached. Well-designed health incentivizing programs, though, are crucial in the 9-1-1 center due to the highly stressful work conditions to which 9-1-1Pros are exposed, and the high level of obesity. (See Chapter 12 for a thorough discussion of risks related to obesity and concrete steps that leaders and employees can take towards improvement of this problem.)

Conclusion

Leaders in the 9-1-1 industry are increasingly aware of the stress risks facing our nation's telecommunicators. The establishment of national *Recommended Minimum Training Guidelines for the Telecommunicator* is a heartening case in point. National and state NENA and APCO (Association of Public-Safety Communications Officials) conferences feature topics related to wellness and stress management. Now, with the resources provided in this chapter and throughout The Resilient 9-1-1Professional, hopefully all 9-1-1 centers will take steps forward to build and run their Comprehensive Stress Management Programs.

While the pursuit of your center's CSMP can seem like a big undertaking, the benefits are even bigger: improved employee health, resilience, morale, better retention and performance are all possible outcomes. My hope is that this chapter makes the task clearer and less daunting.

In the next chapter we'll define how your center can build its own Peer Support program, as called for in the NENA Stress Standard. If you can't afford to implement all the eight Stress Solutions immediately, this may be one you'll want to pursue first. It's *that* important!

ଓଃଦ

Questions for Reflection
To get the most from this chapter, you are encouraged to write your reflections here (in both the Kindle and paperback versions of this book).

- What was your main take-away from reading this chapter?

- What specifically made it valuable to you?

- How can you apply this take-away concretely to improve some aspect of your personal life and or efforts to support the wellbeing of 9-1-1Pros?

Additional Resources

- Troxell, R. (2008). *Indirect Exposure to the Trauma of Others: The experience of 9-1-1 telecommunicators.* (Doctoral dissertation). Retrieved from ProQuest Dissertations and Theses. (Accession Order No. AAT 333542).
- For a full set of tools to help build your center's Comprehensive Stress Management Program, visit **https://www.911training.net/911-wellness-toolkit**. This free 9-1-1 Wellness Tool Kit includes…
    - The link to download the full PDF version of the NENA Stress Standard
    - Access to a full PowerPoint™ presentation, developed by Jim Lanier, Alachua County Sheriff's Office (FL) and me. This resource was presented at the National NENA conference in 2017. It provides condensed descriptions of each of the eight solutions (elements) of care called for by the standard and suggested feasible steps that 9-1-1 directors and their personnel can take, even with little or no funds to begin building their CSMPs.
    - 911WF **NENA RESOURCE A:** This is A Guide Sheet for Building Your PSAP Comprehensive Stress Management Program (CSMP). This document serves as a grid to help you focus, organize, and record your agency's implementation efforts.
    - 911WF **NENA STRESS RESOURCE B Helpful Links**. This PDF document provides you with hyperlinks to key resources you can use to create and fulfill each of the 8 elements of your PSAP's CSMP. For example, you'll see handouts on free stress education info you can print and

display in your center to fulfill CSMP element 3: providing your personnel with "Onsite educational materials."

Works Cited

Department of Veterans Affairs & Department of Defense (2017). "VA/DoD Clinical Practice Guideline for the Management of Post Traumatic Stress." *U.S. Department of Veteran's Affairs*, 2017, **www.healthquality.va.gov/guidelines/MH/ptsd/**

"National NENA Standard on 9-1-1 Acute/Traumatic and Chronic Stress Management." *National Emergency Number Association (NENA)*, 5 August 2013, c.ymcdn.com/sites/www.nena.org/resource/resmgr/Standards/NENA-STA-002.1-2013_9-1-1_Ac.pdf.

End Notes

[1] One of the goals of the 911 Training Institute is for every 9-1-1Pro in the U.S. (and beyond) to have access to trustworthy, empirically supported resilience training, like our course *Survive and Thrive Together in the 9-1-1 Center: Comprehensive Resilience Training*. However, understaffing and funding struggles make this impossible for many PSAPs. Since *The Resilient 9-1-1 Professional* teaches a great deal of the content required by the NENA Stress Standard, 911 Training institute is working to make it possible for PSAP personnel to gain continuing dispatch education credits for reading this book. This provides an affordable and more convenient option to onsite training compared to online and onsite training. Visit **www.911Training.net** and see the Training tab for updates on this opportunity. Feel free to also email my team for **info@911Training.net**.

[2] "The National 9-1-1 Program is housed within the National Highway Traffic Safety Administration at the U.S. Department of Transportation and is a joint program with the National Telecommunication and Information Administration in the Department of Commerce." (Source: https://www.911.gov/about_national_911program.html)

[3] The national pilot of the Certified Emergency Mental Health Dispatcher was launched in 2017 in partnership with Alachua County Sheriff's Office, Gainesville, FL. To inquire about the CEMHD training or about the status

The NENA Stress Standard

and availability of software version of the LifeBridges FlexProtocol, request information at the email above.

CHAPTER 16
The Power of 9-1-1 Peer Support: The First Line of Care and Prevention for the Very First Responder

Jim Marshall

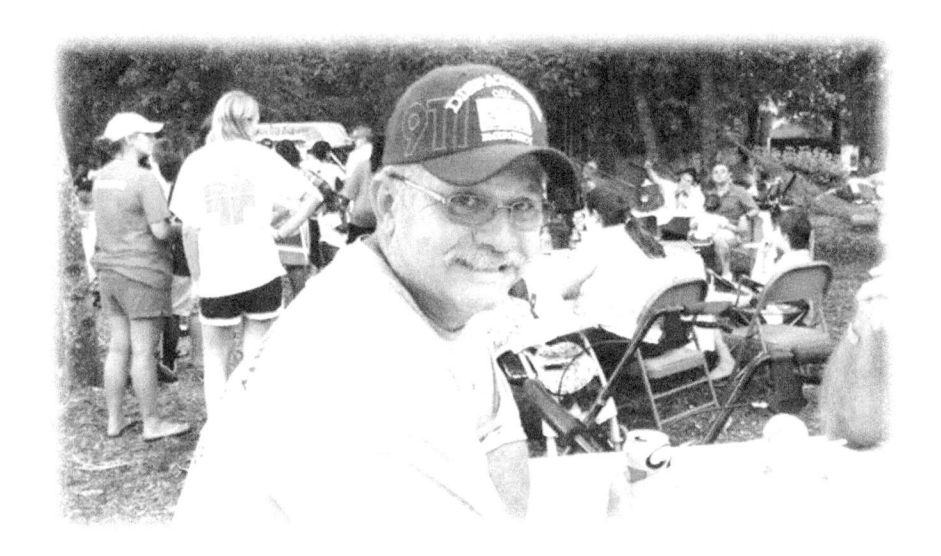

Michael Stanley
Born September 19, 1956
Deceased February 7, 2018

Introduction

The Need for Peer Support

If you've turned to this page, you may well be in the good company of many of our 9-1-1Pros, at all levels, who are feeling the climate change in America, their communities, and their PSAPs. Our dispatchers and their leaders are encountering (or bracing for) an increasing number of high impact events in the line of duty. All while they deal with 9-1-1's version of business as usual: the steady, high volume of 'regular' emergency and non-emergency calls, long

work hours, understaffing, and constant adaptation to new systems. And many employees face their own serious personal struggles which they are trying to manage along with their 9-1-1 stress. In combination, these factors can tug hard at their mental health. Without venting all the stress constructively, they're more at risk of struggling with depression, negativity, and gossip that can eat into the center's quality of life and morale.
Center leaders and their frontliners are looking for solutions. As we've already discussed in other chapters, there's certainly a role for professional mental health care for 9-1-1, but not every struggle requires professional care. And there really is no one who can come alongside a 9-1-1Pro like another 9-1-1Pro who totally 'gets it'. That is, in fact, what Peer Support is all about. So, it comes as no surprise that I have had more requests from 9-1-1Pros and their leaders for help in building 9-1-1 Peer Support Teams in the last two years than I did in the previous ten.

There are at least two levels of peer support you can deliver at your center:

1) *Informal,* real-time support that all personnel can provide to each other, supported by basic training. As all members of a PSAP invest in each other, and are more prepared to provide this organic support, their shared sense of unity as a team can increase. So, morale and attitude can improve. In Part 1 of this chapter we will look at the essence of good informal peer support: what it is, the blocks that get in the way, and how to remove them so that 9-1-1Pros can just 'be there' more helpfully for each other. To bring this to life, I will share the story of a 9-1-1Pro, and personal friend, Michael Stanley—one of the most inspiring people I've ever known.

2) An *official* Peer Support Program, delivering strategic support as the comm center's first line of preventive care available to all PSAP members. So, in Part 2, I will introduce and describe key elements of the national pilot, 9-1-1 Certified Peer Support Program (CPSP), launched in Wisconsin in early 2018. We will explore …
    - The unique value of a formal Peer Support Program
    - The Foundations on which it must be built
    - The steps you can take to build it, and
    - Key considerations in building the program to achieve *best practice*

Let's get started…

Part 1: The Heart of 9-1-1 Peer Support *The Charleston County 9-1-1 Family*

At the 2011 National NENA conference, I met Jim Lake and Allyson Burrell, the director and deputy director respectively, of the Charleston County Consolidated 9-1-1 Center (CCC). They participated in four sessions that I led—all related to 9-1-1 stress. Their investment in caring for their people was clear throughout the day. Many of their 9-1-1Pros had worked on the day in 2007 when nine firefighters perished in the Charleston Sofa Super Store fire. And, like so many comm centers in the United States, they had been hit by more highly stressful events since. So, Jim and Allyson asked me to come to Charleston to provide a hybrid form of support to their team: combining resilience training with supportive group experiences led by their Peer Support Team and me. Our goal was to enable all four CCC squads to process the traumatic experiences they had traveled through and how it had impacted their teams, while gaining new insights and skills to protect personal resilience and heal as a team. Jim and Allyson have brought me back several times since, as they have encountered more high impact events including the AME church shooting in 2015 (see Chapter 23). Through these experiences that my friendship with Michael Stanley came to be.

Michael Stanley, ENP: The Heart of 9-1-1 Peer Support

You may have noticed that this book is dedicated to Michael Stanley (and two other people to whom co-editor Tracey Laorenza and I owe the greatest debts of gratitude). "Mike" was born on September 19, 1956. Sadly, he passed away, far too soon, on Wednesday, February 7, 2018, from injuries sustained while working under his car. As I write this, it has not yet been two months since his death, and he is deeply missed by so many. Fortunately, he lived many years longer than he might have, thanks to peer support.

A Man on a Mission

Mike was a man on a mission, and he made one of the most profound impacts on my life of anyone I've known.

Twenty 9-1-1Pros sat with me in a large circle in comfortable chairs in the clubhouse on Dewee's Island. This location was offered in gratitude by the island's residents for CCC's part in saving this natural preserve from decimation when a huge fire spread through its interior years ago. Jim and Allyson had arranged for every squad to have one day on the island. They were away from the comm center, where they could do intensive resilience work: small group discussions, full group training, and solo times for self-care planning. We went around the room on day one doing our personal introductions. Everyone was appropriately polite, some were funny. Then it was Mike's turn to speak.

He didn't pull any punches. CCC's leaders and their people had been to hell together in the line of duty in the past many years. And trainees were trying to find their footing on their squads. Through it all, they had excelled. Mike knew how strong they had been, and how much people needed to recognize the opportunity they had in these special days on the island to do a hard reset, emotionally and as a 9-1-1 family. And, as at any comm center, many may still have felt they had to live by the old 'Suck-it-Up' Emotional Code. Jim and Allyson were working hard to change that, and Mike wanted his co-workers to know two things. First, was that there, in that room, on that island, it was safe to say anything. There was no pressure to speak whatsoever; but they would have his complete support if they chose to share openly. The other thing he felt strongly they should know, was his story. Some of his newer peers had not heard him share this history before, nor had I. I'm quite sure that what we heard that day was a gift to many of Mike's peers. I know it was to me. His story more clearly, more powerfully, conveys the heart and the power of Peer Support than any other example I can imagine.

Mike's Story: Extraordinary Loss, Extraordinary Resilience, and How Peer Support Matters

I'll lead you through his story, with discussion along the way, much as Mike and I talked about it when he told me. In this way, we'll identify the mission and heart of peer support. But, before we begin let me emphasize something. I've shared this story with emergency responder groups for several years now. However, I thought twice about sharing it here in the book, so soon after his death. Then I recalled what he had said to me just a few months ago when I asked, yet again, for permission. Mike had a way about him when he spoke. He slowed his speech, lowered his voice, added some gravel to it, and then told you how things ought to be. "Jim. You can stop asking for permission. I've already told you. You can share my story whenever and wherever you want. As long as there is the chance that it will help someone, do it." So, with his direct order ringing in my ears, here goes...

Mike served for seventeen years in the US Navy Submarine Service and retired successfully at the highest enlisted rank. For twenty-five years, Mike was as a volunteer firefighter with many certifications. He also served for fourteen years as a NREMT/paramedic crew chief for Berkeley Co. EMS.

That all came to a full stop, like a ship out of fuel, in 1997. *And that's where his story begins…*

When Mike was still a paramedic, he experienced the tragic loss of his ten-year-old son, Nathan, to drowning. Three months later, Mike was called to the scene of a ten-year-old boy pulled from water. CPR was not successful.

What Makes Peer Support Difficult

After they did all they could to care for the deceased boy, Mike went to the back of his rig and began to weep. Most of the members of Mike's EMS team that day probably knew that he had lost his son. Yet, none of his coworkers came to his side to offer comfort. Here, we need to pause the story (as we will along the way) to make our first reflection on peer support.

When I got to this point in sharing Mike's story once in a classroom with 9-1-1Pros in Florida, I said, "we need to wonder compassionately what kept these peers from going to Mike's side. It is easy to judge…" Before I could finish my sentence, one of the veteran 9-1-1Pros, who is also an officer, slapped the table and erupted, "That's bullshit! They should have been there for him!" I was leading up to an important point about peer support when she interrupted me, but I wasn't offended in the least. In fact, her protest was driven by precisely the kind of heart for her peers that we need!

Wondering Compassionately & Removing Blocks to Good Peer Support

Plenty of other dispatchers have also been baffled by the lack of support that Mike got from his peers in that moment. He clearly needed someone alongside him, even if they said nothing. Yet, they may have known that just as well as we do. Most of us have 'failed' to act with compassion, too. So, we need to gain insight about what blocked Mike's peers, by *wondering compassionately*. This means pulling out of our immediate inclination to judge based on what we think we know and reaching to understand what may be at play when humans fail to step up, or throw bad advice, into the pain of a coworker. We wonder this way not to make excuses, but to gain insight about our mindset to remove mental blocks. By the way, wondering compassionately is perhaps the practice *most essential* to doing great peer support. So, before we go on with Mike's story lets wonder together about his peers. What do you think might have been their mindset—their emotional state and thought process—that drove their inaction? We can't know for sure, but I, and your 9-1-1 peers in my classes, have wondered about the following possibilities:

- It is possible that Mike's peers, with whom he had worked for many years, had *also been struggling* in their grief for him, related to the loss of his son. On scene that day, they may have been in shock as they recognized the magnitude of this experience for their friend. In other words, they *may have been frozen* by their own empathy.
- They *may simply have not known what was best to do*. They may have been immobilized by the fear of doing or saying the wrong thing *because* they knew how painful this was to Mike. So, they may have reasoned, the better choice was to do nothing rather than something that would be hurtful.
- Knowing that Mike was inclined to be stoic, 'Mr. Tough Guy' (as he called himself looking back on this event), they may have sincerely believed that he *wanted to be left alone*; that he would have felt weak, more loss of control if they acknowledged that they saw him crying. This would mean their inaction was a choice (however wrong in hindsight) out of respect, not a lack of caring.
- Finally, Mike's friends may have, like many emergency responders, learned to cope over the years by disconnecting emotionally from tragic scenes as a way of survival. They may have practiced the 'Suck it Up' Emotional Code, which we explored in Chapter 5.

I think, somehow, Mike may have wondered compassionately himself. Because he told me that he didn't judge, blame, or resent his co-workers for their lack of support that day—even though his life almost ended within the next hour as a swirling, tangled mess of painful thoughts and emotions pulled him down…

Mike continues his story, "I…left the medic station at the end of my shift and started thinking. Big mistake! After a short period of time, my mind went blank and I had my truck pointed at a large pine tree in an upcoming curve with the speedometer buried. At the last minute, I suddenly realized that this was not what Nathan would have wanted. And I still had two other boys to think about. I hit the brakes and managed to keep the truck on the road. I still don't know how I missed that tree. Had to be divine intervention. I was that close. I got it stopped, walked about 5 miles back to the Medic Station and called a friend for a ride."

Swapping Emotional Codes: A Key to Peer Support, and Saving Your Own Life

This is a striking detail in Mike's story. Why did he call a friend? He needed transportation because he realized two things. Killing himself wasn't the answer to free him from his pain. There had to be another way, and he was going to stick around to find it. That led to the second reason for calling his friend. The way beyond his pain had to take him on a different route than he and his EMS peers had followed for so many years; sucking up their pain as they rescued everyone else. He realized in that moment that he wasn't meant to bear the load alone. Not anymore. He could have called a taxi, but instead he called a friend. Mike's Emotional Code changed that day from Suck-it-Up to Ask-for-Help. I'm not guessing at this, as you'll see in a second. This is probably the decision that saved his life—with a little help from his friends.

He continues, "My truck sat there overnight. The station was in a rural area…absolutely no traffic. During my walk (close to an hour), I spent a lot of time thinking and listening to the bugs and animals in the woods. How was I going to deal with this? I always thought I was Mr. Tough Guy and could handle anything. I mean, I had already buried two of my siblings, both younger than I was, one of my sisters-in-law, also younger than me, my father, both of my in-laws and many friends without any major issues. That was when I realized I needed to talk to others about what had happened. I could not do it alone."

By Mike's own account, his SOP for coping with emotional pain prior to this turning point was to submerge and disconnect from his feelings. This is nothing to judge. It is the way in which military and emergency response cultures have historically learned to cope with distress. Fortunately, though, Mike now recognized that was no longer working for him.

What is your Emotional Code? What do you believe you should do with what you feel? If it is captured in those classic three words that Mike had embraced, 'Suck-it-Up', wonder compassionately about what has made it feel important, probably even essential, to keep your pain distanced from others, even from yourself, perhaps?

While true listening is paramount to peer support, and we will explore this later, the first job of those striving to excel in peer support is to evaluate their own Emotional Code. I emphasize this for three reasons:

- The future of your own mental health and quality of life depends on respecting, releasing, and seeking support for serious emotional distress

- Your investment in the bigger picture of emotional self-care will depend on giving yourself the permission that Mike did, and
- If you want to officially serve your peers as a Peer Supporter, you've got to be committed to living out a real self-care plan to offset the extra load of stress they will place on your kind shoulders.

Mike gives us a fourth reason to give up this old Emotional Code and for leaders to champion peer support: *retention* of good employees. He explains, "After that call, when I called my supervisor, it was like he was telling me to just suck it up. I could not do that anymore."

Mike is not blaming here. He is simply saying that the job was no longer bearable, especially not without good emotional support. Would he have stayed if such support was there for him at work? That I don't know. I do know that good peer support has the power to help people stay in emergency response (if it is the right career for them) and grow stronger through traumatic experiences. Peer support can promote *Post Traumatic Growth* (Chapter 9).

There's more to gain from Mike's story. As a mental health professional, I've always gotten a kick out of Mike's next statement:

"I started going to counseling and was placed on Prozac. Prozac was not good to me, and my counselor was a jerk…I went off the meds, stopped seeing that counselor…"

Clearly, Mike just throat-punched my entire profession and is not the poster boy for success with psychotropic meds, either! But don't you wonder what he meant when he said his counselor was a jerk? From Mike's account in our discussions, I gathered that in his opinion, the therapist did far more talking and doling out solutions than actually listening to Mike. He failed to connect on a basic human level and did not give Mike room to release his pain so he could heal.

Mike had done his part. He got his butt to these professionals and was even willing to start on some meds (which by the way, for other folks, has been a life-saver). This treatment failure points precisely to the need to help 9-1-1Pros connect with clinicians who truly 'get it'; who understand what 9-1-1Pros go through, and what their work demands of them. And these clinicians must use evidence-based treatment that works. Bridging peers to such qualified therapists is also a vital piece of doing great peer support (more on this in Part 2).

Yet, Mike didn't just give up on himself when he discontinued professional care. He wasn't' finished with his last sentence…

"…*and* [I] started to openly talk to my peers and friends. I asked them questions, talked about God, His plan, what were their thoughts. I actually asked them why this happened to me."

Mike made a choice to begin opening up and talking to others about the loss of his son, Nathan. He chose to grieve with others alongside him, and to look for spiritual help. But did you notice that he posed one of the trickiest questions a friend or peer could ever be asked by someone in great distress, "why did this happen to me?"

Sometimes Questions are Really Statements: A Key Principle of Peer Support

When Mike asked this delicate question, those who listened were able to avoid a common pitfall to good listening: answering questions we shouldn't try to answer. One of the cardinal principles of good peer support is that we do our best by *not* offering answers to questions that are unanswerable, especially *Why did this happen?* Have you ever asked that question in the midst of huge emotional pain? Many 9-1-1Pros have heard this painful question on the phone in the worst moments of callers' lives. It activates within us a troubling combination of empathy and helplessness. And it is precisely when we feel this combination of emotions that we are most apt to spill out some kind of an answer. But consider this: when someone cries out, "Why did this happen?" are they actually asking for an answer, or is it a guttural cry of helplessness and pain? Sometimes it's another way of proclaiming, "This doesn't make sense! This pain is unbearable, and I feel utterly helpless to change it."

Removing another Block to Good Peer Support: The Compulsion to Fix

One of the most common blocks to effective peer support is the compulsion to explain why someone is suffering. If they want our advice, they can ask for it. The most helpful response we can usually offer to the *Why did this happen* question, is the most honest one, combined with empathy and a simple assurance, "I don't know why. But I'm so sorry, and I am right here with you."

Our bent to fix our peers when they are hurting is not wrong in its intention. We usually do this because we care and want to give relief to our peer's pain. 9-1-1Pros are paid 'fixers'. That's the job. Which is precisely what makes it so hard to switch gears when comforting a peer; to not *fix*, but just be alongside them with empathy. Fixing is also, often, an effort to relieve our own anxiety connected to our feelings of helplessness. It feels more empowering to have answers than it does to witness pain without any explanation. Yet, it is here, in the quiet of sitting alongside a friend without any compulsion to fix, that they experience our presence most powerfully.

Mike's Big Break Through

It turns out it wasn't only his peers that Mike asked why. As he continued his story he said, "I had asked God this also. This helped immensely."
Mike's peers didn't have to answer the big *Why* question. While God doesn't seem to always answer when we call out to Him, He's the only one who can answer some questions (even if He doesn't do it the way we think He should).

After crying out this question to God on many occasions, one day he received an answer he couldn't have expected. Mike said he heard Nathan speaking clearly from heaven, assuring his father, "I am okay, dad. Live your life and be happy."

The Gold Center of Peer Support for the Thin Gold Line

Mike found the peer support he was looking for within a group you might find pretty danged surprising. "Three months after this incident…I left EMS and started a new life in construction. Many of the friends I made talked openly to me about their families and problems. And I openly talked about mine. I think I out trumped them most of the time, but *they listened*."

I hope you can join me in seeing the humor and irony in Mike's experience. We don't usually think of construction workers as the most sensitive, empathic and attuned bunch. They've been stereotyped as a tough macho group. How could they do a better job of listening than professional communicators? No insult intended here, but this really gets to the point of one of the biggest challenges for 9-1-1Pros in doing peer support.

The way you, as a professional emergency telecommunicator, have been trained to listen and communicate with callers flies directly in the face of the kind of listening Mike needed. 9-1-1Pros aren't just *paid fixers*…You are also *paid interrupters*. I say this with the utmost respect. Think about it. Callers in distress may be talking quickly; they can be very hard to guide as they ramble, overwhelmed and unsure of the information that you as a 9-1-1-Pro need. So, when they're ziggin' you zag 'em, and when they're zaggin' you zig 'em, right? They don't know the information you need to intervene in that moment to get your assets rolling, but you do. You do your best to stay in charge of the call from one second to the next, seeking only the key information needed as the clock ticks. So you interrrupt strategically and often.

All this works wonderfully at the console. The problem is that it doesn't work so good face-to-face with the peer who really needs you to listen with full attention. 9-1-1Pros must do what I call a "manual override of the automatic tendency" when a peer is seeking your support. Rather than interrupt, fix, or offer solutions, all Mike needed was simply attunement and sincere listening. For 9-1-1Pros this is very difficult because it seems as if you're doing nothing at all, and nothing at all in an emergency call leads to an even greater emergency. Yet, the most powerful thing in peer support is to notice your own tension when you are about to jump into the fix-it mode. Experiment with the power of simply listening. For Mike this had an enormous value, "To me, that was the biggest help. Being able to openly remember the good times and share those experiences. If I had not been able to open up, I probably would not be here today." This is an enormous statement and brings us to the core of peer support.

Listening without fixing was, for Mike, perhaps a major factor in saving his life. As he finished his story he hit the bottom line. "I just needed someone to listen to me. Not offer any advice, just listen. Ask me about my kids now and you will have a hard time getting me to shut up."

During my years as a therapist, I have seen what Mike describes here as a hallmark and evidence of healing. With the freedom and the support to share his story of loss, he found himself reconnecting with positive experiences about his kids. So much so, that his new construction worker friends may have been reaching for the duct tape!

Less is Often More in Peer Support

It could be easy to dismiss this bottom line about peer support as common sense and unnecessary, "Okay, Marshall, we get it. We need to shut our mouths, avoid fixing, and just listen." Yes, that is it. However, when your brain has been trained to do just the opposite, for very good reason, this is far more easily said than done. The other reason it is much more difficult to just simply listen, is because many of us have not experienced its power in our own lives, as Mike had. Have you ever personally experienced a friend or loved one come alongside you, in a time when you were greatly hurting, and just listen this way? If you have, you will know its power and be more easily able to do it for others. If you haven't, you will still believe that more is *more* (fixing, giving advice, etc.) when in fact the opposite is true. I would encourage you to experiment the next time someone you care about opens up. Less is often more.

One final note (which is actually a bit funny): your 9-1-1 brain is trained to multi-task and you're inclined to operate according to that same software when you communicate face-to-face with your family and your friends. So, the next time you're sitting with them, or with a peer who is finally opening up to you, remind yourself: *they can see me!*

Closure about Mike's Story & Living out His Legacy

You already know that, many years after the story captured here, Mike passed away. But the thing that I celebrate, as his friend, is this: from the moment his recovery began, though imperfect for sure, he continued to heal and live many more years with much fulfillment. In fact, it was inevitable that Mike, being Mike, driven to serve, would decide to return to emergency caregiving. While he chose not to reenter work as a paramedic, he became a 9-1-1 professional. He served for seventeen years at the Charleston County consolidated 9-1-1 center, ascending once again, into leadership. And I believe his fellow Peer Supporters would say, he was the heart of their peer support program. I believe his service to his peers, through this program, represents a significant part of Mike's legacy.

෴

Part 2: Building a 9-1-1 Peer Support Program

When Listening is not Enough: The Need for Advanced Peer Support

In a comm center there are many times when 9-1-1 Pros need peer support that moves beyond 'just' active listening. Doing peer support should never place a clinical burden on a non-clinical person. That's rule number one in my book. Yet, if one of your peers is struggling in the moment with a more serious problem, you may need to move into *active engagement*--helping problem solve; or even *active rescuing*--bridging them to emergency care to prevent suicide, domestic violence or other life-threatening risks. And that is the reason our comm centers must consider launching a formal Peer Support

Program (perhaps with other area PSAPs). All PSAP personnel need to be trained to provide the informal, 'organic' peer support we've describe thus far in this chapter. Yet, the magnitude of 9-1-1 stress necessitates equipping a select group of employees on each shift to be specially trained Peer Supporters. This was the message from 9-1-1 leaders and their frontliners that led to the development of the 9-1-1 Certified Peer Supporter Program (CPSP).

The Dane-Waukesha National Pilot: The 9-1-1 Certified Peer Support Program

John Dejung and Gary Bell, long-time colleagues, have been on the cutting edge in the pursuit of resilience support for their PSAP personnel since we met years ago. In 2016, after I trained their personnel in *Survive & Thrive*, they joined together to take their wellness initiatives to the next level. John and Gary, directors of Dane County 9-1-1 and Waukesha County (WI) 9-1-1 centers (respectively) asked me to move my 9-1-1 Peer Support model off the science bench and prepare it for action as a pilot project at their PSAPs.

One of the maxims John leads by is captured in a quote from General George Patton (which he unpacks in Chapter 21), "Bring me an adequate battle plan in time for the battle, not the perfect battle plan a day late." Gary reads from the same play book. So, with the hard work of a highly invested core group of 9-1-1 employees, these two PSAPs worked with me over the next two years to build out the CPSP model. They proudly gave their own name to their finished local product *SWIPST*, the *Southern Wisconsin Peer Support Team*. *SWIPST* officially launched into service in January 2018. Their goal, as a team, is to assure that every 9-1-1Pro knows one of their specially trained 9-1-1 peers is available 24/7/365 to come alongside when they need support and bridge them to more help if needed.

Building and Replicating 9-1-1 Peer Support Programs: A Crucial Need

The greater goal of this pilot partnership and the 9-1-1 CPSP is to establish a best practice model for peer support in the 9-1-1 industry. This will be achieved by continuous improvement of the model as it is replicated at other PSAPs; a process that is already underway in response to demands to meet this immediate and critical need. The effectiveness of this model will ultimately be determined as we gather data along the way. In the remainder of the chapter, I want to offer a sketch of the 9-1-1 Certified Peer Supporter program, to provide our 9-1-1 leaders with the information they need to consider building their own program. We welcome you to use this information for this purpose, whether you choose to partner with 911 Training Institute or not; our shared mission in the 9-1-1 family is to safeguard and equip our telecommunicators. And any effort in that direction is worth supporting!

The information provided here represents the principle and practices upon which the 9-1-1 Certified Peer Supporter Program is built.

Purpose and Value of 9-1-1 Peer Support Programs & the Role of the Peer Supporter

In addition to the rationale for advanced peer support provided above, adoption of a Peer Support Program serves a powerfully preventive role for the PSAP. One of the greatest threats to the mental health and morale of those in the center is the cumulative build-up of stress from the multitude of demands, frustrations and irritations over the course of weeks, months, and years. Certified Peer Supporters (as defined in 911 Training Institute's model) can mitigate this cumulative stress. They are fellow 9-1-1Pros who are specially trained to listen without fixing, and yet can support constructive brainstorming and problem solving. They can come alongside their peers to help them find relief and fresh perspective. This support can often resolve the problems before they escalate requiring professional help. These Peer Supporters are also prepared to encourage coworkers in practicing key resilience concepts.

The Importance of Self-Care for Peer Supporters

One important premise of the program is that all Peer Supporters must first be trained in effective psychological *self-care* and show a willingness to actively practice this. One of the greatest risks in volunteer roles, such as peer support, is that good and caring individuals may burn themselves out in the effort to help other people. So, training in self-care must be the foundation of training to assure that candidates practice good preventive physical and mental health and are attuned to 'cues' when their own stress is accumulating. All candidates for Certified Peer Supporter in the 911 Training Institute model must first participate in the sixteen hour *Survive & Thrive Comprehensive Stress Resilience* course. Then once they begin the CPSP training, upon selection by their directors (which we will discuss in a moment), they are each required to build a self-care plan, based on their *Survive & Thrive* training, and commit to practicing that plan throughout the duration of CPSP service. All team members must also sign their commitments to honoring *Our Shared Responsibilities*, a document which includes agreement to seek professional help as needed (along with peer support from other team members).

Selection of Peer Supporters for the 9-1-1 Peer Support Program

The 9-1-1 Training Institute has developed a list of criteria for CPSC candidates. Among other qualifications, they must:

- Have a strong reputation within the com center as being a trustworthy and mature individual who has shown the ability to honor confidentiality and does not participate in gossip.
- Possess the respect of their peers as highly competent in the core duties of dispatching—a matter of credibility increasing the likelihood that peers will seek their help.
- Be perceived by their PSAP leaders as being emotionally healthy. This is essential to assure that the work of peer support will not place them at risk of greater problems, and unmanaged personal problems can impede a Peer Supporter's ability.

I encourage directors partnering in the implementation of the Peer Supporter program to use the criteria provided by the training Institute, yet also consider input from others about candidates. Leaders are not always fully aware of how a specific employee is regarded by their peers.

Once selected, and CPSP candidates have completed the prerequisite training (*Survive & Thrive*, and the introductory one-day *Power of Peer* support course), they take part in a three-day certified Peer Supporter training.

Qualifications of the Peer Support Curriculum Developer and CPSC Trainer

The very nature of peer support involves the use of *lay-people* (those who lack clinical training) providing support to those who may have serious mental health problems. In this model, if candidates are not properly trained, there is greater risk that they may practice peer support in a manner that is beyond their scope of competence. Accordingly, it is critical that the training process be developed, and directly overseen, by a licensed mental health professional with thorough knowledge of the unique stressors faced by emergency telecommunicators.

The CPSP Training Curriculum and Real-Time Training Experience

Curriculum must be designed to minimize the risks that can result from the improper practice of peer support. It must also address the proper management of risky peer support situations that they could foreseeably encounter while serving in this capacity to their co-workers.

The CPSP training process must also be more than the transmission of facts and information to candidates. Training should be designed to blend clear instruction of key concepts with in-depth conversation among candidates and the instructor. This format (and the spirit of this discussion) assures thorough exploration of the peer support concepts discussed below.

Training Content and Process

Certified Peer Supporter training covers topics including, but not limited to, the following:

- Defining the essence of peer support (as described in the Mike Stanley story in Part 1 of this chapter)
- Terms of confidentiality between a 9-1-1Pro and their Peer Supporter
- Identifying *personal* blocks to effective peer support
- Defining and practicing elements of effective listening
- Understanding the thought process of peers struggling with clinical depression, suicide risk, and other of mental illnesses
- Management of crises, including suicide risk
- How to access mental health professionals
- Extensive enactment of possible peer support scenarios to assess and improve conceptual and practical grasp of the topics listed above, and to optimize real time use of emotion management and resilience strategies (Chapter 6) for best peer support and self-care.

The 911 Training Institute's model of CPSP instruction recognizes that while preparation in all these areas (and others not cited here) is essential, candidates facing the curriculum could assume that their excellence requires mastery of it in its entirety. This is not true. Peers are generally forgiving of imperfections in Peer Supporter's efforts when considered sincere. The expression of sincere caring for a peer is ultimately *more* meaningful to those struggling than competent *technical* practice. Candidates must also be assured that the support relationships they create with their peers will each be unique. Each Peer Supporter brings their own distinct capabilities and style to each one-on-one experience. These candidates can gain confidence and reduce their performance anxiety as they launch into their role by remembering a truth affirmed during the Dane/Waukesha Pilot Project training, noted earlier, *You already are the somebody that someone needs.*

An Underlying Instructor Responsibility

Effective instruction and guidance of CPSP candidates requires psychological expertise to effectively oversee the above instruction. Such expertise is also essential to monitor and assure the well-being of all candidates during the training who may be triggered by course discussion and content.

Continuing Education

According to the 911 Training Institute, success in the role of Peer Supporter requires continuing education (CE). The Institute has developed content addressing a variety of issues and struggles that peers might bring to a Peer Supporter. Delivery of such continuing education is also an ethical obligation of the organization contracted to instruct candidates. While, as in dispatch training, these candidates cannot be prepared for absolutely every scenario, guidance in management of predictable high-risk scenarios should be provided. Leaders of the agency, along with their peer support project coordinator(s) are encouraged by 911 Training Institute to collaborate with the Institute in developing continuing education materials.

Logistical Considerations in Building, Launching, and Operating the Peer Support Program

There are considerations in developing and launching a peer support program that cannot be addressed within the scope of this chapter. My intent here is to address just a few of those that are most critical.

- *Project Coordination.* The training Institute encourages selection of a project coordinator or lead Peer Supporter to oversee the tasks related to launching the program. In addition, a lead group selected from among the full group of candidates can be designated as coordinators who can help achieve the administrative tasks required. (This is how the Certified Peer Support Program pilot program (SWIPST) chose to organize their project.). The Institute has prepared step-by-step guidance defining and tracking the tasks required en route to launching the CPSP program.
- *CPSP Standard Operation Procedures.* Each 9-1-1 center that launches a peer support program will need to develop standard operating procedures approved by their agency. The SOP designed by SWIPST, in collaboration with 911 Training Institute, is provided to other partnering PSAPs to serve as a helpful template.

- *Joint Peer Support Programs.* 9-1-1 centers can choose to join with neighboring PSAP's to form a joint 9-1-1 peer support team. This minimizes the costs and work involved in launching a program. Joint peer support programs also create a very valuable choice to employees considering seeking help: they may choose to talk with someone *outside* their own comm center, since it can lend a greater sense of anonymity.
- *The Clinical Liaison's Role.* In the 911 Training Institute model of peer support, all programs engage a local mental health professional (with assistance of the Institute) as the program's Clinical Liaison. This liaison plays an important role by providing consultation and support, as needed on a case-to-case basis, to members of the peer support team. The clinical Liaison of the Wisconsin SWIPST pilot program is Randy Kratz, whom I interview in the next chapter.
- *The Peer Supporters' Resource Guide.* Since the Peer Supporter is never intended to be in a clinical decision-making role when risk is present, the Institute has developed a Peer Supporter's Resource Guide. This guide contains instructions and information about resources they can use in real-time to manage their peer support cases, and to effectively bridge their peers to professionals for 24/7 assistance.
- *The One-on-One Nature of the CPSP Model:* The 9-1-1 Certified Peer Supporter Program as designed by the Institute provides one-on-one support. For reasons explained in Chapter 15, this model is preferred to group processes unless CPSP activities are led by a licensed mental health professional.
- *Internal Marketing of the Program.* This activity is equally as important as the selection and training process to the success of the Peer Supporter program. It does not do any good to develop a peer support program if leaders and members of the team do not continuously educate their peers and encourage use of the program. These ongoing awareness efforts are also crucial to changing the culture, so that it no longer follows the old 'Suck It Up' Emotional Code. All PSAP personnel must recognize that their leaders and their Peer Supporters highly value and heartily encourage its use as integral to the organization's success.

Conclusion

Leaders of emergency telecommunication centers in and beyond the U.S. are striving to find the means by which they can support and equip their personnel to withstand the extraordinary demands of their work. As Dr. Michelle Lilly stated in her interview in Chapter 4, peer support programs, like the CPSP model, show great promise in prevention of more severe struggles with PTSD/PTSI. And because such a program utilizes peers to serve peers, employees can experience a level of empathic connection and support that helpers in other roles cannot deliver. The role of Peer Supporters, in bridging peers at risk to professional counselors, can assure that 9-1-1Pros, who would not otherwise reach out for help, can find the care and healing they need. Our 9-1-1 family has lost members to suicide. We cannot know what difference a formal peer support program might have made in their lives. But we can dedicate our efforts, as 9-1-1 stakeholders, to doing *all* we can to prevent as many suicides as we can in the future. Finally, 9-1-1 Peer Support Programs recognize that not all stressors must be big or traumatic to deserve support. By offering 9-1-1Pros relief on a day-to-day basis with the "little" stressors, the risks of cumulative stress conditions are decreased and quality of life, morale, and performance are safeguarded.

Questions for Reflection

To get the most from this chapter, you are encouraged to write your reflections here (in both the Kindle and paperback versions of this book).

- What was your main take-away from reading this chapter?

- What specifically made it valuable to you?

- How can you apply this take-away concretely to improve some aspect of your personal life and or efforts to support the wellbeing of 9-1-1Pros?

Additional Resources

- See www.911training.net for a full explanation of 911 Training Institute's peer support curriculum, services and resources available to help build, launch, and maintain 9-1-1 peer support programs.

CHAPTER 17
Choosing and Using Your EAP: How Employee Assistance Programs Can Help 9-1-1Pros

Randy Kratz and Jim Marshall

Part 1: Can you Imagine This?

Jim Marshall

Tom is a new telecommunicator, just six months out of training. He's wondering if he got into the right field. He's afraid of making major mistakes on the job that could result in someone's death. He hasn't gotten close enough to any of his peers or supervisors to feel comfortable admitting this. His wife doesn't understand either and he doesn't know what to do.

Kelly is on night squad B, at her com center. After seventeen years she's starting to feel burned out and is getting sick of what she describes as "these young whiners who wait for somebody else to answer the phone, so they can just keep gossiping."

Andy is a veteran telecommunicator with twenty-six years on the job. He was telecommunicator of the year in 2014, but he confided in me on break during a class that his "give a damn is very busted" and he's been written up twice in the last year for blowing up at callers. He can't retire for several years, because he lost a lot of his seniority after his old center was consolidated into his current PSAP. He's afraid of being fired, even though his boss has made no mention of this.

Sue has been a 9-1-1Pro for seven years. She took to the job quickly and was soon highly respected by her older peers as one of the very best telecommunicators. She could rock almost any call without seeming to ever be ruffled, until this past week when she took a really bad one involving the death of an infant. While she has mentioned nothing about her distress to her peers, this call triggered a flashback of her own child's passing ten years ago. Sue hasn't slept much at all since the call, because of panic attacks. Still, she's been gutting it out, because that's just what folks at her 9-1-1 center have always done.

Can you relate to any of these 9-1-1Pros? Maybe you're thinking of one of your work peers or perhaps your own challenges. The obvious thing that all these 9-1-1Pros have in common is that they could benefit from a bit of good mental health counseling support. The less obvious thing is that each of them could seek that help at no charge from their government agencies' Employee Assistance Program (EAP). But it's not likely that they will. Few of our telecommunicators in the U.S. know about those programs or have recognized their value to get some support. That's why we're writing this chapter for you!

But what about Sue? Her situation is more challenging. Her emotional struggles are driven by more severe traumatic experience that has taken a toll such that she now needs immediate attention.

If Sue is willing to get help, should she go to her EAP or should she go directly to a therapist who specializes in treatment of trauma? And how would she know which choice to make? While discussing struggles of this intensity with telecommunicators, I've heard from those who have tried their EAP, and others who went directly past the EAP for specialized trauma therapy. Unfortunately, most often when the 9-1-1Pro brings serious traumatic stress to an EAP, they discover that the counselors are not prepared or qualified to provide treatment that would resolve their symptoms. But once they've taken this vulnerable step of opening themselves up to tell their story, they don't want to start over with a second, more qualified therapist because the EAP had to refer them. At this point, Sue might just drop out of therapy and struggle on her own with her anxiety and sleep problems. Fellow co-author of this chapter, Randy Kratz and I want to help you and your 9-1-1 peers avoid this tangle and get to the right help the first time.

To be clear, good EAP counseling can help with a variety of less serious problems you or a peer might be dealing with that are not directly related to traumatic stress, complex high risk mental health, or relationship problems. And that's a great resource to know about! However, most 9-1-1 professionals either have not learned thoroughly about these programs or have not used them. Throughout this book we've emphasized that the resilience of the telecommunicator depends on such supports and resources to offset their experience of stressors at work and at home. But the Emotional Code of most emergency responders and telecommunicators in the past has been to "Suck it Up" (Chapter 5). So, seeking professional help from mental health clinicians is not an option that typically comes to the mind of our 9-1-1Pros, unless they are in extreme distress or crisis.

So many of our more severe struggles can be prevented by getting earlier help along the way—before we reach the crisis point or face major struggles such as clinical depression, PTSD, or severe compassion fatigue. As a 9-1-1Pro you need to know that a good EAP is an incredible benefit. You can get free counseling for several sessions that can bring great relief for many more common emotional and relationship struggles and keep you on track in your personal health.

So, why do so many of our 9-1-1Pros hold back from using their EAP? We have no national study that can help us answer this question with certainty. However, I am convinced, through countless discussions with 9-1-1 leaders and their frontliners, that there are two primary reasons. First, EAP programs could do much more to actively and regularly connect with 9-1-1 leaders and frontline personnel. Of course, 9-1-1 leaders share responsibility for employee awareness of, and encouragement to use the EAP. However, EAP providers should take the lead in building these relationships with center personnel by taking the following initiatives:

- Providing them with plenty of good on-site printed materials including information about how to access services
- Offer a link to their website for good Q&A about how and when to use the EAP, and what challenges they can help you with.
- EAP clinicians should work to establish relationships with employees by spending time in the communication centers and doing "sit-alongs" to build trust with 9-1-1Pros—the essential condition for them to trust EAP providers.

This last recommendation is a must for EAP providers to honor. In my classes on domestic violence and helping callers with mental illnesses and suicide risk, I ask the question, "Can you imagine how hard it is for someone who struggles with huge shame and sense of worthlessness to even press that 9? How long does it take before they can then muster the courage to press that 1, and the 1 again? How hard is it for them to reach out in such circumstances and then wait on the line to talk to a complete stranger about problems that may be very embarrassing and shameful?" Do you see my point? Because of the ingrained notion among emergency responders that admitting emotional pain is weakness, telecommunicators also may struggle mightily to reach out to a professional. It's a very big deal for a 9-1-1Pro to call and finally walk into the office of a mental health professional.

The Good News: Meet EAP Pro Randy Kratz!

Some of our centers still don't have EAPs. That must be remedied ASAP, as an ethical issue and because it is a glaring liability. Yet, there are already outstanding EAP programs serving our 9-1-1 centers. Randy Kratz works with one of them, FEI Workforce Resilience. Our friendship began two years ago when he agreed to serve as the local Clinical Liaison to 9-1-1 Training Institute's U.S. pilot of the *9-1-1 Certified Peer Supporter* project. This project, initiated by Dane County 9-1-1 director John DeJung and Waukesha County 9-1-1 director Gary Bell, launched in early 2018 as the Southwest Wisconsin Peer Support Team (SWIPST). Randy "gets" the stressors and psychological needs of 9-1-1Pros and had already worked to establish a strong relationship with them locally. His efforts reflect a mindset that all our PSAPs need and should expect from an EAP provider. That's why I asked Randy to join me in writing this chapter.

We have three goals:

- To equip 9-1-1 leaders with the knowledge they need to have about a truly effective EAP, so they can advocate for EAP services that truly meet their employees' needs
- To prepare frontline and supervisory telecommunicators with what to expect from an EAP, when to seek an EAP, and to encourage use of this service when it fits their needs
- To provide this chapter as a resource that 9-1-1 leaders and telecommunicators can both share with their EAP providers to influence and shape the best possible services. In essence, Randy and I are trying to define the elements of *best practice* Employee Assistance Programs to help all three groups to succeed. We'll begin by describing what that best practice EAP should look like, then we'll wrap up with steps 9-1-1 leaders can take to gain such services locally "in the real world." Enjoy!

ೞ∞

Part 2: Interview with Randy Kratz

In Pursuit of a Best Practice in EAP Care for 9-1-1

Jim: Randy, could you just explain in a nutshell what an EAP program, at its best, has to offer 9-1-1 personnel?

Randy: First, it should offer them 24/7 access to support. This is essential when you're working with first responders. And telecommunicators are the *first* first responders! On the most fundamental level, we need to be available to see them according to their work schedule to be adequately responsive to them. Even a Saturday or Sunday is just another day of the week for me, because availability to 9-1-1 personnel is that important. In terms of what we should offer as the substance of our programs, the EAP counselors must be able to recognize signs that a 9-1-1Pro is possibly struggling with traumatic stress and compassion fatigue. They need to be prepared to screen for these conditions since dispatchers are affected by trauma related injuries. Once the EAP counselor screens and identifies such risks, they need to bridge the 9-1-1Pro to counselors who can offer evidence-based treatments (see Chapter 9). The EAP provider should participate in (and offer support related to) any type of diffusing, debriefing provided to 9-1-1Pros after critical incidents in which they have been involved.

Jim: Randy, the reality is that many of our centers across the country don't get that level of customized care (and we'll tackle that challenge in the second half of the chapter). But I agree that all these services are essential for an EAP to provide. You're setting the bar pretty high for what an EAP can and should do, and we've just gotten started. That means the EAP leaders and the counselors they assign to 9-1-1 have got to know what 9-1-1 really does, doesn't it?

Randy: Absolutely! To offer the services that 9-1-1Pros need, the EAP provider needs to be the student first.

Jim: Okay, so if you were to design a 101 level class, we'll call it *The EAP Provider's Introduction to 9-1-1*, what would it include?

Randy: That's a seriously great idea! We EAP providers need to learn what an ordinary day in the life of the dispatcher actually looks like. It is really helpful for me to spend time in the comm center sitting next to a telecommunicator as they are doing his or her work.

Jim: You're talking about what folks in the industry call a 9-1-1 "Sit-Along." The 9-1-1 Training institute has made this a requirement for therapists who want to serve dispatch centers as part of the *Registry of EMDR Therapists for 9-1-1* (Chapter 9). Can you explain more about the Sit-Along and what makes it so important?

Randy: Being a part of that experience in the comm center, staying out of the dispatcher's way, but putting on a headset to listen and observe, immersing myself in their nitty-gritty work really helps. It helps as I think about their ups and downs, and what their work life is really about; this includes the variety of calls that they might experience. This Sit-Along is the only way I can truly "get it" and be prepared to deliver the highest possible value to them as a helper. By being in the PSAP, I can also experience the *culture* that 9-1-1Pros live in and shape together (for better or, sometimes, for worse). And, finally my Introductory 101 Class on 9-1-1 for EAPs should include taking time to learn from the center's peer support team if they have one. These peers deeply understand how their colleagues are being impacted by 9-1-1 stress on the job and when they go home.

By studying the 9-1-1 center and getting to know their personnel this way, I, as an EAP provider, have been able to identify the types of counseling support and resources most helpful for them. Jim, the bottomline is that, as EAP providers, we must recognize the unique nature of their work and help create a safe space in our offices where they can regenerate and reinvigorate to get ready for the next shift.

Jim: Absolutely. As I've taught our mental health colleagues about the unique role and stressors of 9-1-1 work, most all of them have admitted that they hadn't thought of the telecommunicator as an emergency responder—until that moment. Then the lightbulb always turns on! Now, let's assume the EAP provider is tuned in to 9-1-1 and they "get it." Can you give us a couple examples of issues that a 9-1-1Pro could bring to an EAP for help?

Issues You Can Bring to your EAP

Randy: There are a number of issues that we could help a 9-1-1Pro with, if they'll give us a chance. Most of them are related to personal wellness, struggles with peers and performance, and common family concerns. They might be seeking help with a game plan to manage the stress. A good stress management program takes a look at exercise, fitness, mindfulness and relaxation to help slow down strategically. It also looks at nutrition and diet. We help explore those things with them. Often 9-1-1Pros will talk about the challenge of eating right, because they work such a crazy schedule. Research shows they're in good company, amidst other workers who struggle with high overtime hours, frequent shift changes, or those who work nights. Those folks tend to eat a diet high in processed foods, fats and sugars which puts them in more of a high-risk category for medical risks. That also then affects their sleep, right?

Jim: I think you're spot on. Many of my students have defined these same concerns. What else should EAPs offer related to wellness?

Randy: We can help them look at sleep-related issues (which could result in a referral to a physician to rule out medical factors). And a good EAP needs to help them improve their work/life balance—how to wisely manage both sides of their world: life at work and life at home. We can also offer basic counseling support as telecommunicators travel through tough life transitions or to sort out career decisions.

The 9-1-1 Director's role in Gaining Great EAP Support

Jim: When I step back and look at the services EAP should provide, as you've described, I can see that many of our centers are lacking. So, our 9-1-1 center directors must go to bat for them—take an active role in the selection and design of EAP services their people receive. The challenge is that their standard involvement in this decision-making process depends on who their centers are operated and governed by. Some 9-1-1 centers are consolidated and are run by their own governing boards; others are "secondary PSAPs" run by, for example, an ambulance company. 9-1-1 managers of these two groups may automatically be positioned to have the most clout in that decision-making process. But, most of our centers are operated under the auspices of law enforcement agencies—police departments, sheriff offices or regional state police headquarters. The 9-1-1 managers of these centers are typically not included as stakeholders in the EAP selection and design process. What can these 9-1-1 managers do to have a say?

Randy: They need to initiate or request involvement in meetings with their governing bodies, to influence the shape of currently contracted or potential EAP providers. 9-1-1 leaders can then explain to the decision-makers the services their people need as outlined in this chapter, even share a copy of the chapter to support the need for this more robust EAP model.

Jim: Randy can you give us an example of an issue that a 9-1-1Pro should pursue specialized mental health care for *rather than* standard EAP counseling?

Randy: Dispatchers are trying to constantly be on top of their game, giving and giving, thinking of others beyond themselves. Reaching out to mental health providers is not easy for them to do. They may struggle with serious depression, anxiety, traumatic stress and major relationship problems, because they are exposed to the worst that life can bring—incidents involving homicide, suicide and other sad and violent deaths. As with other first responders, they're apt to experience traumatic events far more often than the average person. To survive, they can become desensitized to the most awful cases amidst a career full of more minor, but highly frustrating, experiences serving the public.

9-1-1Pros may struggle with a variety of more severe issues for which we might want to screen to identify these needs, then bridge them to a specializing clinician. These struggles would include: traumatic stress, serious depression, suicide risk, major relationship and parenting crises, or major grief and distress in the aftermath of a bad divorce or other major losses or deaths. In all these cases, our primary role would be to facilitate a really good referral. Then the proper helper—a specialist therapist or physician, or both in some cases, can conduct a thorough evaluation, including (in some cases) the need for medications. Those things won't be resolved with just a few sessions in an EAP, so it would be better to refer them from the start, when possible, to clinicians who can provide the level and quantity of care the 9-1-1Pro needs.

Jim: You mentioned traumatic stress as one of the issues you'd refer to an outside clinician. We have a suspected PTSD rate in the 9-1-1 industry at about 24% (using civilian cut-off scores, Lilly, see Chapter 4). So this hits a real nerve. Can you say a bit more about your role in helping with possible PTSD?

Randy: Yes. Sometimes it isn't just the recent traumatic event the 9-1-1Pro experiences that is impacting them. Those events may trigger past trauma. EAPs provide only a limited number of sessions (usually between one and ten) as a free benefit from the sponsoring agency. A few sessions may not be enough to effectively resolve traumatic stress. We want to be sure that the telecommunicator receives the three elements of great care for trauma:

1. Evidence-Based Treatment like EMDR delivered by...
2. A qualified therapist who can provide...
3. Longer-term treatment if needed.

These are the three elements of a safe place in which a 9-1-1Pro can really heal.

Jim: How would you respond to a telecommunicator in need of intensive alcohol and drug services like detoxification?

Randy: We'd certainly want to help bridge them to a program that provides that help. They may need to start with an inpatient program or an intensive outpatient program. For the dispatcher with less severe struggles, that may not require the diagnosis of alcoholism or other addictions, the EAP counselor could offer support to strengthen their ongoing recovery.

Jim: Randy, you've counseled and led countless debriefing sessions with emergency responders. You know they are often hesitant to even call to set up an appointment for an EAP counseling session, because they may think their problem isn't a big deal or that asking for help makes them weak. What do you want them to know, to help them push through this old mindset?

Randy: First, it's imperative that the Employee Assistance Provider pave the way for 9-1-1Pros to the front door of the EAP by educating every PSAP team member about the program. And I don't mean by just passing out pamphlets and business cards once a year. I need to put my boots on the ground at the PSAP, as a real person, so that telecommunicators can put a real human face on the "EAP support" they'll receive when they call us. They need the chance to get a first-hand sense of who I am as their assigned EAP counselor. Otherwise, how can I expect them to feel comfortable and trust me for support or as a safe bridge to a safe place for more special help?

Jim: Good point! Sometimes the harder we try to just "gut it out" the worse we make it. But it's so counter-intuitive for Extraordinary Care Givers like 9-1-1Pros to say, "Okay, it's my turn to get care for myself!" Plus, they're often busy nearly every square foot of their daily lives.

Randy: You bet. To those hesitant to reach out, I'll also say this: it can really pay off. Sometimes if we can just get the words (about our struggles) out of our mouths, the whole issue feels better—maybe not all at once, but over time. Still, because it often feels impractical to take time out for counseling, we may not ask for help until it is too late. Per what you're saying, Jim, 9-1-1Pros are certainly at risk of waiting too long; given how mentally consuming their job is, the hours they work, and because so many people are depending on them for so much. They may feel like they can't take the time or let down to reach out for counseling as part of their self-care. Well, fair enough. Yet, also consider this: if you leave your emotional struggles unresolved, your ability to fulfill all your responsibilities at work and at home will be undermined. So, if you want to be on your game personally and professionally, it's really important to make that call for EAP support. Do it before others have to be highly concerned for you and your fitness for duty. Please realize that EAP is here for you as a free, agency-sponsored program to use proactively to get the help you need. And we, as EAPs, are an entirely confidential program. The only way others will know that you're using the program is if you tell them yourself.

A Big 9-1-1 concern about EAPs: Will they Really be Confidential?

Jim: Randy, one of the biggest apprehensions about EAPs that I've heard repeatedly among 9-1-1Pros is this, "can we really trust them to be totally confidential? Will they have my best interest in mind since they're paid by employer?" It's been discouraging to hear how much mistrust 9-1-1Pros often have toward EAPs. And sadly, in a few cases reported to me, they have actually experienced a breach in confidentiality when their 9-1-1 leaders wanted information about their care. How should EAPs secure the confidentiality of their programs so 9-1-1Pros can be legitimately reassured that it's safe to seek their help?

Randy: We need to earn the trust of frontline 9-1-1Pros by clearly defining how we will honor their trust, and then live out those terms of confidentiality as our very first commitment to them. Without protecting the confidentiality of their counseling experience, EAPs put themselves out of business. Why would I, or anybody, call a counselor if I thought it would get back to my workplace or my manager? So, this is of importance above all else. In every state there are confidentiality and privacy laws that should be explained by the counselor to the client before they begin sharing any personal information. The only instance in which we are obligated to share information is when there is risk of imminent danger—when we feel that anyone's life would be in danger and we must do all we can to assure their safety. Other than that, everything stays private and confidential.

Jim: But doesn't an EAP Program provide client information to their contracting agency to prove the program they're paying for is actually being used?

Randy: We never include any personal identifying information in our EAP program utilization reports. These reports only note the number of total contacts, not who has used the program.

Jim: One purpose of an EAP, though, is to provide remedial counseling to an employee struggling with performance, to help save their job. When an employee has been required to pursue such EAP counseling, 9-1-1Pros may believe that their boss has the right to detailed information about their counseling sessions. Is this correct or incorrect?

Randy: I'm happy to say that this is incorrect. The information provided to an employer, when remedial counseling has been mandated, must be limited to include only a status report; an acknowledgement that X number of sessions have been held, and that the employee is complying with our treatment recommendations. But never, ever should the EAP Program share the nature of a personal problem or details of a session. Any diagnoses given to the client would not be included in that simple status report. Also, even though it isn't required to do so, my best practice approach includes asking the employee for their authorization to share even this limited information with the employer. This is an extra effort to show my respect for how vulnerable it feels to do mandated counseling.

Jim: This is a remarkable gesture of respect, for sure. I would support this as part of a best practice in EAP delivery in the 9-1-1 industry. It does raise an important question though. The employer is trying hard to keep a good employee by sending them for EAP help rather than just going the disciplinary route toward termination. And I know you want to help this process succeed. But what do you do when the employee refuses, for whatever reason, to give you permission to share that status report about their mandatory counseling?

Randy: That's an important question. In my 25 years as an EAP professional, probably less than five people have ever chosen to refuse sharing information in that situation. When somebody clearly understands how limited information is in these status reports to the employer, they are usually comfortable providing permission. On that rare occasion when the client withholds authorization, it's my opinion that the EAP should stop the counseling process to honor that request. At that point, the employee would be referred back to the employer indicating only that the employee elected not to provide any additional information and that the EAP is required to honor that request. It would then be the responsibility of the agency to determine how they would proceed with the employee from there.
Ultimately, as an EAP, we are trying to support the 9-1-1 client's *success* as an employee and as a person. When we treat them with respect, and honor these terms of confidentiality, they usually understand that. The bottom line is that the EAP must conduct their care professionally and ethically. That means they must always protect the confidentiality of their clients above all else.

Summing it all Up: What to Look for in an EAP for 9-1-1

Jim: You've done a tremendous job defining the elements of what I consider to be a *Best Practice EAP*. I want to wrap up this chapter by summarizing those elements. Thank you, Randy, not just for your EAP expertise, but also for your personal investment in serving the 9-1-1 Family.

Randy: My pleasure, Jim!

In Pursuit of a Best Practice in Delivery of EAP Service to 9-1-1: Five Essential Elements

- The EAP must be committed to learning the special counseling needs of 9-1-1 Professionals and assure that their contract includes provision of services needed to meet those needs.
- The EAP counselors assigned to serve the 9-1-1 center and its employees must be qualified to deliver the services to meet those needs, either directly or, for more serious conditions, by effectively screening and bridging the employee to the care they need from specialists.
- The EAP counselor must put in their time as a student of 9-1-1; doing Sit-Alongs to truly understand and show respect for the 9-1-1 professional's work experience and the culture in which they live their work life.
- Honoring confidentiality is at the core of the EAP's integrity and the basis of 9-1-1Pros' ability to entrust them with personal issues; so the EAP upholds the highest standard of confidentiality in accordance with all applicable laws.
- Finally, the success of the EAP, in service to 9-1-1Pros, requires the 9-1-1 leader to actively take part in their governing agency's EAP selection and contracting process. In essence, to act as an advocate for EAP services and qualified therapists to meet the specific needs of the Very First Responder.

Jim: Randy, thank you first for thinking so thoroughly as a mental health professional about the needs of 9-1-1Pros. The EAP you have shaped and defined in this chapter serves as a Best Practice model I hope will be replicated everywhere. In support of our directors' efforts to secure such services, I've included a supportive document in this chapter's appendix (end of book) about best practice EAP for 9-1-1 that can also be shared with EAP providers. (See Additional Resources for more information.)

Questions for Reflection

To get the most from this chapter, you are encouraged to write your reflections here (in both the Kindle and paperback versions of this book).

- What was your main take-away from reading this chapter?

- What specifically made it valuable to you?

- How can you apply this take-away concretely to improve some aspect of your personal life and or efforts to support the wellbeing of 9-1-1Pros?

Additional Resources

- In addition to this chapter, 911 Training Institute has prepared a document entitled *Assuring Best Practice in 9-1-1 Employee Assistance Programs*. This is offered as a resource that 9-1-1 directors can share with their governing bodies and current or potential EAP providers to assure the criteria for effective EAP services to 9-1-1 are secured. This is found in the Appendix to this chapter in the Appendices section at the end of the book.

SECTION IV

LEADERSHIP THAT GROWS RESILIENT 9-1-1 PROFESSIONALS

CHAPTER 18
How to Inspire Employees to Stay and Excel: The Power of Servant Leadership

Lora Reed

Editor's Introduction

All 9-1-1 leaders want their organizations to excel, but what does that really mean? Certainly, success must be tied to 9-1-1's mission to deliver rapid, effective emergency services to citizens at-risk. But it's possible for a comm center to succeed technically at this mission, for a while, even as employees are becoming overwhelmed with work-related stress that threatens the center's future success. Throughout the U.S, 9-1-1 centers face serious retention and recruiting problems resulting in chronic understaffing and overtime, leading to employee exhaustion and poor morale—further fueling retention problems. But what primary factors drive those retention problems? APCO's *Update to Project Retains* shows that one major factor is employees feeling undervalued and un-appreciated. All these challenges lead us to Servant Leadership.

In this chapter, Servant Leadership scholar, and friend of 9-1-1, Dr. Lora Reed reveals the five leadership characteristics that 9-1-1 managers can develop to help produce resilient, high-spirited employees who foster strong team morale, and are personally invested in the organization's success. These leadership characteristics are: Interpersonal Support, Egalitarianism, Moral Integrity, Building Community, and Altruism. She will share specific examples of what each of these characteristics looks like in action and the results they can produce in your comm center.

When you finish reading this chapter, you will be invited to engage in Lora's online *Servant Leader Scales for 9-1-1 Emergency Communicators* to help identify your strengths and needed growth related to each of the five characteristics. This is a great first step to building a customized strategic plan for personal leadership development.

The Interview

Jim: Lora, as you know, the term "Servant Leadership" can seem strange and awkward to non-scholars. If a leader were to refer to him or herself as a *Servant Leader*, I'd be inclined to wonder if they were bragging or acting self-righteous. Folks could also interpret this term to suggest weakness versus strength. So, if leaders are unfamiliar with this concept, they might ask, "You want me to become a door mat for my people to walk on, so I win their approval? No way!" Can you give us a nitty-gritty definition of what it means to be a Servant Leader? What's the big distinction here?

Lora: Great question, Jim! According to Robert Greenleaf, one of my favorite authorities on Servant Leadership, the main difference between a Servant Leader and a leader of any other style is *motivation—what drives the leader to lead* (Servant 7). By that I mean, most people pursue a leadership role because they want to lead others. But the greatest desire of those with the Servant Leader style is to *serve* others. So, their pathway to leadership is different. Their co-workers and superiors identify them as leaders because their influence on others serves the highest order needs of followers, the organization, and society. They are sought out to become leaders.

Ironically, the last people on earth to call themselves Servant Leaders are those who truly are Servant Leaders! They are quite humble and are not likely to behave in a self-righteous manner. (They would be put off by this behavior.) I have heard that some people are offended by the term Servant Leader because they associate the word *servant* with servitude, or slavery. That is not at all the meaning of the term. Servant Leaders lead by example, not by being a "doormat." They are typically people who care about their followers but are also willing and capable of having difficult conversations with them when necessary.

The Servant Leader recognizes that sometimes caring about people means standing against them as well as with them. This is an especially important leader attribute to help develop resilient, long term relationships with work associates. These are the types of relationships that are most valued by the Servant Leader. They want to help develop others as a part of serving them. Ultimately, Servant Leaders serve an idea that is bigger than just an organization. So, in a 9-1-1 emergency communications center, the Servant Leader recognizes the value of their employees, their followers, and the organization. Yet, they know that all members of the organization exist to serve a purpose for the community above the organization or any individual.

Jim: What is the Servant Leader's bigger idea and greater purpose?

Lora: They are motivated by much more than their own career or personal goals. In the 9-1-1 center, the greater purpose they serve is to help save lives by delivering the best possible emergency services as a communications team in collaboration with the caller and field responders. All while protecting the lives and well-being of responders in the comm center and in the field. The Servant Leader realizes big ideas are not the property of any one person—everyone has something to contribute, so they seek employee's ideas. This leader knows that excellent service and goal achievement hinges on developing and empowering followers so they too can lead by serving. To paraphrase Greenleaf, the best way to identify a Servant Leader is by how they develop the gifts and potential of their people, at all organizational levels, to help them become Servant Leaders too. Ultimately, employees at all levels are leaders. They lead other first responders, as well as individuals who call in emergent situations, if only for a short period of time (Servant 7). Perhaps, most importantly, the Servant Leader ensures that anyone being served actually benefits, including callers, coworkers, other first responders, and the community at large, and is not deprived or harmed in the leadership process. As a result, others often become Servant Leaders too.

Jim: So, what positive differences can it make for a 9-1-1 center if leaders possess these Servant Leader qualities?

Lora: According to my research over the past couple decades, there are some great benefits to Servant Led emergency communication centers. Let me just list a few here.

- Servant Leaders inspire followers to be proactive instead of passive, to take initiative to assist in problem solving and making suggestions for organizational improvement.
- Several studies show Servant Leaders have positive influences on employee attitudes toward work and job performance. (In my national study of 9-1-1 communications centers, I also found this was the case.)
- Where employees perceived their centers as Servant Led, they perceived themselves as empowered and their ideas as appreciated— they were engaged as stakeholders whose voices mattered in pursuit of the organization's outcomes.
- Servant Leaders create an organizational culture where followers (other employees) emulate the leaders' behaviors.

In 9-1-1 work cultures like this, other benefits can occur: more Servant Leaders emerge, and employee retention improves along with employee morale.

Jim: These are huge benefits. Our 9-1-1 leaders throughout the country struggle chronically with employee retention. So, if you have evidence that practicing Servant Leadership boosts retention, you can expect a lot more leaders lined up at your door! Our leaders also want to avoid preventable PSAP failures. What negative fallout happens when leaders don't practice Servant Leadership?

Lora: The most negative impact when Servant Leadership is not practiced is on the followers—the employees. One key finding of my research study was that when Servant Leadership is not practiced in 9-1-1 centers, followers see themselves as having a more passive role in the center; they aren't inspired to be as proactive. So they are *less* likely to:

- offer suggestions to improve the organization or its work processes
- engage in decision making beyond what is essential
- perceive themselves as accountable for organizational performance
- perceive themselves as leaders or contributors to how work gets done.

These are certainly not attitudes any leader would intentionally cultivate in their employees. Did you notice what they all have in common? When 9-1-1 leaders don't strive to practice Servant Leadership, their followers are not encouraged to fulfil their best potential. This not only limits the employee, it can inhibit the center's ability to achieve its greater purpose, and it can also increase the likelihood that employees will leave. Or worse yet, they may stay, but check out mentally.

Jim: Those are significant impacts. How can 9-1-1 leaders *practice* Servant Leadership? Do they have to do a complete overhaul of who they are and how they approach their work?

Lora: No, a total overhaul of personality and work approach or ethic isn't necessary. And while Servant Leadership is not a quick fix, leaders can identify steps of growth to take immediately from where they stand right now. Then it's an ongoing learning and development process continuing to develop five of the many key characteristics. As the Servant Leader develops, so do his or her followers. With time and effort, anyone can develop these characteristics. But most 9-1-1 leaders have risen to their positions because of their passion for the emergency response mission, so they are already positioned and motivated to further develop these characteristics. And this kind of development not only improves a person's work life, but also their life overall.

Jim: That's encouraging. Our 9-1-1 leaders are already quite accustomed to hard work—no pain, no gain, right? They just need to know their time and effort is worth it, and you've already shown that it is. So, what are those five characteristics of Servant Leadership?

Lora: They include:
- Interpersonal Support
- Egalitarianism
- Moral Integrity
- Building Community
- Altruism

Jim: Can you define each one and give us an example or two of what that characteristic looks like in action? It would help our readers if you would describe how each one positively impacts employees and the 9-1-1 center.

Lora: The first characteristic is *Interpersonal Support:* This is the extent to which a person helps others, regardless of their level, to grow and develop. Interpersonal support as practiced by leaders includes providing the resources and the environment employees need to do their best work and for such growth to occur. In a 9-1-1 center, this support, practiced among peers, might be as simple as call takers learning the 'how' supporting callers with emergencies and/or other first responders to ensure smooth and effective job performance from all as part of a team. It might also include ensuring the call taker knows the outcome of the emergency response, whenever practicable. The difference it makes for employees involves them realizing that the work they do matters and they are valued as individuals and as team members. This can be the difference in whether or not good people stay and contribute to the center as a great organization.

Jim: The second characteristic of Servant Leadership is what you call *Egalitarianism.* That's a mighty fancy term. Can you tell us what it means, share an example of how it might look like in action at a comm center, and what positive impact it can have?

Lora: *Egalitarianism* can be seen when leaders are open to learning from anyone (at any organizational level) of the agency. Sometimes it shows up in the way ideas are debated or in how constructive criticism is perceived. Even though most 9-1-1 centers are paramilitary in structure, it is important for Servant Leaders to demonstrate egalitarianism. It acknowledges the leader realizes all employees in the center lead by serving, whether it is a caller, another first responder, or a co-worker in the agency. *Egalitarianism* is what strengthens employees, so they can achieve the goals of serving and leading when such challenges arise…and they will. An example of egalitarianism in action is a leader asking the person or persons closest to a task how it might be improved. The advice might not always be taken, but it is thoughtfully considered. It can make the difference of whether or not employees are engaged in their work or just going through the motions and doing the minimum.

Jim: The third characteristic is *Moral Integrity*. Can you define it, give examples, and tell us from your research about how it makes a difference?

Lora: This is so important in the 9-1-1 centers. *Moral Integrity* is related to trust building, transparency, and valuing integrity above personal gain. This is often the area in which 9-1-1 leaders score the highest of all the Servant Leadership characteristics. Leaders, at any organizational level, who score high in Moral Integrity can admit and learn from their mistakes, and from mistakes made by others. Greenleaf described the moral person as conducive to the moral society (Institution 4). The moral person is the individual who does the right thing, even when it is not popular; a person of character or integrity. Employees that experience their leaders as being trustworthy and possessing integrity are more apt to endure hardship at work and stay on board, despite the other employment options that may open to them. For followers, doing meaningful work for a leader with moral integrity is a *big idea* often more inspiring and valuable than being paid a higher wage doing less meaningful work.

Jim: Lora, when you say that Servant Leaders work to "Build Community" what does that mean?

Lora: Since Servant Leaders value every employee at every level, these leaders inspire their team members' commitment to the organization. And with this commitment, a spirit of cooperation spreads; people help one another more. Everyone is valued for their contribution to the organization. In a 9-1-1 center, team members show care to the peer who has just had a tough call or an especially trying personal experience. The Servant Leader in the 9-1-1 center builds Community by recognizing that each employee's individual differences, and the job they perform, help make the organization a strong community. When workers feel the leader's care and concern, and realize they are part of a vibrant community, the positivity can spill over into their families. It can even be felt by the larger community the center serves. This is part of a big idea that cannot be neglected. In the real day-to-day life of the center, it is priceless.

When employees work together in a 9-1-1 center that has become this kind of community, morale, retention, and team performance are all improved. Anyone who has worked in a 9-1-1 communication center for even a year or two knows that different shifts can live as different organizational cultures. Some shifts are vital communities as we've defined here, and some are not.

Jim: It's ironic that you would propose that Altruism is a key characteristic of leadership that produces real results in the 9-1-1 center. As you know, cynicism is common among veteran emergency responders because they've experienced so much lying, crime, and ugly human behavior as part of their job serving the public. What do you mean by altruism, and how can it actually make a difference?

Lora: Altruism is about doing the right thing, helping others, because it is the right thing to do. It is at the very heart of the Servant Leader. In a 9-1-1 center, you see it when individuals serve others with no expectation of reward or being served in return. It is quite prevalent in 9-1-1 centers by the very nature of the work. Leaders demonstrate altruism when they fight for what their employees need, despite the consequences; this is an unselfish act of service. You see it when the 9-1-1 leader or another employee goes the extra mile to help the team, assist a caller, and or another first responder. It shows up in terms of fruit, as organizational outcomes, as improved work performance, person-job fit (having the right person in the right position), and stewardship in community.

Jim: So, let's assume all of our readers would like to take a first step to build up their Servant leadership characteristics. Obviously that step is to explore how they are functioning right now related to those characteristics. Fortunately, Lora, you've created a very cool instrument, *Servant Leader Scales for 9-1-1 Emergency Communicators*, that helps leaders learn how their employees see them living out these five Servant Leadership characteristics in the workplace.
I know your tool produces super valuable information for any of us seeking growth; it helps us see where and how we need to target our personal development efforts. But, let's face it, offering employees the chance to comment about us as a person can seem mighty vulnerable and a bit scary.

My father always said, "If you don't want the answer, don't ask the question!" What can you offer to help leaders rally the courage to take this step?

Lora: Another great question, Jim. Asking others for feedback can make any of us feel vulnerable, for sure! Yes, you're right. However, such feedback is important to make progress, help us grow, and achieve positive change as individuals and organizational leaders. Let's face it, leaders make themselves vulnerable by daring to influence others. In this case it's sort of like stepping on the scale the day before we finally start that diet, as well as at various milestones when we are attempting to change our lifestyle. That baseline allows us to glimpse our reality in order to define our goal and make real progress toward it. Although it can feel threatening, it is far more threatening to never step on the scale and make a change. We're more apt to rally courage to do an assessment like this when we realize how much help it can give us, *and* we can trust the process involved.

9-1-1 leaders can feel secure in choosing to do the *Servant Leadership Scales for 9-1-1 Emergency Communicators*, because we ensure both anonymity and confidentiality in all our data collection. The identity of those evaluating their leaders remains totally anonymous and confidential. In fact, an organization can have the leadership (as a team) evaluated without any one leader being named, if they want to begin with examining their organization as a culture. We safeguard the assessment process and data so everyone involved as a participant is treated with professionalism.

Jim: Could you share an example of Servant Leader Scales for 9-1-1 Emergency Communicators results for one anonymous leader, so our readers can clearly grasp what the results would really look like?

Lora: Jim, I can tell you that each report is individualized in that it provides a 360-degree perspective of the leader in the five dimensions of servant leadership (interpersonal support, moral integrity, altruism, egalitarianism, and community) from both employees and other stakeholders (anonymously) and the leader him or herself. This is because, often the perceptions of the leader are quite different from those of the employees with whom they work. For example, a leader might perceive his or her motives for behavior as representing support of employees, but the leader is not really aware of what the employees need in terms of support, so they perceive the behavior differently. What I typically do with the information is provide insights as to how the differences in perception are impacting the center as an operation, as well as employee job satisfaction, morale, and commitment to the organization/work. Then we begin to build a strategy for improving the situation for all. When someone contacts me about this type of consultation, intervention, or collaboration, I give them specific ways in which this could best work for their organization prior to engaging in any data collection and/or interpretation.

Jim: what results do leaders get from doing the assessment?

Lora: We pose the questions and write our reports so that leaders gain meaningful feedback about their leadership style as an individual leader and/or as part of a leadership team. The results point the leader to their areas of strength and areas they can improve, as well as how the improvement might be measured in the center itself. The leadership instrument can also be combined with other instruments, such as the *Big Five Personality Inventory* that was used in my 2005 dissertation study. This can be tremendously helpful in leader development, individual coaching, and development of teams and/or the organizational culture as a whole. Initially it can take a little bit of courage to embark on this journey, but it's always valuable for leaders to learn more about ourselves, our followers and our organizations. That way we can better pursue achievable meaningful changes, and then celebrate milestones achieved.

Jim: As the editor of this book, let me make a point. My goal in asking you to teach our readers about your Servant Leadership tool is not to sell products. Throughout the book, we make the recommendations to help our readers support our shared mission: peak performance and optimal wellbeing of our Very First Responders. I became convinced that your tool helps empower our leaders to achieve this mission unlike any other available resource. (We've already defined those benefits.) It has evolved from your work over many years learning about the life of our 9-1-1Pros and supporting leaders.

While there is a minimal cost to use your tool, I'm not apologetic; I'm very grateful. We all have to be paid for our life's work or we couldn't do it. With that, how can leaders obtain the *Servant Leader Scales for 9-1-1 Emergency Communicators?*

Lora: First, Jim, if a leader has gotten this far in reading the chapter and has interest further in Servant Leadership in his or her center that is wonderful news! It shows a desire to make a positive difference for everyone–the leader, their employees/followers, their organization, and for the first responders and other stakeholders who interface with their agency. Second, as you can imagine, money was not my motivation for creating such interventions, but it is essential for being able to offer most any service in our society, even 9-1-1, so that we can continue to do research and add to the body of knowledge in what we do.

If a leader wants to engage in the assessment process, he or she can contact me directly by email (**Lreed7@tampabay.rr.com**) or phone (941.705.0042). I will be happy to guide them as to how they can best use the assessment tool and analysis of the results for an individual, a team, or an organization. I can also point the leader toward additional resources that are specifically focused on the needs of the individual, team, or organization at that time. (See also *Additional Resources* at end of this chapter.) In addition, my team and I are in the process of making several resources available to 9-1-1 communications center leaders through Amazon which is especially convenient for people who want quick references that are e-reader friendly.

One of those resources (see below) is titled, *Servant leadership, followership, and organizational citizenship behaviors in 9-1-1 emergency communications centers: Implications of a national study.* The article, which can be accessed online for free, includes a variety of tables of information that describe how Servant Leadership is different from similar leadership styles. It includes tables that list the five characteristics I have discussed here, along with how those dimensions pertain to employee (including leader) competencies in the comm center. For example, *Building Community* can have a positive impact on team multi-tasking and *Egalitarianism* can contribute to morale or esprit de corps.

Jim: Thank you very much, Lora, for investing with us on this project. You're making a contribution unlike anyone else can make, because you've applied your expertise about Servant Leadership specifically to empower our 9-1-1 leaders. Any closing thoughts for our readers?

Lora: I want to say that developing one's Servant Leadership characteristics is not a quick fix and the five dimensions I have explored with you here are much like facets of a diamond, the diamond being the personality of the leader and the culture of the organization. These are just a beginning, but they are a fine place to begin when a person is attempting to become their best as a leader and developer of others. In addition to the option of taking the *Servant Leader Scales for 9-1-1 Emergency Communicators* to build their development plan, there is also a short list of books and articles at the end of this interview. The leader might want to enjoy those as additional food for thought.

I have very much enjoyed this interview. Thank you so much for your interest in this work. Like you, I have a special place in my heart for 9-1-1 professionals, at all organizational levels. They are often unsung heroes.

Questions for Reflection

To get the most from this chapter, you are encouraged to write your reflections here (in both the Kindle and paperback versions of this book).

- What was your main take-away from reading this chapter?

- What specifically made it valuable to you?

- How can you apply this take-away concretely to improve some aspect of your personal life and or efforts to support the wellbeing of 9-1-1 Pros?

Additional Resources

Popular References

Blanchard, Ken & Broadwell, Renee. "Servant Leadership in Action: How You Can Achieve Great Relationships and Results." *Berrett-Hoehler*. *Available in Kindle Edition only, 2018.

Jennings, Ken & Stahl-Wart, John. "The Serving Leader: Five Powerful Actions to Transform Your Team, Business, and Community." Berrett-Koehler 2016.

Annotated Scholarly References

Dannhauser, Zani and Andre B. Boshoff. "The Relationships between Servant Leadership, Trust, Team Commitment and Demographic Variables." www.regent.edu/acad/sls/publications/conference_proceedings/servant_leadership_roundtable/2006/pdf/dannahuser_boshoff.pdf. Retrieved 3/7/2018, 2006.
This academic proceeding article discusses how Servant Leadership has been shown to be related to developing trust and commitment in work teams.

Drury, Sharon L. "Servant Leadership and Organizational Commitment: Empirical Findings and Workplace Implications."
www.regent.edu/acad/sls/publications/conference_proceedings/servant_leadership_roundtable/2004pdf/drury_servant_leadership.pdf. Retrieved 3/7/2018.
This academic proceeding article discusses how Servant Leadership contributes to employees caring more about their work and organizations as demonstrated through their commitment to the work.

Greenleaf, Robert K. *The Servant as Leader.* Robert K. Greenleaf Center for Servant Leadership, [1970] 1991.
This is the original essay by Robert Greenleaf. He discusses ten aspects of the Servant Leader.

Greenleaf, Robert K. *The Institution as Servant.* Greenleaf Center for Servant Leadership, [1972] 2009.
This is the original essay about the Servant Led organization and what that can mean for stakeholders.

Reed, Lora. "Personality and Leadership as Dispatcher Retention Tools: A Study of the Big Five Traits & Servant Leadership Characteristics for Motivation, Job-fit, and Employee Retention in Emergency 9-1-1 Call Centers." *VDM Verlag Publishers*, 2008.
This is Lora's published dissertation on relationships between personality and employee retention in Servant Led 9-1-1 Emergency Communications Centers.

Reed, Lora. "The Big Five Personality Traits as Tools for Retention of Florida e9-1-1 Telecommunicators" *Dissertations Abstracts International,* 2005. This is Lora's dissertation referenced above.

Reed, Lora. "Servant Leadership, Followership, and Organizational Citizenship Behaviors in 9-1-1 Emergency Communications Centers: Implications of a National Study." *Servant Leadership: Theory and Practice*, Volume 2, Issue 1, February 2015.
This journal article contains various information tables pertinent to Servant Leadership in 9-1-1 Emergency Communications Centers.

Reed, Lora et al. "A New Scale to Measure Executive Servant Leadership: Development, Analysis and Implications for Research." *Journal of Business Ethics.* DOI 10.1007/s10551-010-0729-1, 2011.
This is a journal article demonstrating the research process on the scales from which the Servant Leader Scales for 9-1-1 Emergency Communicators is based.

Trade Publications

APCO "The Compiled Report Synthesizing Information from the Effective Practices Guide & Retains Next Generation." Project Retains, 2009.

Work Cited

APCO. "The Compiled Report Synthesizing Information from the Effective Practices Guide & Retains Next Generation." *Project Retains,* August 2009, **www.apcointl.org/doc/conference** documents/personnel-human-factor/282-project-retains compiled-report-2009/file.html.

Greenleaf, Robert K. *The Institution as servant.* Greenleaf Center for Servant Leadership, 1972.

Greenleaf, Robert K. *The Servant as Leader.* Robert K. Greenleaf Center for Servant Leadership, 1970.

Reed, L. "Servant Leadership, Followership, and Organizational Citizenship Behaviorsin 9-1-1 Emergency Communications Centers: Implications of a National Study." *Servant Leadership Theory and Practice,* vol. 2, no. 1, 2015, pp 71-94. www.sltpjournal.org/uploads/2/6/3/9/26394582/servant_leadership_foll wership_and_organizational_citizenship_behaviors_in_9-1 1_emergency_communications_centers-_.pdf.

CHAPTER 19
The 9-1-1 Leader as Stress-Risk Manager: Recognizing Your Role as the Center's SRM

Jim Lanier and Jim Marshall

Introduction

Research conducted by Towers Watson and the National Business Group on Health shows that that stress in U.S. organizations is "the number one workforce *risk* issue, ranking above physical inactivity and obesity" (U.S. Employers Rank Stress... 1). 78% of the 199 organizations in this survey ranked stress as the top risk.

That statistic may not blow your socks off, but perhaps the next one will. "...only 15% of employers identify improving the emotional/mental health (i.e., lessening the stress and anxiety) of employees as a top priority of their health and productivity programs" (U.S. Employers Rank Stress...1). That's not to say they didn't have Employee Assistance Programs (EAP), and other resources, but these typically do not target stress reduction or address needed changes in work conditions promoting stress. Here's the kicker: the survey authors discovered a big discrepancy between what leaders and followers of these organizations see as the chief stressors. Employers believed the greatest stressors included lack of work/life balance, inadequate staffing, and technology making them available beyond work. However, survey authors concluded differently, "Employees' message to employers is clear: Pay me adequately. Support me on the job. Guide me on my job priorities" (2013/2014 Staying@Work Report...6).

So, here's the first take-away: leaders of the studied organizations generally were concerned about the well-being of their employees and invested in health and wellness programs. But they were missing the mark. They didn't accurately identify the stressors faced by their employees. Thus, they didn't have plans in place to address these stressors. 9-1-1 telecommunicators may not rank their stressors as the survey respondents did. But we know that their work is far more stressful than most other professions. In addition to the long list of common stressors, they also experience another entirely different dimension and magnitude of stress with their life-saving responsibilities and exposure to traumatic events. With a PTSD rate estimated to be four to five times higher than the general public (Chapter 4), the risks and the urgency of strategic stress management planning for 9-1-1Pros is even greater than for those in the study. And with chronically low retention rates in the 9-1-1 industry as we move into the NG9-1-1 era, the time couldn't be more perfect to heed the study's caution, "Employers that fail to understand employees' views on stress risk diverting time and resources to fixing the wrong problems and, at the same time, alienating employees" (U.S. Employers Rank Stress...1).

This chapter is built on a premise: our 9-1-1 leaders want to do right by their employees; yet, they're not stress experts and they have many demands competing for their attention. There's also an inescapable principle of management: if no one is designated to do a task, it's not likely to get done. If the task is trivial, no big deal. But if it's vital to the health and core mission of the organization, and it goes undone, that's a bit of a problem. We've clearly established that stress is a major issue for 9-1-1Pros. We believe that comm center leaders, supported by their governing agencies, must serve as their PSAP Stress-Risk Managers. And this means identifying the specific risk factors their 9-1-1Pros face. This chapter is divided into three parts, each designed to help leaders prepare for this role.

In Part 1, Jim Lanier, a veteran 9-1-1 manager will share his personal story about what he experienced that led him to prioritize stress resilience for his PSAP. In Part 2, I interview Jim about his mindset and approach to 9-1-1 stress-risk management. Then in Part 3, we provide you with our conclusion, recommendations, and guidance to help you succeed as your PSAP Stress-Risk Manager (SRM). Finally, at the back of the book you'll find the Chapter 19 Appendix with a tool that provides concrete guidance as you work to implement your PSAP resilience plans. Thank you for taking the time to travel with us and enjoy!

PART 1. Jim Lanier's Story

Every leader's approach to management is shaped by their experiences both personally and professionally. I'm no exception to this rule. What I believe most about managing 9-1-1 professionals, what works best for me in leading a comm center, has grown from my own journey in the trenches.

Early Attitude about 9-1-1

I worked "the street" for quite a few years as a paramedic (more on that later). Then I mulled over trying out the role of telecommunicator, not because I respected 9-1-1; just to gain comm center experience so I could qualify for a field supervisor position. I passed the communications aptitude test and was transferred over to the 9-1-1 center. I swaggered in there as a cocky field medic armed with all my predispositions, stereo-types and biases about dispatch. I mean, how hard could this be, sitting all day inside a nice air-conditioned office, eating whenever I want, talking to responders on the radio, and reading patient care instructions from silly card sets to the callers? That sounds a lot better than being spit on and swung at on scene, right?

Okay, now cue up the first 9-1-1 call I handled solo, without all my EMS co-workers and equipment around me, and without being on scene to see and interact directly with patients. It was a cardiac arrest. I was lost--a stammering fool. I learned very quickly that this 9-1-1 work was much more challenging than I had bargained for. But I soon discovered it could also be very enriching. This initial experience as a call-taker is something I will never forget. It cemented in me a deep recognition of the skillset required to succeed as a telecommunicator, recognition of their unique environment, and that supporting these professionals is a cause worth championing.

As my career progressed, I stayed on the Communications Center pathway. After a few years at the console, I became involved in training and quality management. Eventually I was selected to lead the Communications Center. The Communications Center was run by a private EMS agency contracted to provide ambulance transport, EMD call processing, and dispatch to the community. The company worked under very strict contractual requirements, with a razor thin profit margin. So, unfortunately, their leaders' focus was on contract compliance and profit. This often took priority over a focus on the well-being of the employees in the field and in the Communications Center.

Lack of Understanding Fuels Lack of Needed Support

I remember one conversation vividly: the Vice President was gleefully congratulating me as the Communications Center Manager on coming in under budget for the year. I wanted to point out to him the simple fact: there was no way we could have spent all our allocated personnel funds! We were too short-staffed and under supported in the dispatch center; and the agency either would not or could not transfer any employees to us. Under pressure to focus on micro-managing my staff's dispatch processing times, I felt quite helpless to lessen their stress as I watched them toil away admirably.

Yet I quickly learned how to fight and defend them as we struggled, understaffed, to fulfill certain contract terms. Agency leaders would ask, "How come we are late to all these calls and paying penalties? Why didn't the right units get dispatched?" The Communications Center had historically been a target on a leash. Managers responsible for scheduling would understaff field units during shifts on which we had clearly identified spikes in call volume. So, when my people couldn't dispatch units to the scene, they were blamed for the resulting service failure. I took these attacks on my staff seriously since I had once been a whipping boy as a field responder.

While some of those attacks on the PSAP staff could have been driven by ignorance about what it takes for a 9-1-1 center to do their job, some represented a form of bullying—intimidating and blaming subordinates to produce desired outcomes. I have a passionate hatred for bullies. As a leader, I had to learn to temper my gut reactions to what I first interpreted as unfair criticism of my staff. In some cases, the agency leaders' or customers' concerns were legitimate, and I could only recognize this by withholding judgment and listening carefully to them.

Core Value #1

My point is not to bash or villainize agency managers, promote a victim mentality among our rank and file, or make excuses for their performance failures when they're at fault. But in my agency our employees were expected to do too much with too little. Those experiences helped me form what I'll call *Core Leadership Value #1: As leaders we must do all we can to assure that the demands placed on our staff do not exceed their personal and team resources.* During that time period, my agency's field responders and telecommunicators organized to gain representation by a labor union. Some of our executive leaders didn't see this coming and asked, "Why did they do this?" I was surprised it took them so long. Negotiating with unions can be stressful, but I believe there is a way to prevent these contentious, often exhausting processes.

The cooperation of union representatives, and the morale of our frontliners they represent, doesn't depend on giving them everything they want. That's a darned good thing, since even when we recognize their demands are fair, this kind of total wish fulfillment is often just not possible. So how can we avert the most stressful employer/employee relationship struggles, including those that will otherwise end up unionized? By instilling confidence in our followers that we are *doing all we can to make the demands they face manageable*. This means putting Core leadership Value #1 into practice. We also need to communicate with our followers about these efforts so they are aware of the steps we are taking. Granted, there will always be those who thrive on negativity, refusing to believe us even when given the evidence of our good will. While we can't please everyone, even when we walk the talk, *most* of our employees will see that we are sincerely trying to live out this core value.

Game-Changing Event

But let me go back to one event in my work life prior to becoming a leader that fueled my passion for prioritizing employee well-being, to take on the SRM role. Sparing you the gory details, I was in my 5th year at the 9-1-1 console and going through a contentious divorce with custody arguments. At the height of these struggles, my father was diagnosed with an aggressive esophageal cancer. Despite living in the same town, he and I had been estranged for years. Now I was experiencing massive guilt because he had never met my three-year-old daughter, his own grand-daughter. I was also working huge hours in the Communications Center, for two reasons: I was up to my neck in debt and needed the overtime money; and, the center was one place I could go to feel some sense of control when everything else in my life seemed out of control. I thought I was handling all these stressors okay, so it didn't occur to me to let anyone else know I was struggling or to seek support.

One day during this period, I was filling in at the Supervisor position. A long-time colleague came out of the QA office into the Communications Center and literally grabbed me by the collar. He rolled me in my wheeled chair away from the console and swung me into his office against the wall. I was shocked to say the least and was honestly ready to punch him in the face. I shouted at him, "What the #$%*!?"

He shot back, "What the hell is wrong with you?"

"I don't know what you're talking about. I'm fine!"

"Listen to yourself on this call you just took!"

So, I pulled up the call on the recorder and listened. I was mortified. The caller was very cooperative, and he had a legitimate issue for calling 9-1-1 and requesting an ambulance. I sounded like an uncaring jerk. I prided myself on being an excellent and empathetic call-taker, but in this moment, I realized that the one thing I thought in my life I could count on--doing my job well-- was no longer a sure thing. Without realizing it, the stress of my personal hardships had combined with the cumulative stress of all my 9-1-1 and paramedic years into what I would now call Compassion Fatigue (see Chapter 10). But back then I had no idea what this term even meant.

This co-worker and I had been through a lot together. I knew he had my best interests at heart. So, when he laid into me with this caring 3rd degree interrogation, it really hit me. I tried to fight back the tears at first. But then I just let all the emotion packed inside me for so long flow out. It was embarrassing, but as I emptied out all these feelings, it felt like a weight had been lifted. After that incident, I sought out counseling through our EAP program. My therapist was able to provide me with good support and assistance to get through all the personal drama.

This personal experience with Compassion Fatigue was a big catalyst for my resolution as a leader to support my 9-1-1 staff not only related to their work-life and careers, but also when they are going through hardships outside the PSAP. Can you relate to how stress from the home-front swirls together with stress from the workplace? I had been a classic example of someone whose job performance was suffering because of their personal life. If leaders had responded to my performance issues just by writing me up and reviewing employee policy, I would have struggled even more. Without my peer noticing my struggle, and reaching in to help, I may not have regained my footing at work or faced my personal life. We're all in this together.

PART 2. *The Interview*

Jim M.: Jim, your story here offers a number of great lessons. One is about how crucial it was for you to realize your own need for support and self-care. This isn't easy for managers, especially emergency response leaders accustomed to taking care of everyone else. Yet an organization can be only as healthy as its leader. Still, this is exactly where the work of boosting resilience in the 9-1-1 center should begin. Can you speak more to this?

Jim L.: As emergency responders under constant demand to take control of scenes where danger threatens lives, it's hard to admit to each other when we're facing circumstances beyond our personal control or mastery. We're conditioned to just disregard our pain and push through. We often don't even know what we feel or what to do with the struggle within ourselves, or what to do when we see that distress in others. We as 9-1-1 leaders need a new flight plan. First, to succeed in handling all the stress of our leadership work, we need to be attuned to our *own* distress and be willing to ask other leaders for the support we need. We also need to become each other's wingmen, looking out for each other and checking in to offer the same support we seek.

Jim M: Another strong theme of your story was your recognition of just how incredibly stressful the work of the frontline telecommunicator is. So, you realized that assuring their wellbeing was one of your core responsibilities as a leader. But put some meat on the bone here. What concrete action steps are you advocating for leaders to *do* to fulfill this SRM role?

Jim L.: We need to be attuned to the distress of our employees and offer them the support they need through two paired initiatives that are ongoing: 1) commit to providing them with the resources called for by the NENA Standard on Acute/Traumatic and Chronic Stress (Chapter 15), and 2) systematically assess how stressful their current working conditions are, then strategically optimize those work conditions. This second initiative must include preparing them for added stressors to come with NG9-1-1 (per guidance offered in Chapter 22). By fulfilling these two initiatives we can *assure that the demands placed on our staff do not exceed their personal and team resources* (Core leadership value #1).

Jim M.: Jim, your twin recommendations here are spot on with what current research says can pay-off in huge ways for the organization. Stock wellness programs that fail to target the specific stressors and needs of employees end up being very expensive nods to risk management that fall short. By contrast, there is plenty of evidence that a process that defines and then directs resources to meet specific group and individual needs of personnel, clearly improves the major organizational benchmarks: retention, attendance, sick leave, performance, and morale. So, your recommendations flow from your core leadership value above?

Jim L.: Yes. Consistent with the role of the Stress-Risk Manager, we are the proverbial "shepherd of the flock". To be successful as the PSAP leader and SRM, we have to be strategic in how we look out for our people. We need to be prepared to invest in them and the organization at the professional *and* personal levels. We will invest in our people this way when we value them highly and care about them as people of worth. I know (and have been on the receiving end of) leaders who were very professional and on top of their game operationally and strategically. Yet, they were ultimately not successful because they didn't cross over to the other side of the tracks and invest in personally supporting their employees. So, their people never invested in their leadership agendas.

Jim M.: It really struck a chord in me when you emphasized the importance of leaders seeing and connecting with their employees as "people of worth." Dedicated PSAP leaders are often pushing non-stop amidst a myriad of responsibilities; clawing their way through the incessant demands of their work. So, there's the risk that even the best leaders may feel that they and their personnel are like cogs in the gears turning the emergency response system ever forward. Your mindset can offer a refreshing encouragement to step back, take a deep breath, and wipe the road film from their glasses: to notice with fresh eyes who their team members are as people with unique value and a need to feel validated. This kind of investment in your employees is highly effective in motivating them for success.

You also urged leaders to "invest in *personally* supporting their employees". But that requires a leader to become somewhat personally vulnerable; and leaders of emergency response centers, like those leading military operations, need to uphold a very clear chain of command. So, doesn't it take some wisdom for 9-1-1 directors and managers to invest at the "personal level" with employees without becoming over-involved and blurring the employer/employee boundary?

Jim L.: Yes. There is a fine line to walk here, but to succeed at stress-risk management it is essential. If you are too distant and "professional" relating to your frontline staff on a daily basis, you can come across as aloof and disinterested in their basic yet important needs. If you are too "personal" with all staff then you can cloud the chain of command. This can also cause perceptions of favoritism, and potential loss of respect for your role as leader. But the line can be walked as long as the leader is flexible, investing in a level of general day-to-day personal contact with their employees they can sustain; and by being mindful about how and why they choose to engage in one on ones to provide more intensive support to employees. Learning how to strategically connect in more personable ways with staff is a smart risk worth taking.

Jim M.: You also said that you believe the 9-1-1 leaders, at their best, are a sort of shepherd for their employees. This triggers an image of the manager intent on looking out for their people, to help keep them safe amidst the threats that could damage or destroy them. To follow your analogy, the wolves and steep cliffs endangering the telecommunicator are the 9-1-1 Stressors. Some of these stressors are external, such as demands from the field and the public. Yet work conditions within the center also factor in heavily. So, in continuing with your analogy, 9-1-1 leaders as shepherds will look vigilantly to identify and improve their employees' day-to-day work conditions that complicate their efforts to meet those external demands. Jim, all your comments here point to a *mindset* that can help our directors succeed as their PSAPs' Stress-Risk Managers. Can you just expand on that a bit more?

Jim L.: The way we live out the SRM role calls for a big picture view of how we think about and do leadership. We need to know our people, actively participate in their work life, openly communicate with them, intervene when trouble stirs, and support them in fulfilling their responsibilities. That's the essence of it to me. And I really need to put this into a "real life" context! Currently, the PSAP that I am responsible for is experiencing some challenging times. This past year has been one of our hardest ever, with a tragic death of one our people. We are also down a considerable number of telecommunicators. Some employees have transferred to administrative positions within the agency. Some are pursuing careers as law enforcement officers. Others have left the profession completely. Unfortunately, we have not been able to maintain a large enough trainee and candidate pool to offset the losses of experienced staff. We are at the point of mandating overtime on occasion; as much as this is an anathema to me, it has to be done so we can meet minimum staffing levels.

I realize that it's our turn in the PSAP staffing challenge "barrel." We will grit through this and get back to a better place because we are not accepting this as a new normal. My point is that we as PSAP members live through these things together. And we as leaders need to redirect our attention to attend to suffering in our own teams when it occurs. I think it is also important, whenever possible, to do some sort of a retrospective forensic analysis of root causes of our struggles so we can better understand what might have led to the changes in circumstances.

My summary of this chapter is offered in light of this difficult last year at our comm center: we as leaders are hopefully striving for excellence in leading and supporting our amazing telecommunicators and those that they serve. Yet, we and our employees are sharing life in the real world. That life can change on a dime and derail our very best plans and intent. Sometimes we just have to put our heads down and pull the proverbial plow to get what needs to be done, done. Even during those roughest seasons, we must always be on the lookout for those opportunities that will present themselves if we keep our eyes open! When we are in the proverbial sludge, we need to remain optimistic, so we can recognize the pathway out of crises; breathe a little more deeply, and pursue proactive, strategic planning like we're going to propose below.

Jim M.: This mindset is certainly not easy, and as you said earlier, leaders may at times need to ask for the support of their colleagues to sustain it. When I think back to many hours of discussions with 9-1-1 leaders, I think your summary is very important; because it puts this work of stress-risk management in the "real-world" context of 9-1-1 life. And acknowledging the hardship our leaders will face as they pursue this work doesn't place employee wellness on the backburner. You're saying *do all you can do to make things as good as you can for your people*. So now, let's help our 9-1-1 leaders do just that, by offering some concrete direction and tools they can use.

PART 3. Conclusion, Recommendations, and Guidance

In this chapter, we've shared Jim Lanier's story, and our discussion of Stress-Risk Manager, with the hope of preparing you with the encouragement, insights, and mindset you need to embrace the role of the SRM at your PSAP. We believe you can succeed in this role by overseeing two tandem initiatives:

1. Assign a team to help you build your center's Comprehensive Stress Management Program (CSMP). This PSAP program will provide your employees with the resilience resources called for in the 2013 NENA Standard on Acute/Traumatic and Chronic Stress Management (Chapter 15). You will find a downloadable version of this Standard at **https://c.ymcdn.com/sites/www.nena.org/resource/resmgr/Standards/NENA-STA-002.1-2013_9-1-1_Ac.pdf**. Materials to assist you in developing your CSMP are offered in the Chapter 19 Appendix. As you begin this work, we also urge you to visit **www.9-1-1training.net**, for news of any updates to this NENA standard, and to see other helpful resources. Also, please read our second recommended SRM initiative below before you begin this first initiative, since they can be best achieved when coordinated together.

2. While not included in the NENA Standard, we also urge you to engage your morale team (or resilience optimization team) to systematically evaluate and optimize your 9-1-1 center *work conditions* to foster resilience. While providing the resources called for in the CSMP are essential to prevent and resolve stress-related issues, they are not *sufficient*. PSAP leaders must also carefully evaluate work conditions that can continuously produce new stress threatening employee performance and well-being. So, such evaluation of work conditions is *preventive* Stress-Risk Management. Optimization of these conditions serves as primary protection of employee health and will boost

retention and morale (see Chapter 19). To help you conduct such an evaluation/optimization process, we have provided you with *Additional Resources* below.

∽✢∾

Questions for Reflection

To get the most from this chapter, you are encouraged to write your reflections here (in both the Kindle and paperback versions of this book).

- What was your main take-away from reading this chapter?

- What specifically made it valuable to you?

- How can you apply this take-away concretely to improve some aspect of your personal life and or efforts to support the wellbeing of 9-1-1Pros?

Additional Resources

- Chapter 19 Appendix: *A PSAP Project Guide: Optimizing Six Key PSAP Workplace Conditions* (see at back of book).
- For additional information and guidance related to achieving this evaluation of workplace conditions, see: *Tackling work-related stress using the Management Standards approach: A step-by-step workbook*, published in 2017 by The Health Safety Executive, United Kingdom. You can download this resource at no charge at this link: **http://www.hse.gov.uk/pubns/wbk01.htm**

Work Cited

"2013/2014 Staying@Work Report U.S. Executive Summary." *Willis Towers Watson,* September 2013, **www.towerswatson.com/en** US/Insights/IC-Types/Survey-Research-Results/2013/09/2013 2014-stayingatwork-us-executive-summary-report.

"U.S. Employers Rank Stress as Top Workforce Risk Issue: Understanding Employee Views is Key to Addressing Issue." *Willis Towers Watson,* 13 November 2013, **www.towerswatson.com/en** US/Press/2013/11/us-employers-rank-stress-as-top-workforce-risk issue?webSyncID=a7599718-2049-874d-6ba3 50b765ba676d&sessionGUID=60c4a620-22d1-400d-385e bdcc322a1b53.

CHAPTER 20
How a 9-1-1 Director Engaged His Employees to Boost Morale and His PSAP's Major Metrics of Success

Ivan Whitaker, Interviewed by Jim Marshall

Editor's Introduction

Ivan Whitaker is now with the Priority Dispatch Corporation™, but he was once the director of a larger 9-1-1 center in serious trouble. Those woes included low morale, high turn-over, budget problems, and over-use of leave time (sick and personal). His novel yet systematic approach to overcoming these problems involved launching a set of initiatives to target the wellness of his employees. He was convinced that if he attended to issues impacting their well-being first, the PSAPs other critical indicators of success would also improve. It turns out that Ivan was right. In our interview that follows, he never made reference to the Servant Leadership model; yet, his story offers a great example of a 9-1-1 director driven by a Servant-Leadership mindset (Chapter 18), who put this mindset in action in the role of the Stress-Risk Manager (Chapter 19). So, this story will help you put more "meat on the bone"; it will help you flesh out how the key concepts of Servant Leadership and stress risk management can be put into practice in your PSAP.

One important note: we don't offer Ivan's case study as a model of perfection or one that can serve as a canned template for every center. Every PSAP is different, even if two are the same size and serving the same demographics. And every manager's style and skill set are different. As I've emphasized throughout the book, *there are no cookie-cutter solutions*. Yet I'm confident that leaders and their teams from every type of PSAP will gain from adapting Ivan's ideas to fit their centers. Enjoy!

JM

૭૩✵૭

The 9-1-1 Director's Challenge

Jim: Ivan, when I first heard your story, I was struck by how well it represents the situation many of our 9-1-1 directors find themselves in. You were tasked with launching a consolidation under tight timelines and with limited resources. This meant placing even more demand on already stressed-out employees.

Ivan: Right! One of the major reasons I was hired into the position was to reduce our turnover rate, which was 44%. Nearly half of the individuals hired were being lost for various reasons, within one year. Even from my initial, informal conversations, it was clear that morale was poor. I learned then that there was no path for employees to advance in the organization.

Jim: This sounds like a perfect storm for a 9-1-1 director! Can you describe your mindset—how you looked at this challenge, and settled on the best way to face it?

Dealing Head on with Existing Challenges

Ivan: As 9-1-1 directors under pressure to consolidate, we are inclined to be so absorbed in pursuit of the consolidation that we may be tempted to put aside existing PSAP problems until after that big process is complete. My gut told me if we didn't resolve major issues, like morale, prior to that change process, the consolidation would just intensify them. And, as is often the case, I knew there could be critical issues not even identified yet that could get the best of us if left unattended. My first goal was to identify and address all major pre-existing deficits. And we had to move those mountains quickly, because I had mandates to clear the path for the consolidation within one year.

Jim: Your approach strikes me as wise risk-management and fits the mindset that Jim Lanier set forth as he described the Stress-Risk Manager in Chapter 19. You're placing the priority on addressing existing PSAP problems first, to the fullest extent possible, before placing more demand for change on your personnel?

Ivan: That's it. We must first gain key insights about the *true status* of our organization *as the basis* for changing it. This includes identifying all challenges and liabilities as well as the agency's resources and strengths. We can gain this insight two ways: through analysis of key data and by engaging our employees.

Jim: Can you unpack these approaches for us?

Dealing with Dark Matter

Ivan: Sure. *Analysis of key data* is about paying attention to the *dark matter*. Dark matter includes those variables affecting PSAP success that we as leaders often do not see clearly or quantify, so they remain unknown; in the dark. Yet they deeply impact morale and all the major metrics of PSAP success. Every 9-1-1 director must deal with these variables, such as sick leave usage, FLMA, turn-over, etc. If we can define, as *hard data*, the status of those variables, they are no longer dark matter. This step enables us to then prioritize initiatives to identify and improve underlying issues driving the disturbing statistics, such as low morale and under-managed stress. And we can learn a great deal about those issues by listening closely to our employees. (They, like us, are not always right, but all their perceptions are valuable!)

Listening to and Empowering Employees

I learned a long time ago that if I, as a leader, walk to the beat of my own drum instituting change that affects employees without their input, I may be walking down the wrong path. We must first gain understanding about how our employees perceive their work experience before we go about changing it (Herrero 66). Discovering and dealing with the dark matter is more than analyzing existing data. It has to include systematically gathering feedback—raw but vital information—from our personnel and engaging them as stakeholders in the agency's future. So, I sought to achieve this employee input and participation by creating three forums. Each of these forums produced crucial data and insights we could use to make our best decisions.

Jim: Could you just define each of these forums?

Ivan: Yes, and as I do, keep in mind that each one produces knowledge that feeds and cross-pollinates the others.

Communication Forum #1: The PSAP Morale Committee

First, to vitalize the relationship between management and employees, and create a conduit for communication essential to this project, we established a Morale Committee. Among those I chose were those perceived by existing management personnel to be the most disgruntled. Some folks thought I was out of my mind for selecting these employees to be on the committee. But my sense was that there was more substance to those employees' struggles than just "bad attitude." I needed their help as allies, not fortification of negativity. But we set forth rules at the beginning for how members were to engage as part of the committee. The first rule was that they had to be ready to offer solutions to any challenges they identified and be willing to work on those solutions.

With those ground rules we sailed a pretty smooth course. Sure, at the beginning, during the first few meetings, folks did tend to push outside those boundaries. But with a little reinforcement of the rules, they came together well. A good friend of mine, Jim Lanier, said that if you approach difficulties like this the right way, reflecting carefully, acting deliberately, you will move from rowing upstream to navigating rapids.

Communication Forum #2: Strategic One-on-One Leader/Employee Meetings

Ivan: I met with every dispatcher in the dispatch center individually. We spent at least one hour discussing the issues and challenges in the agency as they perceived them. I assured them that their input really mattered; that there would be no retaliation for honesty; and their input would be completely anonymous.

Jim: That is a pretty extreme effort for a 9-1-1 director! I can imagine directors, tired and already overworked, reading this right now, groaning, and asking, "Is this guy for real? Are all those hours really necessary? I care about my PSAP too, but I'm already maxed out!"

Ivan: it did take a great deal of time to sit with every employee that way. But the information and the changes that resulted from that time made it extremely worthwhile as I'll explain in a bit. There's one more data-gathering forum we need to explain.

Communication Forum #3: 360° Evaluation of Leadership

We also engaged all frontline personnel in a completely anonymous 360° evaluation of our leadership. This was a powerful tool for gaining understanding of employees' perceptions of those in leadership and the management team. This 360° evaluation allowed all the followers to say exactly what they felt about their leaders with complete safety. The supervisors were also evaluated this way. We didn't single out individual leaders. We looked at what the supervisors as a group needed to change.

Putting it All Together

Once I had gathered all the data from the one-on-one meetings and this 360° evaluation, I quantified it and brought it to the Morale Committee. This group joined with me to become our workhorse for the entire project.

Together, we were able to analyze this information and identify a *Top Ten List of PSAP Challenges*. As a team we then put a plan in place defining how we could improve those issues and prioritized the top three issues. We then set an agenda for pursuit of changes related to those issues. So, as a leader, I was able to report back to all our agency personnel about the research we had conducted and our plan to achieve change. They had all been a part of this through the one-on-one interviews and the 360° evaluation, and they knew their peers on the Morale Committee had represented them in building these plans. So, they were supportive and invested as we pursued changes.

Key Findings

Jim: Can you first tell us about the key findings you, as a leader, gained from your forums about core issues threatening your agency's success?

Ivan: Employees were, of course, concerned about how the consolidation would affect them: moving into a new center, new positions, possible changes in their pay, and other unknowns about their basic work conditions. But they shared much more concern about *existing* conditions at the comm center. They believed that *morale* was poor for several reasons. On a fundamental level, they had come to believe that their voices didn't matter. They had proposed many changes in the comm center over the years that hadn't materialized. As an example, for years the employees had wanted the building painted near the entrance since the paint was coming off the walls and looked bad. Their requests had been denied.

Little Changes Pave the Way for Big Changes

Jim: So, even though this was technically a very small issue, their request for change was reasonable and it represented what they were most discouraged by.

Ivan: Yes. I saw how the morale of the personnel matched the appearance of the building. So, I asked The Morale Committee to write up a proposal for painting this part of the building. This was a chance to show our employees that their voices mattered, that we were listening, and willing to let them participate in change. When I presented it to my boss, he said there was no money. I told him that if we could not approve something this simple, we would, ironically, be demoralizing the morale committee. We'd also be sabotaging the bigger mission we were trying to achieve: improving morale, retention and a successful consolidation. Fortunately, our boss received donations from other county budgets, and the custodial department volunteered their services. You could see the committee light up. They had proposed something as call-takers and dispatchers: now they could see it become a reality.

Our employees saw that they could truly participate, and the Morale Committee saw that we, as a team, could write a proposal resulting in change. It was a huge step for everyone. So, the committee decided to take it one step further. We set up task groups for issues like new uniforms. They decided everything about the uniforms from style, color, even what the icon would look like. The only thing I had to do was approve their decision. They made the decisions and wrote accompanying policies and procedures themselves. I just did some editing and delivered the plan to Human Resources. They did it all. It was this kind of empowerment that actually led to them being engaged as stakeholders.

I had employees who were now invested and involved in major changes in the communication center. This freed me up to engage in the rest of my administrative duties. I didn't feel like I had to have to my phone constantly in my hand outside of work. Often, as directors, we may feel that we have to personally drive and implement every significant change in our centers. That's exhausting and not sustainable as you pursue all the changes needed. The good news is this: if you lay out the canvas, position your people around it as stakeholders, they will usually rise to the occasion and achieve.

Jim: So now you were in good shape as an organization to take on the biggest obstacles to a successful future as an agency. You came to the agency with a clear understanding of the serious *retention* problem. And then through your forums you confirmed serious problems with morale. What did you discover about the relationship between these two problems, and how did you address them?

Tackling the Big 9-1-1 Two-fer: Morale and Retention

Ivan: In those forums, we discovered that morale was so poor, in part, because people did not see a future for career growth at the center. *Workers felt stuck in a dead-end job.* They didn't see their work as a career with stepping stone possibilities. There was no promotional process or ladder. There was just one tier of positions in call-taking and dispatching, and people had been in those same positions for 15 or 20 years without progressing at all. Their wages were flat; they received only their annual base increase, but nothing beyond that. There was no agency process to strategically foster growth and development of employees.

Jim: That would be pretty demoralizing. So how did you tackle this challenge?

Employee Step Ladder to Career Advancement

Ivan: To address the lack of opportunities for advancement within the agency, we took a hard look at what it would take to keep employees for a longer period of time. Since employees saw employment at the communications center as just a stepping stone beyond the agency, we needed to create a step ladder system with real opportunities for advancement *within* the agency. Then employees would be able to see 9-1-1 work as a career in itself, with financial gains along the way.

So, the Morale Committee wrote up *new job descriptions* defining new levels of employment within the agency. I then engaged Human Resources (HR) for help defining the description of acceptable activities at each one of these levels. We made it possible for employees to get to the next level of the job within the center.

Jim: This makes so much sense as you describe this step ladder advancement initiative; you saw that morale and retention are both tied to the employee's ability to wake up in the morning and see a future for them in their current workplace

Advancement Requires Training and Education

Ivan: Exactly. Of course, employees must be *capable* of success in the new roles now available to them in the agency. Our personnel and I recognized that assuring this capability called for an organizational commitment to *training*. For a number of those positions, that includes supporting employees in pursuit of formal education. Often doors to career development are closed to dispatchers because they do not have a four-year degree. We knew that in order to help them build a career we had to do something to incentivize pursuit of education and growth development. We decided to *give compensation* to those who chose to better themselves. We believed (and I was confident through data on such business practices) that employees would actually stay with us longer the more educated they were--because now they had chances within the agency to use new training.

Jim: So how did this growth development incentive program work for you over the next few years?

Ivan: As employees gained more skills, they wanted to be better employees; the professional standard in the agency increased. So, instead of losing them over that period of time, they were working to be great employees. Even those we lost over a five-year period were better employees during the time they were employed. Those who chose to stay became great leaders; some moved on to leadership positions within the organization.

Jim: How else did you boost retention and morale?

More Strategies to Improve Morale and Groom Leaders for the Future

Ivan: Everyone needs to feel that their talent can be used in their work; and in every PSAP there is a sizeable percentage of personnel who really want to actively contribute to the agency's change process but lacked the platform to do so. Leaders might never know these employees had that interest or ability to contribute. The Morale Committee proved they had both. So, creating such opportunities for participation in the future of the 9-1-1 center can be a major incentive for retaining employees.

Building Supervisors. To incentivize and equip more frontline dispatchers to become supervisors, we provided them with training to build skills that the agency had not developed among non-leadership employees. In addition to conflict management training, we provided them with course work on how to motivate employees, conduct proper evaluations, and write good professional reports.

Budgeting Training for Supervisors: As a director I was, of course, responsible for our comm center's budget. I made sure all our supervisors and managers knew how to run this budget. I engaged them in our budget meetings. We would rotate chairmanship of the meeting, so that each supervisor had a turn leading. They learned how to conduct themselves as a group leader, which required them to gain a higher level of understanding about budgeting concepts and how to manage a budget effectively. We worked to create a great learning environment.

Jim: This is such a powerful example of strategically valuing employees and recognizing their potential for greater contributions. It's also a pretty good approach to succession planning! You mentioned at the start of the chapter that high use of sick leave was really hurting your agency's bottom-line. What did you and your personnel decide to do about that?

Driving Down Costs with an Employee-Authored Sick Leave Policy

Ivan: With the Morale Committee's small initial successes writing new agency policies, they were now capable of writing a new sick leave policy. And they wrote a good one that provided *financial incentives* to the squads with the lowest sick leave use. We looked at how we could reward our team by meeting certain important benchmarks (Key Performance Indicators, or KPIs). Those benchmarks were secondary to compliance and call management. Some KPIs were actually rewarded with cash from the county given to an entire group. But the amounts were so small that if divvied up to each employee, it would result in trivial rewards like a coffee cup or mug. So, we decided to pool that money and hold group events that folks could actually bring their families to, like a cookout. At these events we could pass out awards and engage the families so they all could share in this morale building activity.

We also had shift competition activities based on comparing compliance stats. These resulted in pizza parties as rewards. However, the compliance on all the shifts improved so greatly that they all ended up earning pizza parties.

Pursing Wellness in the PSAP

Jim: Ivan, the initiatives you've describe so far, each helped to boost morale at your center. And better morale fosters healthier employees. How else did you work to support the mental health and resilience of your employees?

Ivan: We know that our telecommunicators often struggle with personal issues in their lives that impact their performance in service to the public. In fact, when I listened to recorded audio of our telecommunicators' communication with citizens, you could actually hear how their emotional distress (unrelated to the call) came across in their voice with the callers—not just what they said, but in their tone. So, we pursued support for *stress management* training with our employees.

Folks were so stressed about getting their tasks done, they weren't aware that the way they were handling conflict as a team was lacking. So, team leaders needed good *conflict resolution* skills. Many of our employees were guarded and had a tough time identifying what was driving the conflicts. So, we also brought our employees through conflict resolution training. This was very helpful. It equipped them to identify their own internal stress that drove conflict.

Jim: I'm wondering if this conflict management training also helped identify and develop more leaders too?
Ivan: Yes, this initial round of training actually gave us the idea to incorporate stress management and conflict resolution training as part of the process for

moving up the career ladder. Supervisors must be equipped to relate skillfully to conflict among, and with their teams. To make this training fully relevant to our 9-1-1 work, we engaged local actors and actresses to enact major mistakes in call scenarios that were driven by stress.

Jim: That actually sounds like a fun process. And you recognized stress as a key factor in performance and helped them deal with it. Nice! How did this training make a difference?

Ivan: Typically, as leaders, we would respond to call performance mistakes with discipline. Before watching a scenario between the actors, the supervisors were asked to imagine that this dispatcher struggling was their *best employee*. After observing the scenario, they were asked to explore how they would manage this employee when such mistakes took place that would typically result in discipline immediately. We wanted to see if they could explore other factors that might be driving the troubled behavior rather than assume willfully poor performance. After the scenarios, the supervisors could ask questions to learn about these factors.

So, in the enactments, the scenario would not finish until the candidate for advancement could identify those other factors driving the struggles. This was productive. For example, they learned that the dispatcher was a mother who had major struggles at home before she came to work. The trainees recognized that their best leadership response, rather than just immediately hammering the mistake, would be to work with the employee to engage in proper stress management, or in some cases, to seek professional help.

Balancing Discipline with Support

Jim: This can be a very powerful approach that does two things at once: it helps the employee address the struggles underlying their problem with performance. And it strengthens their relationship with, and trust in the supervisor. Yet, it could also be perceived by leaders as being too soft and not holding employees fully responsible, after all, directors aren't therapists!

Ivan: When discipline must be issued to uphold performance standards, then it is administered. But jumping to discipline without trying to understand what drove the behavior in an otherwise good employee is a mistake. The first goal is constructive reinforcement and creating a learning environment where employees welcome feedback. We can uphold our standards, and gain insight to restore good employees who might otherwise be lost if only discipline is applied. In fact, we may be able to excel more in upholding work standards by this supportive approach.

More Results

Jim: Ivan, this is really an extraordinary collection of initiatives. Can you tell us a little more about the results they produced?

Ivan: With the morale committee and the rest of those initiatives in place we were able to:
- Drive down sick leave usage by 54%.
- Achieve a 27% reduction in overtime in a twelve-month period
- Make a 22% reduction in turnover in the same twelve-month period
- Collectively, this resulted in a cost savings of $200,000 as a comm center.

So, there was a significant tangible benefit, but also a huge morale and stress benefit as well.

Jim: These are tremendous results, and I hope they are encouraging to other directors still mid-stream in their struggles. Since appreciation is a known factor in sustaining success, I have to ask: was your team given any formal recognition for this success?

Ivan: Well, since you brought it up, the center did receive some nice recognition from our county, what they call the *Golden Standard Award*, for achieving these accomplishments so quickly. I'm proud of our team. Each time I sat down with the Morale Committee with a list of objectives, they would blow them out of the water (exceed my expectations with their efforts).

Conclusion

Jim: Can you just briefly summarize a few of the key elements of the approach that contributed to the success of this project?

Ivan: Sure, I'll state them as objectives that any comm center can apply, irrespective of size or budget:

- Empower your employees and trust them to respond (Greenleaf).
- Shed light on the Dark Matter: quantify those key agency metrics and the human factors that drive those number down.
- Take a hard look at morale and stress factors and then work to boost well-being.

- To do this, establish a Morale Committee and empower them to create solutions and policies to enact those solutions.
- Invest in the personal and educational development of your employees with incentivizing programs.
- Reduce sick-leave usage and use the money you save to fund such incentivizing programs.

Jim: As I look back over your message in this chapter, as summarized by this list, I'm really struck that your initiatives all promote resilience in the 9-1-1 center. And the primary approach you have used to achieve this is to create improvement in six *working conditions* addressed in other chapters of this book. In the guide we provided in the Chapter 19 Appendix we identified these working conditions to include:

- Demand
- Control
- Support
- Relationships
- Role
- Change

You've given our readers great examples of how they can improve these work conditions. Thank you, Ivan!

Questions for Reflection

To get the most from this chapter, you are encouraged to write your reflections here (in both the Kindle and paperback versions of this book).

- What was your main take-away from reading this chapter?

- What specifically made it valuable to you?

- How can you apply this take-away concretely to improve some aspect of your personal life and or efforts to support the wellbeing of 9-1-1Pros?

Additional Resources

- *"It's Your Ship"* by Captain D. Michael Abrashoff gives a conceptual view of how incorporating non-conventional leadership tactics led to what is considered the Best Navy Ship in the Navy.
- *"Developing the Leaders Around You"* by John C. Maxwell explains how servant leadership tactics can ultimately create the desired learning environment and growth development.

Works Cited

Greenleaf, Robert. "What is Servant Leadership?" *The Robert K. Greenleaf Center, Inc.,* 2008.

Herrero, Leandro. *Viral Change: The Alternative to Slow, Painful and Unsuccessful Management of Change in Organisations,* Meetingminds, 2008.

End Notes

[1] Incentive programs may seem less applicable to smaller 9-1-1 centers where there are fewer opportunities for advancement. Yet, it may be that the percentage of employees who choose to participate may hold constant whether from small or large PSAPs. The net result of the incentives may also be a "win" for smaller centers since the agency is preparing to more easily and reliably fill leadership positions from within with dispatchers who are uniquely qualified; have the required leadership training; and are known by the organization and its people.

CHAPTER 21
Eight Reflections for 9-1-1 Leaders Pursuing Resilience, from Forty Years at the Helm

John Dejung

Editor's Introduction

Our authors of the first three chapters in this section were tasked with unpacking major leadership concepts and recommended approaches to optimizing resilience. Lora Reed taught us about Servant Leadership (Chapter 18). Jim Lanier explored the 9-1-1 leader's role as the Stress-Risk Manager (Chapter 19). And in Chapter 20, Ivan Whitaker put meat on the bone; he described how he put these concepts into action to help his communication center improve working conditions and boost morale with minimal resources.

This chapter, written by Dane County (Madison, WI) 9-1-1 Director John Dejung, is intentionally different. It serves as a leadership oasis, of sorts. Take a deep breath and get refreshed as John offers inspiring, easy-to-digest reflections on eight of his favorite quotes. He wonderfully reinforces leadership concepts already presented while also preparing you with the ideal mindset to explore how to shape your best future in the Next Generation 9-1-1 PSAP. Enjoy!

JM

※

Introduction

I learned many things about leadership over the twenty years I was a Coast Guard officer, and many more as a 9-1-1 Director during the subsequent twenty years. The most precious gems I can pass on to you were those mined and polished by others. So, even though some of the following sayings are known by my past and present colleagues as "Dejung-isms," I quickly and gladly attribute them to those who did the real pioneering and phrase-coining.

Sometimes I think there are just too many books on leadership theories, programs and approaches for busy leaders to absorb and apply. So, the use of well-known sayings, to lock in a key concept, belief, or leadership practice, can be more helpful. For each saying I've offered reflections about what they've meant to me and how they might apply to your work as a fellow 9-1-1 leader in pursuit of resilience at your center.

~1~
"BRING ME AN ADEQUATE BATTLE PLAN IN TIME FOR THE BATTLE, NOT THE PERFECT BATTLE PLAN A DAY LATE."
General George Patton

This may be my favorite and most-used principle as a leader. Do you think, as I sometimes do, that you have to deliver a perfect "A+" product on every assignment? Sometimes under such self-imposed pressure our products end up being delivered late, or they don't get delivered at all! So, in some situations I've urged my managers to just "get 'er done." The result may be a "B-product," but by staying on schedule there is apt to be more time to improve it as part of the review process with the support of other team members. At least this way you have a product on time, to use or improve.

Of course, in some cases the project or product's initial quality is more crucial than the deadline and it does need to be "A" quality out of the starting gate. However, if a less-than-stellar product will suffice, use it. That's not to say I promote mediocrity; but I know we as 9-1-1 leaders have more things to do than we can get done in the allotted time, especially if too much time is spent fully polishing a draft product. *Sometimes, perfect is the enemy of adequate.* Just be careful and use discretion on which products can be left rough and which ones need to be polished.

~2~
"A PLAN IS WORTHLESS; PLANNING IS PRICELESS"
President Dwight David Eisenhower

As we all know, plans, otherwise known as Standard Operating Procedures (SOPs), Administrative Policies, Continuity of Operations Plans (COOPs), et cetera, are necessary. But, how often do they really get used? Some SOPs are used many times; some are hopefully followed every hour of every day. Others, perhaps COOPs, may be rarely, if ever, used. So, the temptation may be to avoid developing, maintaining, and practicing implementation of plans that rarely, if ever, get used. Or, conversely, there is the temptation to not mess with policies, such as SOPs, because after all, "they must be OK since we're using them every day." I'd argue, as did Ike, that the value is not the plan or document, but the process of planning that forces the individual, or better yet, the team, to think each issue through. This exercises the neurons in the brain that will prepare the team for what Murphy's Law might bring our way.

Likewise, as when you wipe down and clean a ship's engine room, you don't know where the leaks are until you take a closer look. The planning process forces us to think hard and look more vigilantly. Insight can be priceless. We gain it from the close inspection. Shared insight, gained through a team planning together, can reap many rewards. Recently, my management team engaged in a "risk assessment" process that considered: 1) probability of occurrence, 2) severity of the problem, if it occurs, and 3) the strength of the safeguards built in to mitigate the risk. The multi-day exercise, spread out over a number of weeks, was painful, but yielded precious results.

When we had catalogued the seventy-five or so risks we could dredge up, it was instantly clear that we had a "top 10" from which we could work. Of the ten, there were five that we could couple together and attack with a plan to "accelerate learning." Those risks are being dealt with via five teams. Each team is led by a manager, staffed with two or three supervisors, and designed to draw in engagement from other team members. We don't have a "risk management plan," other than the catalog of risks, but we do have action underway. Much of the risk mitigation has to do with frequent training and continuous learning. If that results in saving one life, then the planning would indeed be priceless

~3~
"SIX MONTHS FROM NOW, WHAT WILL WE WISH WE HAD DONE MORE OF NOW?"
Source Unknown

Or, in the words of singer Bob Seger, "I wish I didn't know now, what I didn't know then." But like Seger, we *will* know more in 6 months. If we think *now* about what might come about *then*, maybe, just maybe, we can take steps to avoid an unfortunate or unplanned outcome. At least once a month, during my weekly huddles with my managers, I ask our team to get out of the foxhole of daily brush firefighting and mentally project ahead six months to determine what we need to pay attention to now. Every once in a while, the exercise yields a tidbit that gets us going in time to produce a positive outcome, rather than to let fate take its course.

And here's another approach that just occurred to me today, while preparing for a media interview for tomorrow. Ask yourself what the media might ask you about in six months that you can prepare for now. This is one that I wish I had thought more about six months ago. I can foresee, just eighteen hours in advance, that the TV story could reflect poorly on our 9-1-1 center. Had I let myself get "hypnotized" into thinking this particular challenge is outside my control? You see, the topic of the TV news coverage will be about the status of PSAPs' wireless phone location technology. The journalists may ask, "When Uber ride-sharing patrons are already capable of narrowing down their location to the front door of a dwelling, why can't 9-1-1 get better locations for emergencies?"

Will the media let me "blame" the FCC since we aren't mandated to comply strictly to their new requirements until 2022? Can we place the blame on Telcos for lobbying to avoid major short-term investments needed to make those requirements a reality? Or will the TV newsies, on behalf of the public, wonder why we haven't taken the bull by the horns and partnered with the myriad of application developers to solve the problem locally? Hmm, maybe APCO or NENA have better answers to that than I have right now, the night before the interview. When other stakeholders that our agency depends on for advance planning aren't doing their part, what is my PSAP's responsibility?

"Six months from now, what will we wish we'd done more of now?" With this working question as a guide, our agency produced a "2020 Vision." This activity involves looking even further ahead to be ready for what the organization will need in and around, the year 2020. We have organized the "vision" into the following four categories:
       1) People
       2) Processes
       3) Technology
       4) Infrastructure

In the category of People, our work to assess future needs includes:
- Staffing studies and efforts to predict how much more labor-intensive NG9-1-1 will be.
- Determining how much labor and time we might save using applications, such as "ASAP to PSAP" (where alarm "calls" are sent directly to CAD without intervention of the alarm company or the

PSAP call-taking personnel). Such savings could help us cover the increased labor associated with NG process time.
- Taking a hard look at training and how to pull off continual learning without breaking the overtime bank.

In the Processes category we're working to assess future needs including:
- Quality assurance
- Hiring
- Call-taking and dispatching
- Supervision and evaluation

Technology looks ahead at a what staff support will be needed to enable:
- Call-taking (whether CPE or hosted)
- Computer-Aided Dispatch (CAD): 5 years from RFP start to cutover!
- Radio: if and how FirstNet will impact our processes

Finally, our assessment of Infrastructure attempts to explore the brick and mortar questions, for example:
- Will we have enough room for additional consoles in our center as may be called for by growth in our local population or if we consolidate with other PSAPs?
- What additional resources will be needed to fully launch text and video?

This 2020 assessment is much more than a budget exercise because before we can budget effectively, we must think ahead to ascertain how the industry practices will evolve. One example: will video to 9-1-1 be handled (with a much-increased process time) in the PSAP or will responder agencies want to have that visual information simply sent to them for their analysis centers to peruse and use for response? We won't find the answer to that question by looking in the "foxhole" of daily work in the current PSAP; we need to look forward and scan the horizon, planning to manage the changes we can foresee. (See next chapter.)

~4~
"YOU CAN ALWAYS SPEED UP, BUT YOU CANNOT ALWAYS SLOW DOWN."
Commander Roger Allison, My First Commanding Officer

Imagine an icebreaking ship speeding toward a pier, a buoy, or a vessel stuck in the ice. You do *not* want to be charging at the pier or ship, because obviously, hitting the same will cause some real damage. We're talking about the proverbial unstoppable force hitting the immovable object. You see, ships don't have brakes, and putting the engines in reverse can take a while. Even when in reverse, ship's engines don't slow all that mass down immediately. However, you *can* speed up a bit if you need more headway to get gently to the pier-side, or to get close enough to the stuck ship to help it through the ice. Ironically, a ship, like a major decision, can pivot much more nimbly when not lunging too quickly ahead. Like a ship piling into a pier or colliding with another ship, you don't want hasty decisions to bring about tragic, avoidable results, nor damage reputations or important relationships.

In the Coast Guard, we call acceleration *putting on "turns" or RPMs* (revolutions per minute). So, I can summarize my point here with the oft-advised message, "You can always put 'em on, but cannot always take 'em off." This truism applies in many ways to leading an organization. While abrupt decision making is sometimes admired and frequently expected, it's important for the leader to resist the temptation of barking out orders too quickly. So, if a decision is not required in the next few moments, *slow down*. In crises, decisions must be made lightning-fast, but as able, it's wiser to methodically gather key data, soliciting the input of your subject matter experts. This more deliberate process will boost the quality of the final decision and your confidence as you implement it. You may upset those whose response is to rush when stressed, and you may be tagged as a plodder. But hold your head high, your speed gauged, and your eye on the compass. Better to be a leader who plods and plots to stay on course than the Captain of the Titanic!

~5~
"CAPABILITY MULTIPLIED BY CARING EQUALS PERFORMANCE EXCELLENCE."
Professor Alan Filley, University of Wisconsin - Madison

The popularity of shaping mission, vision, and values statements has come and gone over the forty years of my adult life. Those mottos that didn't stick, or were ignored frequently, were those that didn't add up to anything other than mere words on paper. Don't get me wrong, some organizational mottos were helpful, and I usually tried (but many times failed) to instill the value of them in our employees. I'm happy to say there's one statement I latched onto and it has guided me well during my twenty years in 9-1-1 centers. It does add up to something. More accurately, it *multiplies* out to something: "Capability multiplied by Caring equals Performance Excellence," or $C^2=PE$. You don't have to be a mathematician to know that anything multiplied by zero yields a product of zero. So, you can guess what my contention is: we and our team may be 100% capable, but without caring demonstrated throughout our organization, we won't get excellent performance as our final product. And of course, caring without developing the organization's competence doesn't yield much either.

Let's put the emphasis on the second "C" in the equation, Caring, applying it to all members of the PSAP.
- We need to care enough to show up for work when scheduled: on time and when co-workers are counting on it.
- We need to care enough to "give a rip," to help and respect co-workers up and down the chain of command.
- We need to show care toward the callers and the responders.

9-1-1 Professionals need the whole care package. And, yes, that means every one of us caring for ourselves to remain resilient in the face of stress and to be well enough to get ourselves to work over the long haul. This self-care includes augmenting training provided by our organization; feeding ourselves a little each day with self-training on professional topics to improve our confidence through greater competence. Some high-flying, super-competent professionals may believe they are so good at their jobs they don't have to spend mental energy *expressing* care for others. That mentality is toxic to a PSAP, like a cancer. If it is left to spread; then attrition, bad press, law suits, to name just a few, can all come down on the organization like a ton of bricks. Leaders need to consistently find ways to express and model actively caring for their personnel.

Now let's focus on the *Capability* of our team members. While we as managers may struggle with huge limitations in funds and support, and with many demands competing for our attention, we must strive to assure that:
- Essential and excellent employee training is provided.
- Staff have the necessary technology to do their jobs.
- Helpful, clear and concise SOPs are established to guide team members.
- Quality Assurance is in place ensuring that processes and procedures are being followed, and that team members are being assessed, encouraged, and re-trained to sustain excellence.
- A tough-love approach is applied as needed with employees who, due to their unwillingness to care or their inability to learn and perform capably, don't measure up.

There's one caveat related to this "tough-love" statement: the decision to confront must be preceded and guided by Caring *attunement* to risk factors that may drive an employee's substandard attitude or performance. As leaders we need to be watchful for burn-out, chronic stress, and Compassion Fatigue dampening or preventing the employee's ability to "give a rip" (see Chapter 10). We also need to be sure to provide the support to those who are sincerely struggling so that they can regain their well-being. Consider the need for additional training and information on stress management; both peer support and referrals for professional care should be "at the ready" to buoy up your people (Chapters 15 and 16). Like most organizations, ours has an Employee Assistance Program (EAP). Many EAPs are not attuned to the needs of 9-1-1 centers. We are fortunate that our county's EAP is very strong: it is staffed with clinicians who understand 9-1-1 stress and are qualified to support our personnel. With the support of our EAP provider, Randy Kratz (Chapter 19), we have established a Peer Support Team; a group of ten telecommunicators to assist the other seventy or so in our center. This team has received excellent training on when and how to come alongside their co-workers with support. They have also learned when and how to reach out to mental health professionals for additional care as needed.

C^2=PE can serve as an invaluable touchstone and a continual reminder of what matters most: getting the job done with excellence and affirming how to get there—by releasing the power of combined Caring and Capability. When we as leaders believe in and are committed to living out a statement of our values or mission such as this one, our employees are more apt to trust us and follow our leadership.

~6~
"NO ONE CARES HOW MUCH YOU KNOW, UNTIL THEY KNOW HOW MUCH YOU CARE"
Source Unknown

This idea may sound cliché, but it builds on C^2=PE and reflects a key expectation that employees have for their supervisors and managers. Certainly, frontline employees expect that those promoted to supervisory and management positions will be basically competent and capable of giving good advice and direction. But, first they want to know that leaders have got their backs and are resolved to treat all employees equitably, carrying out rules and SOPs fairly. Yet, on what basis will they *know* that we are looking out for them and truly have their best interest in mind? There's no question that leaders can be perceived as unfair despite our best efforts, but we can weather those criticisms better when we put forth appropriate effort.

Caring for Employees in Accord with How They Define Caring

Convincing workers that we as leaders care about them can be tricky. Yes, partly because some employees may be chronically unpleasable. But unless we've already worked strategically to evidence genuine caring and they've repeatedly rejected these efforts, it's a big mistake to assume that folks just choose to be critical and untrusting of us. Convincing our personnel that we, as leaders, care is also difficult because most employees spell that four-letter word with a different four letters: T-I-M-E. There's the rub! Sure, supervisors and managers must convey that they care, but we still must all get our tasks completed. Frankly I struggle with this, and I think many PSAP leaders do too.

If you operate a smaller PSAP, you may be spread so thin as a one-person management team that sitting down with your people feels like a huge strain. However, invest the time upfront with new employees to teach them what your job entails. A brief explanation with a new-hire can help them appreciate the extraordinary demands you face daily. This is not an excuse for ignoring employees. It's not intended as a pleasant form of a brush-off: "Hey, this is why you'll never see me." This quick in-service is a respectful investment to empower the employee with the knowledge they need to shape realistic expectations and prevent ignorance-driven judgments that fuel toxic gossip. Then also apply some of the strategies offered below that you consider feasible.

If you run a big PSAP, you may be layers removed from your frontline folks; and spending time with every employee may be difficult. So, as leaders of larger agencies we can strive to assure our employees feel cared about by adopting a "walk-the-talk" approach. We can utilize those in our chain of command to activate what we could call a *care cascade*. So, our message to our managers to put this cascade in motion might be, "Hey, leaders: you know I spend a bunch of time with you. You need to do the same with your supervisors, and then clearly express the expectation that they too will spend plenty of time with their employees."

This care cascade model is a manageable way to increase the feeling among employees at all levels that they are being cared for. Don't forget, however, to do some "meeting and greeting" at every level, both informally, by walking around and chatting a bit, and formally: attend, or organize, a few more meetings than a time management expert might suggest but take their expert advice and budget your time carefully. Many organizations have something akin to a Labor-Management Committee. We have one, even though my employees aren't technically organized within a labor union. We use an agenda, take minutes, report back on progress, and we start and end every meeting with the question: "what are you thankful for professionally?"

You may think this is too "soft" a question to spend time on, especially since I just urged you to budget your time wisely. But there's huge wisdom and organizational pay-offs by practicing this line of questioning. It's part of "Appreciative Inquiry"—a leadership practice that is "revolutionizing the field of organizational development and change" (Quinn 1).

~7~
"SUCCESS IS 90% PERSPIRATION AND 10% INSPIRATION"
Vince Lombardi and/or Thomas Edison

I'm a proud native of Wisconsin. I grew up in Wisconsin in the 1960's when "Title Town" (Green Bay) was really *Title Town*. The Packers won the first two Super Bowls ever played. And I really believed that it was our great coach Vince Lombardi who said, "success is 90% perspiration and 10% inspiration." After all, he was legend for impressing this hard-work ethic upon his players and it seemed to be a big part of the magic behind the huge success they shared. Only much later in life did I come to find out that the credit for this saying really goes to Thomas Edison. Edison surely embodied it too: he reportedly tried something like 10,000 different solutions before he was able to perfect the light bulb.

Yet, the saying *success is 90% perspiration and 10% inspiration*, could seem to conflict with my earlier motto that performance excellence is driven by the swirling combo of Caring and Capability ($C^2=PE$). But Edison's motto actually helps shed light on the stuff of which these two Cs are made! We must exert great care in pursuit of our mission to succeed at achieving it. The organization needs this investment (perspiration!) from PSAP personnel throughout the chain of command. Still, it is true that The Pack needed more than just the hard-work of its players; they needed the other 10% too: *inspiration!* That came in the form of a playbook that was way ahead of its time: Coach Lombardi knew that he had to honor the caring and grit of his players by strategically *developing their capability*. So, he developed game strategies and training that were unprecedented.

We as leaders need to join Vince Lombardi in recognizing our need for a playbook to succeed as an organization. We too need to invest in the capability of our personnel. First, we build the basics—solid recruiting to support adequate staffing, add good training, and a quality assurance process. Then we boost capability by equipping our employees with the best tools we can get: the technological edge to optimize dispatch and call management (up-to-date CAD systems, GPS mapping software, computer-based protocols, and more). We reward our team's sweat, evidence our caring, and inspire them to become champions by equipping them this way. That means that planning our leader's playbook is priceless.

Lombardi's players knew that he loved them. They judged him by the same standard he set for them, and he fulfilled those words, "no one cares how much you know, until they know how much you care." Of course, sometimes it was pretty tough love, but it was love nevertheless. Read a book about "Saint Vincent" (cited in the Additional Resources below) and you'll gain more insight about how he loved his players, and how that love translated into motivating them to work harder and achieve greater excellence than any other team.

~8~
"SEMPER PARATUS" (ALWAYS READY)
The Coast Guard Motto

We lived and breathed this Latin maxim in the Coast Guard. And I know that *being prepared* is a fundamental value of public safety professionals. However, despite our best intentions we can lose our Semper Paratus grip when/if we're overtaken by the High Frequency/Low Risk (HF/LR) "brush fires" of every day PSAP operations. With our minds full of these steady demands, we may forget the need to prepare the extra training and preparation needed to manage the Low Frequency/High Risk (LF/HR) incidents. We definitely want to "practice" our response prior, rather than during, for those high-risk events. Yet the responsibility is not all ours as leaders. We need to teach our followers as 9-1-1 professionals to share responsibility for preparedness by instilling in them the value of personal accountability for self-training and continuous learning on the job. But don't stop there. There must be a formalized program to ensure that we regularly drill our teams on management of HR/LF incidents. Maureen Wills was fortunately already a believer in this kind of preparedness when her 9-1-1 team responded to the mass casualty event at Sandy Hook Elementary School in 2012.

Practicing HR/LF Incident Preparedness

Many have heard of Gordon Graham, former State Trooper (California Highway Patrol, CHIPS) and risk management expert. Gordon suggests a very simple, yet effective approach to ensuring that HR/LF training is conducted routinely. He suggests a method he practiced while at CHIPs: a simple calendar for each month that includes crucial HR/LF training. This

training was repeated at set intervals, every X weeks or Y months to ensure repetition, and thus help personnel "lock-in" the essential mindset, strategies and tactics. Active shooter training might be a quarterly event; practice drills at the PSAP's back-up center might be conducted bi-monthly, and a CAD Down drill might be practiced monthly. Decide locally about the types and frequencies of training and drills your center will conduct. Signing off on receipt of the training is necessary to ensure all hands are covered.
During my entire Coast Guard career, I never had to abandon ship and never had a shipboard fire on my own ships. But I can tell you, we drilled for those HR/LF events innumerable times, *just in case*.

Semper Paratus!

Conclusion

I hope you find my eight favorite quotes and these reflections helpful. Perhaps a couple will become "old saws" you use often, as I have. Perhaps mine will just catalyze you to reflect more deeply on those you've already collected, or to be on the look-out for new ones that offer you the direction and inspiration you personally need as a leader. Ultimately, what matters is that we're "all rowing in the same direction"—supporting excellence and the well-being of our people. Let me lead you into one last quote as we conclude the chapter.

We as emergency response leaders often need a strong word of encouragement when things don't work out for us in quite the same way as the storybook, textbook, or *playbook* intended. Despite our best efforts, it seems there is always someone disappointed in, or critical of us: the Chief misconstrues your motives; your employees think you are not the epitome of caring because you "haven't shown it" by spending enough time with them lately; or, the local media publish negative reports about your team's response to incidents because they don't understand the technical backstory.

I don't ever impose my faith on others, but it's part of who I am, and it guides my approach to leadership, however imperfectly executed. In my view, we as emergency response professionals are doing God's work, and we're shepherding our teams as they strive to do the "Public Good." I see this as a mission God would have us do as we sojourn here on Earth. Whether we do it as part of the military or as 9-1-1 professionals, we're all operating within what Teddy Roosevelt called *the arena*. So, as we wrap up the chapter, I offer you his words (which, of course, apply to any gender) as a final encouragement:

"It is not the critic who counts. ... The credit belongs to the man who is actually in the arena; whose face is marred by the dust and sweat and blood; who strives valiantly... who, at worst, if he fails, at least fails while daring greatly; so that his place shall never be with those cold and timid souls who know neither victory or defeat."

Questions for Reflection

To get the most from this chapter, you are encouraged to write your reflections here (in both the Kindle and paperback versions of this book).

- What was your main take-away from reading this chapter?

- What specifically made it valuable to you?

- How can you apply this take-away concretely to improve some aspect of your personal life and your efforts to support the wellbeing of 9-1-1Pros?

Additional Resources

- Maraniss, David - *When Pride Still Mattered: A Life of Vince Lombardi.*
- For more general information about Appreciate Inquiry, see **https://www.centerforappreciativeinquiry.net/** and **http://www.davidcooperrider.com/ai-process/**.
- For specific training in Appreciative Inquiry customized to the 9-1-1 leadership role, consider Communication Center Managers (CCM) offered annually by Fitch & Associates' and the International Academies of Emergency Dispatch (IAED). For more information, visit: http://www.emergencydispatch.org/CertCCMCourse.

- Vroom-Yetton decision-making model: The Vroom-Yetton model is designed to help you to identify the best decision-making approach and leadership style to take, based on your current situation. It was originally developed by Victor Vroom and Philip Yetton in their 1973 book, **Leadership and Decision Making**.

Works Cited

Graham, Gordon. "High Risk, Low Frequency Events in the Fire Service." *BCFPD Training*, 17 September 2012, training.bcfdmo.com/2012/09/17/gordon-graham-high-risklow frequency/.

Quinn, Robert. "What is Appreciative Inquiry." *David Cooperrider and Associates,* www.davidcooperrider.com/ai-process/.

Roosevelt, Theodore. "Citizenship in a Republic." *The Man in the Arena,* 23 April 1910, www.theodore-roosevelt.com/trsorbonnespeech.html.

Seger, Bob. "Against the Wind." *Against the Wind,* Capitol, 1979.

End Notes

[1] A lesson like this is so much better to learn in advance. Maureen Wills, the 9-1-1 director at Newtown, Massachusetts when the Sandy Hook massacre occurred, has said: "Just the week before the shooting took place, we had reviewed our Active Shooter training and drilled again. I don't even want to think of what it would have been like for my people if we hadn't done that." Source: M. Wills. October 5, 2016. *Sandy Hook Elementary School Shooting: Lessons Learned, December 12, 2012.* Presentation to the Michigan Communication Directors Association, Traverse City, Michigan.

CHAPTER 22
Leading the Next Generation 9-1-1 PSAP: Managing the Risks of Real-Time Video Interactions

Jim Marshall

Part 1: Facing Challenges: Nothing New to 9-1-1!

Next Generation 9-1-1 represents a robust package of solutions to improve delivery of 9-1-1 services, inevitably resulting in saving more lives. One capability that NG9-1-1 will afford is interaction between emergency telecommunicators with callers and field responders via real-time video (RTV). Yet NG9-1-1 enables our emergency system to achieve much more. So, it is essential to explore our concerns related to RTV in the context of NG9-1-1's greater purpose and anticipated benefits. This is important information, too, for readers who are not in the 9-1-1 industry.

Next Generation 9-1-1 technologies will...

- Enable 9-1-1 calls from any networked device.
- Provide quicker delivery and more accurate information to responders and the public alike.
- Incorporate better and more useful forms of information: real-time text, images, video, and other data.
- Establish more flexible, secure, and robust PSAP operations with increased capabilities for sharing data and resources, and more efficient procedures and standards to improve emergency response.
- Enable call access, transfer, and backup among PSAPs and between PSAPs and other authorized emergency organizations that are geographically separated.
- Enable 9-1-1 callers to quickly send more accurate and more useful forms of information about traffic incidents and crashes to 9-1-1 emergency call centers. For example, the NG9-1-1 system will be able to handle a 9-1-1 call from a personal digital assistant (PDA) or computer, receive photo images, data sets, and medically relevant data that can be routed to appropriate emergency medical services.

- Provide a tool for sending location-targeted hazard alerts and evacuation guidance to motorists and other mobile device users through reverse messaging.

Facing NG-9-1-1 Development Challenges

Industry leaders have worked now for years toward the realization of all these benefits, and they continue pressing forward achieving incremental gains toward the goal. With pursuit of any such massive and transformational change there are a myriad of sticking points: gaps in knowledge or technology to be transcended and unforeseen problems to be solved. Private and public-sector Subject Matter Experts (SME) have joined together, for thousands of hours, to address a vast array of technical challenges en route to making the full capabilities of NG9-1-1 a reality.

The success of NG9-1-1 also requires exploring how its roll-out in PSAPs will affect telecommunicator's experience of job stress. Change is always stressful, and the bigger the change, often the greater the stress response. So the roll-out of NG9-1-1 technologies in each center will require the education, involvement, and buy-in of all personnel to help manage the stress involved. It is beyond the scope of this chapter to evaluate the extent to which adaptation to all NG9-1-1 features will or will not impact dispatchers psychologically. My immediate interest is to support consideration of one specific feature enabled by NG9-1-1: live video streaming. It is now possible (when this feature is installed and activated in 9-1-1 centers) for callers to communicate with dispatchers using any device with live-streaming capability; and for field responders to stream video (with audio) to the dispatcher's monitor in real-time from body or car cameras.

The Working Question about RTV...

This RTV capability raises a pair of questions shared by many 9-1-1 leaders and their frontliners as they work to build and connect to NG9-1-1 capabilities:
  1) *What possible psychological impacts might dispatchers experience as they interact with callers and field responders in crisis via real-time video?*
  2) What planning must be done to optimize the 9-1-1Pros psychological adaptation to use of RTV in light of these expected impacts?

First let's explore some of the potentially positive benefits of 9-1-1 interactions via RTV.

Possible Psychological Benefits of RTV

In discussions with 9-1-1Pros, we have identified several possible ways in which seeing actual live images on scene could possibly buffer acute or chronic stress impacts. A few are described here:

- Communication from callers or field responders utilizing real-time video could in some cases increase the quantity and the quality of data. Dispatchers must currently rely only on spoken descriptions to determine what is taking place on scene.
- When those on scene are overwhelmed emotionally or physically incapable of answering questions, dispatchers' stress rises as the likelihood of failed response efforts increases. 9-1-1Pros cannot, for example, currently monitor if the caller is performing CPR on an unconscious person in accordance with the emergency medical protocol instructions. The ability to see this on-scene intervention (when a third party is there to capture the video) could enable the dispatcher to redirect the caller for better success.
- Callers confused about or unfamiliar with their location could show landmarks to the dispatcher to help identify it. Such video guidance can expedite and enrich scene assessment and data collection, resulting in greater likelihood of better outcomes for all involved on scene. And the better a 9-1-1 call's outcome is, the less tragedy a telecommunicator experiences. With each tragic outcome there is the likelihood of a 9-1-1Pro being exposed to traumatic stress. So, to the extent to which RTV increases chances for less tragic outcomes, this technology could actually decrease the telecommunicator's experiences of intense fear, helplessness or horror.
- As many 9-1-1Pros in one of my most recent classes (with a wide range in years of experience) emphasized, sometimes the pictures they *imagine* are worse than the reality. Without the chance to rectify those emotionally charged images, they may carry more distress into the future with them. One telecommunicator explained what several then confirmed: rectifying those images may be one form of "closure"—the chance to square up with the reality on scene to gain a better sense of resolution.
- Even when calls result in poor outcomes, the ability with RTV to gain richer data from the scene could enable the dispatcher to feel increased sense of call mastery, "Even though it didn't turn out well, I know more of what was actually happening, and I know I did all I could." This sense of mastery can (as discussed in Chapter 6) increase how the dispatcher's brain and body work to positively modify production of stress hormones; with greater confidence in the face of

a stressor, cortisol production may join with production of DHEA, known as the "vitality hormone" resulting in less physical and emotional drain.
- These hormonal changes activated by a sense of increased confidence through call mastery can buffer 9-1-1Pros from traumatic stress impacts. Increased sense of call mastery can also boost *compassion satisfaction*, —the intrinsic reward derived from successful caregiving.

Frontliners' Anticipatory Anxiety

Yet dispatchers in my classes often express strong concerns about potential exposures via RTV, including: watching live, possibly violent scenes unfolding in real-time such as suicide attempts and completions, homicide, abuse, or severe injuries at accident scenes, among others. More commonly it has been the 9-1-1Pros with the longest careers in dispatch that state the most emphatic concerns, often with this (or very similar) phrases, "I didn't sign on for that…If I wanted to see all that on scene, I would have been an officer…The day that comes to my center, I'm gone!" We cannot know if this high level of distress about RTV will sustain in actual use upon implementation, or if these most anxious 9-1-1Pros will successfully adapt psychologically. Certainly, their chances of success adapting will be increased by identifying not only the possible benefits, but the possible negative impacts. Clarity about such risks can produce planning steps to ease the adaptation to RTV.

Evaluating Predictable RTV Risks

Our current understanding of factors producing serious traumatic stress impacts can equip us to predict some of the psychological risks of 9-1-1Pro's exposure to potential traumatic events via RTV. Possible risk factors include:

- *Increased Emotional Labor.* Experiencing callers through real-time video will represent an increase in multisensory input by the telecommunicator. Whereas traditionally they are listening to the caller and using their visual imagination, they would now be directly observing the caller's distress. This more intense emotional input could increase the emotional labor required of them. (Emotional labor has to do with the amount of psychological drain experienced in response to a task.) The greater the energy drain from increased emotional labor, the greater the likelihood of burn out (Troxell 137).
- *Increased Risk of Traumatization.* Call mastery can buffer the impacts of traumatic stress as discussed earlier; yet the greater the intensity of

the exposure, the greater the likelihood of traumatization may be for an individual. The real-time image of a person completing suicide with a fire arm who appears (through the monitor) to be only a foot or two away, may be a significantly greater intensity of exposure than if only heard as gunfire on the phone. Many 9-1-1Pros may never have such a call in their careers. Yet, a high percentage of telecommunicators have managed calls from individuals on the verge of completing such a suicide attempt. Seeing the individual in such moments lifting and lowering a weapon can be traumatizing since the 9-1-1Pros are anticipating the completed suicide. This traumatic information may be stored despite a positive outcome.

- In cases like this, there may be *less likelihood of positive hormonal changes*, discussed earlier since the telecommunicator may have now internalized vivid gruesome images of the person's completed suicide.
- *Increased Triggering of Previous Traumas.* Those with a history of traumatization are generally more at risk of developing PTSD in response to later traumatic exposures (Halligan and Yehuda 1). And we can expect that the greater the intensity of these later exposures (as through RTV) to people in dangerous or tragic circumstances, the greater the likelihood of triggering prior traumas. More frequent triggering would then produce greater risks of compromised ability to concentrate and think optimally during such calls.
- *Greater Loss of Control.* Another stressor related to RTV depends on the degree of participation dispatchers have in determining its use at the PSAP, and what those terms of use are. If telecommunicators do not have any option in how to manage use of RTV (e.g., to turn the function on or off on specific calls), their sense of control will be greatly diminished. The less control or influence a person feels they have in the face of a stressor, the greater the likelihood of serious stress impacts. Therefore, industry leaders and 9-1-1 directors must therefore engage frontline dispatchers as they define the terms by which RTV will be used.
- *Potentially Unrealistic Scrutiny.* Additional stress for the telecommunicator is anticipated if they are held responsible for maintaining visual contact with the caller. The nature of dispatching a call requires the telecommunicator to interact with multiple monitors often while communicating with field responders and their coworkers at the same time. Maintaining constant visual contact with a caller on scene is impractical. Yet, if the 9-1-1Pro's performance is evaluated by such an expectation, their stress related to RTV will likely be significantly higher.

9-1-1Pros need assurance that stress risk factors related to RTV will be strategically evaluated with their input, prior to and throughout implementation of RTV. Failure to explore such risks with their involvement could result in lower retention rates among those most anxious. However, I strongly believe that risks related to RTV can be managed to decrease them. Anxiety about future 9-1-1 stressors is driven in part by compounded current 9-1-1 stress. So, RTV stress assessment and planning needs to take place within a more comprehensive PSAP stress management effort. In Part 2 of the chapter, I offer an approach to this effort.

Part 2: Strategic Planning to Manage RTV (and other NG 9-1-1) Stress

Begin with Recognition of Current 9-1-1 Stressors

In the last decade, 9-1-1 Leaders at all levels have gained increasing awareness of *past and current* stress risks associated with the duties of the 9-1-1 telecommunicators. Those risk factors were defined in Chapter 3. In Chapter 4 researcher Michelle Lilly shared her findings substantiating rates of PTSD and clinical depression among our 9-1-1Pros at rates four to five times higher than the rate experienced by the general public. Again, these high rates among 9-1-1Pros are based on their *current* job demands. Current stressors must be strategically addressed to reduce the level of struggle among 9-1-1 personnel before introducing new major stressors such as real-time video. Accordingly, I propose a three step model:

Three Steps to Reduce Stress Related to RTV

STEP 1: *Provide Fundamental Resilience Resources to PSAP Personnel.* 9-1-1Pros can be buffered from the impacts of new stressors such as RTV, when a solid foundation for management of *current* 9-1-1 stressors is already in place. The NENA Standard on Acute/Traumatic and Chronic Stress Management guides the development of this foundation. It defines the eight *resources* that 9-1-1 centers are required to provide as part of their *Comprehensive Stress Management Programs* (CSMP). You'll notice that many chapters of this book have been designed to help support your efforts to build this CSMP:

- ✓ In Chapter 15, I provided a full explanation of these "Eight Solutions" in CSMPs and offered guidance that 9-1-1 leaders and their personnel can follow to build these programs. Then, additional guidance is provided in other chapters related to several of these eight resources…

- ✓ Chapter 9 describes EMDR, one of the Evidence-Based Treatments for traumatic stress called for in the CSMP.
- ✓ Chapter 16 fully defines, and guides PSAPs in developing 9-1-1 Peer Support and *formal* Peer Support Programs.
- ✓ Chapter 17 provides complete information to guide in securing the best possible Employee Assistance Program (EAP) services for your employees

STEP 2: *Identify and Manage Current Work Conditions. While the 9-1-1 center's CSMP will provide needed resources to manage stress,* PSAP's also need to know how employees are impacted by six *work conditions* in the current 9-1-1 workspace (pre-NG9-1-1). I will list each one and give an abbreviated description of how it can be managed to de-stress employees rather than increase their stress levels, according to the Health Safety Executive (Chapter 19):

1. Change: must be well communicated and managed
2. Demand: workload must be realistic and not consistently exceed the resources of the worker
3. Control: the worker is able to have appropriate input into policies that define their work
4. Role: the worker's role is clearly defined and does not clash with the other roles that they are given
5. Relationships: open, honest and respectful communication is welcomed between and within all levels of the organization
6. Support: encouragement and needed resources are provided to manage stress (Mackay 91)

If left unmanaged, these conditions can significantly worsen stress and major performance and costs metrics (including worsening retention and increased costs related to sick leave and FMLA). But the *good news* is that systematic evaluation of these six conditions can lead to effective management of each condition; and this can result in reduced worker stress and improvement in all major metrics of PSAP success including improved personal well-being, morale, performance, and cost containment. Implementation of this systematic evaluation is urged. The contributors to this book provide concrete help to pursue this effort:

- The Chapter 19 Appendix is a tool designed for you to use (along with other resources noted there) to conduct this evaluation and write your plan for successful management of those six conditions.
- Ivan Whitaker's case study in Chapter 20 shows how he achieved those major PSAP metrics by conducting a similar evaluation and planning process.

Note that these first two stress management steps enable PSAPs to build their foundation of support in managing PSAP stressors related to *current 9-1-1 demands*. Without such a foundation, current risks are apt to compound the impacts of new stressors in the NG9-1-1 workspace such as RTV. Yet, with a 9-1-1 center's CSMP in place, along with their plan for effective management of *pre*-NG9-1-1 work conditions, new stressors in the NG9-1-1 workspace can be managed more successfully.

STEP 3: Once you have accomplished Step 2, you will be familiar with the Six Conditions and how to plan for improved stress management related to each *current* condition in the 9-1-1 center. In Step 3 we can use the Six Conditions model again; but this time as a tool to predict and plan specifically for optimal management of RTV as a *future* stressor.

Below, I propose an approach you can take to manage each work condition to optimize RTV use in your PSAP. My goal here was not to create a definitive list of the best steps, but to provide examples of how you can use this model. You can arrive at the best plans for optimizing management of RTV by using this method in team discussions involving personnel from all levels of your agency.

1. Manage **Change** *related to RTV*

Approach: PSAP Leader and personnel explore risk factors associated with RTV prior to implementation. This exploration enables better management of Change by more carefully pursuing three activities:
- *Planning* to effectively manage foreseeable psychological impacts of RTV use
- *Communicating* a message to all personnel regarding plans for RTV use recognizing their concerns, and assuring willingness by managers to listen and carefully consider concerns
- *Checking-in* with frontline dispatchers intermittently after launch of RTV to gauge how they are adapting (stress levels); invite input and recommendations for improving RTV management

2. Manage **Demand** *relatedto* RTV:

Approach: leaders work with frontline 9-1-1Pros to manage rollout and terms of use relating to RTV to assure that demand does not exceed their resources. Leaders also accommodate individual differences among their telecommunicators recognizing that some will manage RTV exposure better than others. This points to one of the challenges with implementation of

RTV in the center; even those who are less impacted on a call by call basis may, if too heavily relied upon, eventually be at higher risk of burnout. So, demand on all employees must be strategically monitored upon implementation regularly. Related steps:
- Education about stress risks, symptoms and skills to self-identify and manage stress
- Assist each RTV user in recognizing their personal threshold for management of RTV. Such a threshold is not easy to identify. This task will require the telecommunicator's self-awareness and a high level of comfort to openly discuss stress with supervisors as it occurs.
- Create tracking tools to help dispatchers and the supervisors monitor the frequency and intensity of RTV calls experienced on a weekly basis as a trigger for check-ins. Consider utilizing your peer support team for this purpose if your agency has one.

3. Manage the Dispatcher's experience of **Control** related to RTV:

Approach: leaders work to increase the telecommunicators' sense of control as the end-user of RTV:
- Actively involve frontline telecommunicators in decision-making about how RTV will be used; consider creating a committee (or using your morale team if you have one) to help build RTV management guidelines.
- Define choices they will have in using or not using RTV on calls. For example: will dispatchers have autonomy in deciding when to turn on or turn off the RTV feature? Will there be guidelines or requirements for call-types with which it must be used?
- Invite 9-1-1Pros to confidentially express their concerns about anticipated RTV experiences prior to launch, and about actual calls on an ongoing basis after implementation.
- Work to support ways of increasing dispatchers' sense of closure after RTV calls within legal limitations.

4. Manage the Dispatcher's **Role** relating to RTV:

Approach: define who will manage RTV calls to assure fit and prevent overload. (You will notice that this concern ties directly to management of Demand as described above.)
- Consider each dispatcher's prior work-exposures to traumatic stress and their impacts. When such impacts have been extensive or intense, privately discuss any concerns you and they may have, how

they expect to experience RTV. Leaders can opt out of assigning those who appear to be at higher risk of negative impacts.
- For all employees using RTV regularly, an option can remain open for re-assignment at intervals or on an as-needed basis to prevent overexposure to RTV, manage stress and avoid overload. Consider rotating assignments between Fire, Police, EMD assignments to dilute the intensity of RTV exposures.
- Leaders are discouraged from assigning personnel to full-time duty engaged in RTV interactions with callers or feel responders as a permanent assignment. Maximum duration of assignment to RTV can be defined, including process for evaluation of employee's well-being as a condition for any additional RTV duty. (Consider use of Professional Quality of Life screening tool for this review purpose. See Chapter 10.)

5. Manage **Relationships** related to RTV

Approach: recognize that if call-takers experience greater stress interacting with callers via RTV, their residual distress may fuel more conflict with their peers. Three leadership activities could help 9-1-1Pros to manage conflict and preserve the health of their peer relations with co-workers:
- Require use (by all personnel) of stress resilience and conflict management skills (assuming training has been provided in these areas).
- Prepare telecommunicators to recognize cues that they are struggling with attitude or negativity; urge them to seek out peer support informally or through a peer support program (if the center operates one).
- Meet with employees struggling with attitude or negativity to explore stress factors (including RTV) before issuing discipline.

6. Manage (assure) **Support** related to RTV

Approach: assure that the center's Comprehensive Stress Management Program is in place and running prior to launching RTV per Step 1 of the three-step plan defined earlier. (This approach assumes a 9-1-1 center is working to establish its CSMP.)
- Regularly encourage all PSAP personnel to use the resources provided for by the CSMP.

- Encourage preventive use of the agency's EAP program for clinical support to monitor RTV emotional impacts. (Inform and recruit EAP Providers about this objective to assure success.)
- Urge all personnel to pursue periodic treatments with EMDR therapy (Chapter 9) to "clear out" traumatic stress from RTV experiences to prevent accumulation.

Conclusions and Recommendations

The three-step model above was offered to assist PSAP leaders in their local efforts to help employees optimize management of current 9-1-1 center stressors and reduce future stress impacts related to RTV. Yet, national leadership is needed to guide and support these local efforts.

Setting a New Standard of Care

Our 9-1-1 associations have provided effective platforms for bringing together local PSAP personnel with 9-1-1 stakeholders from the public and private sectors to build the *technological* functioning of NG9-1-1. This same association-led approach could now be used to prepare our 9-1-1 Professionals to manage the *psychological* aspects of NG9-1-1 demands. In 2010, NENA established the workgroup that wrote the Standard on Acute/Traumatic and Chronic Stress Management in effect since 2013. This original standard was the result of evaluation of traditional 9-1-1 stressors. Therefore, I would encourage reconvening the NENA Stress Workgroup as the forum in which stakeholders could engage in an evaluative process with the goal of updating this existing standard as ANSI (American National Standards Institute) standard. This updated NENA Standard could define how centers can best address RTV and other NG9-1-1 stressors. The Three Step model proposed in this chapter could be considered as a resource for the workgroup as it addresses current and NG9-1-1 stressors.

Any pertinent data from existing workgroup studies about dispatcher perceptions of RTV and adoption NG9-1-1 should be evaluated and considered by the stress workgroup; and, as needed, a large-scale survey to gain more such information is encouraged. Frontline impressions and recommendations about the use of RTV will be an essential part of this assessment. Frontline involvement and cooperation in the design of this interface and terms of use will optimize functionality of this human/machine interface. It will likely boost the dispatcher's confidence as the end-user of RTV.

Funding for Management of NG9-1-1 Stress

Funding for NG9-1-1 implementation should include line items designated specifically to support the three steps of PSAP stress management proposed in this chapter. Stakeholders should also determine how NG9-1-1 funds will be ensured to include training in stress management for all personnel given the current rates of PTSD and the predictable increases in stress related to RTV and NG9-1-1. Dedicated funds are also needed to support 9-1-1 peer support program development to buffer stress related to adaption to NG9-1-1 changes and reduce risks of PTSD, other stress-related illnesses, and depression.

Questions for Reflection

To get the most from this chapter, you are encouraged to write your reflections here (in both the Kindle and paperback versions of this book).

- What was your main take-away from reading this chapter?

- What specifically made it valuable to you?

- How can you apply this take-away concretely to improve some aspect of your personal life and or efforts to support the wellbeing of 9-1-1Pros?

Additional Resources

- Visit the Resources tab at **www.911Training** for updated information and resources to assist with PSAP implementation of CSMPs and NG9-1-1 stress management.

Works Cited

Halligan, Sarah and Rachel Yehuda. "Risk Factors for PTSD." The National Center for Post-Traumatic Stress Disorder PTSD Research Quarterly, vol. 11 no. 3, summer 2000, p. 1, **www.ptsd.va.gov/professional/newsletters/research** quarterly/V11N3.pdf

Mackay, Colin J., et al. "Management Standards and Work Related Stress in the UK: Policy Background and Science." Work & Stress, vol. 18 no. 2, April-June 2004 pp 91-112, www.hse.gov.uk/stress/techpart1.pdf.

Troxell, Roberta. Indirect Exposure to the Trauma of Others: The Experience of 911 Telecommunicators. University of Illinois at Chicago. 2008.

End Notes

[1] The description that follows was originally gathered from the U.S. Department of Transportation (DOT), **http://www.its.dot.gov/ng911/#sthash.Ty14FEy2.dpuf**. This page is no longer available. However, the DOT has prepared a brief video providing a description of NG9-1-1 benefits consistent with the explanation offered in this chapter. It is available at: **https://www.911.gov/ng911movie.html**

CHAPTER 23
"No One Left Behind": Safeguarding the Mental Health of 9-1-1Pros in the Aftermath of Mass Casualties and other High Impact Events

Jim Marshall

Introduction

The headline read, "'The clock is Ticking': Inside the Worst U.S. Maritime Disaster in Decades." This story retells the sad fate of the 790 foot U.S. flagged cargo ship, the El Faro. The freighter and all its crew were lost beneath three miles of vertical water after it was steered into the wall of a Class three hurricane. The Ship's Master, Michael E. Davidson had a distinguished career among his colleagues for his safety-first mentality, "He was by no means a cowboy. He was a by-the-book Mariner with a reputation for being unusually competent and organized" (Langeweische). So, what went wrong? The results of the Coast Guard's massive investigation of this disaster did not lay blame on him. It concluded:

> It was unlikely that there would be a single cause or culprit, because there rarely is. Most significant aviation and shipping disasters, as well as industrial catastrophes, are eventually determined to be "system accidents"—the result of a cascade of small errors, failures, and coincidences. Absent any one of them, and the disaster would not have occurred—a truth that is not knowable in real time, only in retrospect (Langewiesche).

As individuals in our personal lives, and as members of an industry, we strive to do our best. Yet failures are inevitable as we push the envelope to achieve excellence. It is true that we can learn more from our failures than our successes; if we carefully evaluate the factors that led to them and gain new knowledge to guide future pursuits. There are also opportunities to gain critical knowledge from lessons others have learned the hard way. The El Faro was a disaster involving the wreckage of a ship under extreme conditions. A ship carrying, not only cargo worth millions of dollars, but also Davidson, and his crew of 32, lost at sea. A "20 mile stretch of floating dolls from a container that had burst open" (Langewiesche) pointed to the ship's final location on the ocean floor. But the search for survivors recovered no one. Such is the 9-1-1 industry's opportunity considering this cargo ship's fate.

Transferring the Lesson Learned

We could consider the 5,783 PSAPs (NENA) in the United States as being our country's Emergency Response Fleet. Every PSAP in the U.S. is like a ship with its own crew. Always at the ready, 24/7/365, to serve our citizens with medical, fire and law enforcement assistance. Many 9-1-1 centers and their personnel have sustained heavy damage and personal injuries in the line of duty. We know from the Lilly and Allen study (Chapter 9) that our telecommunicators have experienced far higher rates of PTSD, depression and obesity than the general public.

Yet, our PSAPs are not sailing into a calmer psychological forecast. New tragedies rock our communities weekly, demanding physical and emotional resources at levels that may exceed those possessed by our 9-1-1 personnel. The definition of stress is *demand exceeding our resources*. So, the more that a demand exceeds the resources, the greater the toll we can expect. This concern is not alarmist panic. Some of our 9-1-1 leaders in the U.S., who have experienced such events, already know this toll intimately. They, and their most forward-thinking colleagues, have recognized the imperative to commence strategic planning as an industry, and as PSAPs, to minimize the toll on their people, to keep the 9-1-1 ship upright and on course through these storms. This chapter is devoted to supporting such strategic advanced planning, enabling a best-practice care of 9-1-1 Personnel in the aftermath of incidents I call *High Impact Events*.

High Impact Events

I define High-Impact Events (HIE) as those which, because of their magnitude, are more likely to produce intense fear, helplessness or horror in the involved responders than other events. This emotional response to an event in which there was risk of serious injury or death to self or others, can lead to development of PTSD. Examples of high impact events include the following:
- Acts of Terrorism
- Events involving Multiple Fatalities
- Natural Disasters
- Officers Killed
- House Fires with loss of life
- Child Deaths
- Homicide

- Suicides (APA 271)

Innovators in Caring: Charleston County Consolidated 9-1-1 Center in South Carolina

In Chapter 16, I described my working relationship with the CCC 9-1-1 Center. For a couple years I'd been working with Director Jim Lake and Deputy Director Allyson Burrell delivering and supporting resilience initiatives for their team. Jim and Allyson share a very high level of investment in building core resilience skills at their agency. Then, one day in June of 2015, I received a call from Jim. He told me that I needed to come down immediately. The AME church massacre had just occurred and his personnel were deeply affected. But Jim was not looking for me to deliver critical incident debriefing. His request was different. His eyes were not fixed solely on supporting his people through this immediate crisis. As a 9-1-1 industry leader, he saw this event within a bigger picture. On the phone he said, "Jim, we as an industry have got to do more when things like this happen. It's not enough just to do debriefing and then go on with business as usual. We need to build a system that assures no one is left behind; we need to know how our people really are, not just in the short term but in the *long term*."

With these words, Jim Lake defined a mission. For any responder, there are psychological and physical risks. But those risks are higher for those 9-1-1Pros exposed to High Impact Events (especially if already struggling with serious personal stressors). Without fortification of the 9-1-1 center and its personnel prior to such HIEs, a bigger breach in the hull of the PSAP can be expected, potentially resulting in a devastating toll: low morale, impaired performance and greater proneness to error; increased sick/medical leave; and, amidst such a cascade, increased depression, suicide risk, and the loss of good employees. Yet, these risks can be mitigated by well-planned and comprehensive support. Jim knew that failing to plan is planning to fail. He also knew that the 9-1-1 family has the ability to build a model to assure post-event care for 9-1-1 and EMS professionals. Our work together resulted in a model, still under construction, which I call the Post Event Personnel Care Planner (PEPCP). We will explore the PEPCP in Part 2 of this chapter.

Resounding Concern: The Michigan Communication Directors Association (MCDA)

Of course, CCC 9-1-1 Center of South Carolina is not the only PSAP in our country whose employees have been deeply affected by High Impact Events.

Deaths of officers over the years in Michigan prompted 9-1-1 leaders from the Michigan Communication Directors Association MCDA to request two full days of training for the state's directors at their annual meeting. The morning speaker on day one was Maureen Will, the Director of Communications at Newtown Emergency Communication Center (NECC) during the Sandy Hook Elementary School massacre. Maureen told her story about the December 14, 2012 massacre, and what has transpired since. In the afternoon, I helped the directors in processing how they were impacted by her story. Then on day two, I offered training to these leaders on preparing their PSAPs to minimize and manage the psychological toll of High Impact Events.

It's not necessary in this chapter to set out the heart-wrenching details of what took place at the Sandy Hook elementary school in 2012. I doubt that there is a 9-1-1 Professional in North America who did not personally feel pain for the children who died, the families who survived, and for responders who served them all that day. Newtown is a very small community. We know that 9-1-1Pros' exposure to trauma during High Impact Events is worse if they were serving their own family members and personal friends involved in the events. Maureen and her team members at NECC had close friends whose children died that day.

The Power of Preparation in the Face of Tragedy

A leader can be confident that they are reducing employees' psychological risks in the face of increasing demands if they are equipping employees to manage such tragedies. Incredibly, Maureen had led her nine dispatchers through a refresher of their active shooter training just the week before the Sandy Hook incident. Standing before Michigan's 9-1-1 leaders, she was emphatic about the value of this preparation, "I can't imagine what this would've been like for my people if they had not been through that training."

However, Maureen's comments here, and her preparations prior to Sandy Hook were focused not just on optimizing performance. She and local government officials had worked to prepare a support network for the responders. Maureen was blunt in her bottom-line exhortation to her colleagues that day in Michigan, "You must have the stuff in place." She added, "I had my critical incident stress team in place. A lot of other agencies have nothing. Do you know your EAP people?"

These statements strongly emphasize a key point: establishment of the resources called for in the NENA Stress Standard (Chapter 15) are not only important to support for coping with more common day-to-day 9-1-1 stress.

They constitute essential bricks in the 9-1-1 stress management foundation upon which strategic planning for HIE stress depends.

Maureen also struck a chord with the directors in the room when she pointed out that self-care was not just for frontline staff. She chose to seek it for herself. As most leaders, she deferred dealing with her emotions during the events at Sandy Hook until she had cared for her people and knew they were stable. When it was time for her to finally release all the stress and sorrow that was bottled up inside, she sought peer support. But she had criteria, "As a 9-1-1 Pro, when stuff like this happens I don't want to talk to a cop. I need to talk to a manager of a 9-1-1 center—a peer." If you are a 9-1-1 leader, I hope you will re-read and reflect on Maureen's message. The cumulative impact of stress on 9-1-1 leaders is an unspoken, as yet unmeasured, toll. As you follow Maureen's lead in practicing your own self care, you will protect your own well-being as you set an example for your personnel to do likewise.

Protecting Resilience after High Impact Events

The difficult question facing 9-1-1 leaders, as they strive to systematically plan for stress management is, "Where do we begin?" And this brings us back to Jim Lake's initiative in Charleston. He gained the support and cooperation of the County Department of human resources, the leaders of their county's Employee Assistance Program, their medical director, area clinicians and leaders of the county's emergency medical service. This group represents the needed collection of stakeholders to create the HIE support system that Jim desired. My contribution to the Charleston County group as a consulting subject matter expert was to help define the challenge, the goals, possible solutions, and guide formulation of an approach to systematize HIE care of personnel. The result was the Post Event Personnel Planner.

Expediting Post-HIE Care: The PEPCP as an "Open-Source" Model

The PEPCP model is offered for the first time publicly in this chapter, as an "open source" document. It is offered here, not because it is sufficient or complete in its current form, but because it represents an attempt at planning that is essential. The goal of sharing the PEPCP with our readers is to catalyze immediate and deepening collaboration in pursuit of a best-practice model for post-HIE care of 9-1-1 employees (applicable to all emergency responder groups). Several innovative responder agencies in the United States and Canada have already joined in this collaboration and have much to contribute.

Your active involvement can hopefully expedite the reality of this care system in your community before your personnel face future High Impact Events.

A Precedent for PEPCP

In the same way as employees must maintain physical fitness when their jobs require, it is appropriate to require the participation of employees in mental fitness programs. The intent is not to be "Big Brother" over-reaching by imposing care on employees, or intrusively seeking confidential information about their mental health functioning. In the PEPCP model, involvement of PSAP management and supervisory staff in the employees' mental health is pursued only in direct relation to work-related events. This does not, of course, preclude the employee from seeking out additional support of their peer support team, EAP, or private counseling services as desired.

A Top-Down System Assuring Care

The PEPCP is a system that requires top-down ownership and guidance due to the commitment required to establish needed policies, approve its implementation and allot the necessary resources. Yet, the local adaptation of the model will, at its best, be a very collaborative process involving employee input at all levels. It is preferable that employees assume primary responsibility for their mental health, and the PEPCP reinforces this principle. Once leaders commit to implementing an agency post-HIE care system, employees and other stakeholders should be engaged with a clear announcement emphasizing the agency's commitment. The following message is not offered as a script but to convey the gist of the assurance usually needed by employees you want to invest in the process:

"We, as an agency, are committed to doing our very best to assure your well-being as we face High Impact Events such as…. This means we must be systematic in planning how we will respond with support within the PSAP and with the outside resources available to us. Your input will be very important. So, in the days to come you will be invited to participate in building our 'Post Event Personnel Care Plan'…"

When leaders launch the program with a formal message like the one above, employees will be more inclined to invest. The 9-1-1 leader's investment in the PEPCP system is a statement that a new, healthier Emotional Code is embraced by the PSAP. As employees learn the purpose of the PEPCP, they may feel a greater sense of "permission" to admit and proactively seek help when in distress. In this way, the PEPCP becomes a culture changing process.

The Nuts and Bolts of the Post Event Personnel Care Planner

The goal of a systematic post-HIE care model is to assess and deliver the needed support by accomplishing the following tasks when such events occur:
- Identifying who in the PSAP is most affected by the HIE
- Determing the care they need
- Defining who will provide that care and...
- Who will do ongoing follow-up with those employees to assure the support has been given; and...
- Determine the effects of this support.

It can be very cumbersome to implement such a comprehensive system serving all employees using a paper and pencil version. Such a hard-copy version lacks capacity for dynamic communication between PEPCP team members and record keeping preferable for best results. Still *any* PSAP steps of systematic planning and care will offer a vital improvement over doing nothing of the sort. Therefore, the 911 Training Institute is pursuing partnerships to develop a software version of the PEPCP for optimized functioning. This digital version would help employees build and record their care plans with the assistance of a peer supporter (or other staff members). A software version could also enable data collection and analysis to help 9-1-1 leaders track employees' cumulative exposure to HIEs over time, and PEPCP benefits.

The digital version of a more maturely developed PEPCP would also enable prompts for those involved in the care plan. Such prompts could:
- Verify that care plan elements (e.g., peer support, screening tools) were delivered on time and at specified intervals when planned
- Initiate queries about any difficulties with support delivery, the employee's participation, or to identify any needed increases in support when new stressors are experienced on the job since the plan was developed

A Walking Tour through the PEPCP

Below, I have deconstructed the full model of the PEPCP system so that you can more easily see each component as I explain them. We present the model as it is has been prepared in collaboration with a fictitious employee, Brandon Smith. To simplify the explanation of how a care plan is built and its value with all High Impact Event types, I've chosen an event that typically does not involve a large number of employees—a suicide completed during the call. This is designated an HIE, not because of the number of casualties or number of PSAP employees affected, but because of its predictably high impact on Brandon individually. Using a call involving suicide is important for a few other reasons, too. When a dispatcher experiences callers suiciding, they often receive no follow-up support. Sadly, suicide attempts and completions continue to rise in the U.S (Drapeau and McIntosh 1). Suicides are also among the call types most likely to activate intense fear, helplessness, and horror in 9-1-1Pros, introducing the risk of traumatic stress impacts (Troxell).

You will see six figures below showing you the content of each major PEPCP component. You can review the figure first, and then read the explanation that follows. (Remember that the goal in sharing this model is to inspire your collaboration in its improvement. Your questions, comments and ideas for its development are welcomed.)

PEPCP Component A

	A. What role did this employee have in managing this event? (Psychological Proximity)	High to Low
☐	1. Directly Involved AND Family or close friend of those at risk/believed dead	1
☒	2. Directly Involved OR family or close friend of those at risk/believed dead	2
☐	3. On duty with/assisting those directly involved	3
☐	4. Employed @ agency/Off duty	4

Figure 1

The first component of care planning, displayed in figure 1, involves identifying the employee's *Psychological Proximity* to the high-impact event. In this event, Brandon handled the call directly from an individual who completed suicide while still on the phone. This makes his Psychological Proximity a level 2. Had he also personally known or been related to the caller, it would be ranked a Level 1 proximity, the highest. While this approach to ascertaining possible emotional impact is imperfect, it does, along with consideration of other variables, increase the chances of assuring care to those who need it most. It is possible that care plans such as the one here for Brandon would be prepared for many employees in response to a single event. The work required to achieve care planning in that case calls for an active peer support team (see Chapter 16) or dedicated agency volunteers.

Now we want to see how this factor, Psychological Proximity, combines with other factors to help determine the level and types of support Brandon may need.

Component B: Event Intensity Level

B. Select which Options best fit the Intensity Level of this Event

☐ **ECHO** **Extremely High**
- Mass Casualty/Disaster
- Death of responders >1
- High Damage Natural Disaster

☒ **DELTA** **Very High**
ACTUAL OR ANTICIPATED...
- Death/serious injury
- Of Child/single responder
- Suicide Completion during call
- Other death (espec. violent)
- Other (Specify):

☐ **CHARLIE** **High**
- Severe domestic violence
- All other than Echo, Delta

Figure 2

Figure 2 displaying, Component B, seeks to measure the intensity of an event to which the employee (or employees) has been exposed. In the PEPCP we have created a simple system for ranking the *Event Intensity Level*. You can see that there are three levels of Event Intensity. For Brandon Smith the event involved a suicide completed while he was on the phone with the caller. This falls into the Delta or Very High Intensity level of event. While this approach to labeling intensity of events is admittedly somewhat subjective, we are again striving to err on the side of paying attention and offering support versus assuming the employee is "fine" in response to the traditional, cursory check-in, "You good?" The PEPCP model is built on the well-established premise that emergency responders will almost always minimize their distress when asked about it casually, due to their indoctrination into the old "Suck-it-Up" Emotional Code.

While many factors play into how each person experiences an event, we could probably agree that the majority within any group of one hundred telecommunicators would be inclined to rate the intensity of a mass casualty event higher than managing a domestic violence call where one person was severely injured. Yet, notice that domestic violence (without deaths involved) is still listed among HIEs as a Charlie, or high intensity event. While not as intense as a mass casualty event for most 9-1-1Pros, it could still activate intense fear, helplessness and or horror. So, in addition to the support the 9-1-1Pro may need directly related to this event, we must record it, since a number of such events can have a significant cumulative effect.

There may also be employees who have a personal history involving the same type of event (e.g., domestic violence) encountered while call-taking or dispatching. This history may be reactivated, increasing the intensity of their response to the event and its psychological impact. The employee will therefore have a greater need for help. The employee can choose to note such past events in their PEPCP so that any new calls they take involving significant violence would be flagged, prompting a member of the peer support team or supervisor to offer support.

As you can see, consideration of these first two components is not rocket science. It is simply a way of *trying* to more carefully think about the level of support an employee may need.

Component C: Checking Subjective Units of Disturbance (SUD) (Emdria)

C. Privately ask the employee: *"How distressed about this event do you feel right now, on a scale from 0 to 10?"*	Record Here: " 6 "
D. Specify highest intensity in past ECHO, DELTA, or CHARLIE event for employee: E	
E. Which role did the employee have in this past event? See above: 1 2 3 4	1
F. Clinical Use Only. 911 Center personnel can continue with part F, *Selecting Care Components*	
Was the individual mentally Stable recently prior to the event?	
Any personal History of Mental Illness?	

Figure 3

Figure 3 displays four additional components of the PEPCP. Component C is a quick and unobtrusive check of the employee's level of disturbance, from zero to ten. This is a subjective measure (based on the employee's own sense of their mental state) and does not require a clinician to complete. It can easily be completed with Brandon and one PEPCP support peer during a personal check-in as soon after the event as is possible. If a peer support team is not in place at your PSAP, other PEPCP-trained personnel could be designated, with at least one back-up helper per shift in case the designated helper is sick or otherwise unavailable.

This helper simply asks Brandon, "How distressed do you feel about the event right now on a scale from zero to ten?" This type of inquiry may seem mechanical and awkward, but when a peer supporter or supervisor joins with a fellow 9-1-1Pro with warmth and sincere concern, the peer has reason to be appreciative and cooperative. It is also important to keep in mind that once the PEPCP program is announced and PSAP members understand the process, they can self-initiate the planning. This is a collaborative process.

Again, seeking the peers' SUD is not a clinical action, since no diagnostic or clinical interpretation is performed. A peer supporter is simply helping their co-worker gauge their distress. Since emergency responders are inclined to minimize the intensity of their emotional distress, they often report a lower number, indicating less distress than they actually feel. The helper will simply record that number. Whether the employee reports a number that accurately or inaccurately reflects their true state, they will likely be more attuned to their distress; and "noticing the cues to do something smart for you" can empower the 9-1-1Pro to recognize that they are at a ChoicePoint (Chapter 6)—a moment in which activating the resilience skillset will protect them.

Component D: Identifying the Employee's Past Experience(s) of HIEs and Component E: Employee's Role in Past HIEs

Component D, in Figure 3, seeks to identify the 9-1-1Pro's experience with HIEs prior to the current event; and Component E identifies his Psychological Proximity to these past HIEs. Gaining such knowledge is critical since there is greater likelihood of developing PTSD when exposed to multiple traumatic events. In Brandon's PSAP work history he had been directly involved as the call taker in an incident in which one of their agency's field responders had been killed in the line of duty. This is Level 1 Psychological Proximity—the very highest. So, psychological impact can be expected to be the greatest. And this was a Delta or Very High Intensity Level event. By seeking and officially recording this history, it is possible (if Brandon acknowledges ongoing struggles) that his PEPCP will create a long-overdue opportunity for Evidence-Based Treatment. The history will also produce an extra "flag" (in the software version) prompting immediate clinical evaluation and probable urging to pursue trauma therapy.

Given this fact, the sit-down meeting to complete the PEPCP should (within reason) include asking about the number and level of all HIEs the employee has experienced. Typically, no such record is kept in comm centers, increasing the likelihood that psychological damage has not been adequately accounted for. As a result, the employee will be at an increased risk of stress-related problems. Without the PEPCP, Brandon's peers may have little knowledge of his past exposure to HIEs, especially if he is a new employee or usually works on other squads. The PEPCP provides this information as a basis for intensified peer support and guidance to other resources fitting his actual needs. This brings us to Component F.

Component F: Clinical Use Only

This section of the PEPCP, also shown in Figure 3, is meant to be used by clinicians only. Given Brandon's past and present experiences with HIEs, his PSAP manager will likely require him to seek a clinical evaluation. This directive would be initiated as a best-practice standard for all personnel with similar HIE exposures. The purpose of this clinical evaluation is to assess Brandon's current status related to his exposure to current and past HIEs. With Brandon's permission, *after* the remainder of the PEPCP form is completed, it will be provided to the clinician. Component F conveys an expectation that the mental health professional will, as part of their evaluation, explore two factors: the mental status of the employee prior to the HIE that prompted the referral, and any personal history of mental illness.

This clinical information is of course confidential and none of it is shared with the PSAP. Yet, it upholds another aspect of a best-practice standard for 9-1-1 mental health care: that a clinician is often essential to assure professional assessment of past traumatic impacts and the 9-1-1Pro's history of mental illness. This is not a role, nor is it the business of PSAP personnel in lay-support roles. Still, prevention efforts and effective treatment planning must both be based on this knowledge. The PEPCP supports PSAP personnel in reaching clinical care, helping the employee inform the clinician about their 9-1-1 experience prompting the need, and about the PSAP's effort to provide them with a full spectrum of resources. The identification of such resources is the work achieved in the next section of the PEPCP, Component G.

Component G: Employee Plan Care Options (Resources)

"No One Left Behind"

G. Plan Care Options	1ˢᵗ 24 hrs	72 hrs	Week 1	@ 1 Mo.	@ 3 Mo.	@ 6 Mo.	@ 12 Mo.
1. Leader Care Response	"Leader" may include supervisors, 911 director or designee(s)						
a. 911 Director/Designee: 1:1	X or as able X						
b. 1:1 w/Fl. Spvsr. (after A. thru E.)	X	X	X	X	X	X	X
2. 1:1 Peer Support	*Note:* Peer Supporters operate and are activated for duty in accordance with local PSAP policy or the directive of the director or his designee(s).						
a. Initial 1:1 meeting w/Educ. Info.		X					
b. ProQOL (Screen: Comp. Fatigue)		X				X	X
c. Refer to Director or D.D. (PRN)	X						
d. Seek Peer Supervision		X					
e. Continued 1:1 Support			X	X	X	X	X
d. Make Clinical Referral		X					

Instructions: Place an "X" by options to be included in the care plan. When the activity is completed, circle the "X"

Figure 4

Figure 4 shows component G of the PEPCP, *Plan Care Options*. In the far left column you see two of several care options (or resource) to be considered for every employee after HIEs. In accord with Jim Lake's recognition, that support for 9-1-1Pros after HIE's must be sustained beyond the initial crisis, the PEPCP extends planning through one year from the date of the HIE prompting care planning. Following from left to right (corresponding to the vertical listing of the care options), you can see intervals of time at which these and any available care options (resources) services can be arranged. Additional contacts can of course be made, but this is the bare minimum that Brandon will receive.

The first care option listed in Component G is the opportunity for Brandon to share supportive one-on-one time with *9-1-1 Director or their designee*, and, one-one-one with the floor supervisor. He chose both options to occur within the first 24 to 72 hours. Given Brandon's Psychological Proximity to the current HIE and past HIEs defined earlier, he and his peer supporter agree it would be important for him to take advantage of these one-on-ones. This level of support was especially valuable since he was quite disturbed by the caller's suicide. Of course, it is more difficult for a director of a large agency to provide individual attention to every employee who may be affected by an HIE. Yet, a sincere effort by the director, or their designee, can lend powerful encouragement to struggling employees.

The next resource Brandon selected for support was *Peer Support*. This extends beyond the initial planning help he received building his PEPCP. It refers to official Peer Support assistance (Chapter 16) which your agency may or may not offer as part of a formal peer support program. As Figure 4 shows, with encouragement from his PEPCP helper, Brandon chose to have an initial one-on-one with a Peer Supporter within 72 hours, to talk and get more information about PTSD. At this time, the peer supporter also gave him the name of the vetted trauma therapist to pursue evaluation and possible treatment with EMDR. Brandon also chose to do one-on-ones with his Peer Supporter at intervals beginning within one week of the HIE, then at one month, three, six, and twelve months from the event.

Figure 4 shows that the Peer Supporter also helped him complete the *ProQOL*, the *Professional Quality of Life* screening tool as part of their best-practice HIE care system. The ProQOL can be self-administered and is an empirically-supported measure of possible struggles with compassion fatigue involving burnout and vicarious or secondary traumatization. (See Chapter 10, Additional Resources for more information about this tool and to access it at no charge.)

Instructions: Place an "X" by options to be included in the care plan. When the activity is completed, circle the "X"								
G. Plan Care Options ➡	1st 24 hrs	72 hrs	Week 1	@ 1 Mo.	@ 3 Mo.	@ 6 Mo.	@ 12 Mo.	
3. Clinical Referrals to:	*Note:* Clinical Referrals may be self activated or initiated by the director or his/her Designee(s) according to terms established in PSAP SOP.							
a. Initial Trauma Assess. (EAP)								
b. Initial Trauma Assess (EMDR clin.)		X						
c. Emergency Psychiatric Eval.								
d. Family Physician								
e. Fit-for-Duty Examination								

Figure 5

Figure 5 represents the third category of resources available in the menu of services involving *Clinical Referrals*. Option "a" involves activating an initial trauma assessment through the employee assistance program. Yet, the EAP used by Brandon's agency was not qualified to administer these assessments. (Please see Chapter 17 for more information about EAPs.) For this reason, the Peer Supporter, after consulting with the PSAP manager, requested Brandon pursue option "b" a trauma assessment by an EMDR therapist. Brandon also wanted this appointment for two reasons. First, he knew that the earlier HIE, involving the death of his officer, had deeply affected him and now it was clear he needed to pursue healing. Second, he could have his assessment and treatment from the same person; if he had gone to the EAP for evaluation, they still would (or should) have referred him out for Evidence-Based Treatment for suspected post-traumatic stress struggles. Transitioning between therapists can be emotionally more difficult, especially for a first responder who is hesitant about seeing a therapist.

Option "c" involves assisting an employee in seeking an emergency psychiatric evaluation. Training in the use of the PEPCP program is required for a peer, with support (or directive of the director or designee) to facilitate such a referral. We certainly do not want to rush a peer off to the emergency department when it is not necessary. Yet, a referral to a psychiatrist must be pursued, as when there is a risk of suicide for the employee. Family physicians may also be important resources for an employee to seek when they describe or exhibit physical problems requiring medical attention.

The last care option in this group involves directing an employee to a *fit-for-duty evaluation*. This is not a step that would be prompted by, or the responsibility of, a Peer Supporter or any other employee. This is the decision of the director, or manager, of a comm center when the employee's performance is clearly in jeopardy related to mental struggles; making such an evaluation essential to restoring the employee's ability to work.

Instructions: Place an "X" by options to be included in the care plan. When the activity is completed, circle the "X"								
G. Plan Care Options ⇒	1st 24 hrs	72 hrs	Week 1	@ 1 Mo.	@ 3 Mo.	@ 6 Mo.	@ 12 Mo.	
4. Self-Help Activities	*Note:* "Clinic." indicates that the tool must be scored and interpreted by a clinician. "Self" means that the tool can be self scored and interpreted using instructions.							
a. Initial Resilience Training	Done 2014)						
b. Review/Practice of Resil. Skills		X	X	X	X	X	X
c. Health Incentivizing Program							
d. Support Group:_____							
e. Give SafeCallNow.org #, PRN	X						

Figure 6

Figure 6 shows Self-Help Activities Brandon can choose from (and may be encouraged by his PEPCP helper/Peer Supporter). This list is certainly not exhaustive and will vary based upon resources available in your service area. Item "a," Initial Resilience Training, assumes that employees in his agency have already received such training. It has been several years since Brandon participated in this training, so his Peer Supporter encourages him to review and practice the resilience skills in the course workbook on a regular basis throughout the next year. Because of the intensity of the current event, and Brandon's possible need for care beyond regular working hours, his Peer Supporter gave him the number for a crisis hotline. He encouraged Brandon to call this number anytime, 24/7, if struggling significantly, even if not in an emergency. Brandon was not at risk, but this referral to the crisis hotline was a good interim step before he could get in to see a therapist.

You will notice that the self-help options include use of support groups. Agencies who have established peer support programs or a PEPCP program can create a resource guide including such groups and all other area resources to accompany the PEPCP.

Summary: The PEPCP is built on several premises:

- To assure the value of the PEPCP, each PSAP should seek access for personnel to a full range of resources. These resources, cited in the figures above, are defined in the NENA Stress Standard and are thoroughly discussed in Chapter 15. As you can see from the discussion of Brandon's case, Peer Supporters and a formal 9-1-1 Peer Support Program serve an important role in creating a PEPCP for their co-workers; and they provide uniquely powerful ongoing support that 9-1-1Pros in every PSAP need in the aftermath of HIEs (see Chapter 16 for guidance building a program). When a trained Peer Support Team has not yet been established in a 9-1-1 center, the coworkers helping build and monitor success of the PEPCP can be a small group of peers trained specifically for this more limited yet vital purpose. Still every effort should be made, perhaps in coordination with other area PSAPs, to establish a Peer Support Team in accord with the NENA Stress Standard.
- Support and resources in an employee's PEPCP can extend over any duration of time fitting the intensity of the event, the employees psychological proximity to the event, their history of prior HIE experiences, and their expressed need when planning occurs.
- Establishing the PEPCP care system at your center will require a working relationship between the PSAP, the agency's Employee Assistance Program and other area clinicians specializing in traumatic stress. Such pre-established relationships with clinicians increases their value as a resource, and the likelihood of their availability on an urgent or emergent basis.

Conclusion

Brandon may be fictitious, but his experience with HIEs is a reality many of our 9-1-1 Professionals have faced and by which they have been deeply affected. Hopefully you can see how capturing a visible map of his exposure to High Impact Events serves toheighten recognition of an employee's need for personal care planning; and the likelihood that follow-through will occur, assuring that such care will occur. By contrast, without any system, benign neglect is apt to lead to a failure of support for, and self-care planning by, Brandon. Traditionally, the cursory, "You okay?" check-in may yield little seeking or offering of meaningful support.

The PEPCP model is still evolving and will hopefully continue to improve with input from frontline telecommunicators, whom I call the "Console SME"--Subject Matter Experts, joined by their PSAP leaders, and a wide variety of other subject matter experts. There is a critical need to systematize care of our very first responders in the aftermath of High Impact Events. Just as Maureen Will emphasized, the only way to manage the aftermath of an event is to plan for it effectively before it occurs. This is certainly the way in which emergency responders are trained and maintain preparedness for other predictable scenarios in the field. It is wisest to predict that nearly all of our 9-1-1 Professionals will personally experience an HIE during their career. Their future, and the vitality of our 9-1-1 system, depends on safeguarding their well-being before and after High Impact Events. Innovative 9-1-1 leaders have already begun this pursuit. I hope you will join them so that *no one is left behind!*

ఌఞ

Questions for Reflection

To get the most from this chapter, you are encouraged to write your reflections here (in both the Kindle and paperback versions of this book).

- What was your main take-away from reading this chapter?

- What specifically made it valuable to you?

- How can you apply this take-away concretely to improve some aspect of your personal life and or efforts to support the wellbeing of 9-1-1Pros?

Additional Resources

- All 9-1-1 personnel are encouraged to know about, and consider using (and referring others to use) the National Suicide Prevention Life Line, a fully confidential 24/7/365 help line . Their number is 800-4273-8255. Also consider the Crisis Text Line by texting HOME to at 741741 in the United States.

- Learn more about the Professional Quality of Life (ProQOL) screening tool and Compassion Fatigue in Chapter 10 and at **https://www.911training.net/help-for-compassion-fatigue**.

Works Cited

"9-1-1 Statistics." *NENA,* December 2017, **www.nena.org/default.asp?page=911Statistics**.

"What is the Actual EMDR Session Like?" *Emdria,* emdria.site-ym.com/?120.

American Psychiatric Association (APA). *Diagnostic and Statistical Manual of Mental Disorders* (5th ed.). American Psychiatric Publishing, 2013.

Drapeau, Christopher. and John McIntosh. "U.S.A Suicide 2016: Official Final Data." *American Association of Suicidology*, 24 December 2017, www.suicidology.org/Portals/14/docs/Resources/FactSheets/2016 2016datapgsv1b.pdf?ver=2018-01-15-211057-387.

Langewiesche, William. "The Clock is Ticking: Inside the Worst U.S. Maritime Disaster in Decades." *Vanity Fair,* 4 April 2018, flip.it/30dZv8.

Troxell, Roberta. *Indirect Exposure to the Trauma of Others: The Experience of 9-1-1 Telecommunicators.* University of Illinois at Chicago, 2008, pqdtopen.proquest.com/doc/304351154.html?FMT=AI.

End Notes

[1] Neither Jim Lake nor Charleston County (SC) bear any responsibility for the information shared in this chapter. The PEPCP model is the intellectual property of the 9-1-1 Training Institute. While we retain rights to the electronic version of this model, it is offered to our 9-1-1 industry and interested stakeholders in its current

version as an "open source" document. Readers are encouraged to collaborate in further development of the PEPCP and email correspondence is welcome. Jim@911Training.net.

AFTERWORD

Jim Marshall

The Resilient 9-1-1 Professional is a response to a need for support expressed by many hundreds of emergency responders and their leaders over more than a decade. I recognize that, while comprehensive, this book is far from exhaustive in providing the leadership needed to fully advance 9-1-1 resilience. Nonetheless, the contributors have strived to create for you a type of 9-1-1 resource that did not exist prior to its publication. This volume has sought to offer clear definitions and thorough discussion about the major stress challenges facing our 9-1-1 Professionals. We have also sought to provide solutions to these challenges in several forms: *personal steps* the contributors have taken to overcome individual struggles common among emergency responders; *organizational solutions* that 9-1-1 leaders have used successfully to manage stress, boost morale and improve their organization's success overall; and, finally, we've offered *strategic models* that leaders and their personnel can use to address the most complex challenges our PSAPs now face heading into the future.

In *The Resilient 9-1-1 Professional* we have emphasized that there are no "cookie cutter solutions" to 9-1-1 stress challenges, on the personal or organizational levels. Yet, there is enormous cause for confidence as frontline dispatchers, their supervisors and their directors, joined by other 9-1-1 stakeholders, share responsibility for optimizing 9-1-1 health and performance. This success can certainly be achieved if stakeholders rally the same level of dedication to this cause as has produced extraordinary technological advances in the industry since the first 9-1-1 call in 1968. We hope you have found new insights, concrete examples, and the guidance you need to do your part to support the people upon whom the entire emergency response system depends.

This book is offered not as a conclusive guide to 9-1-1 resilience but as a foundation for catalyzing broader, deeper collaboration between all those who care for our Very First Responders. Be sure to visit **www.911Training.net** for more resources to assist you in your efforts. We also welcome ongoing email correspondence in support of this collaboration:
info@911Training.net.

ACKNOWLEDGMENTS

On behalf of co-editor, Tracey Laorenza and myself, I wish to express a most heart-felt thank you to those who have inspired, taught, and joined in the work that led to writing *The Resilient 9-1-1 Professional*. I am grateful to the dispatchers who have been my teachers all these years; for accepting me into your hidden world and for entrusting me to co-teach with you in the classroom; and to the 9-1-1 leaders in my home state of Michigan who, because of their concern for their people, also accepted this outsider "psychology guy" as part of the 9-1-1 family: Jamel Anderson, Cherie Bartram, Harriet Miller-Brown, Chris Collum, Bob Currier, Rich Feole, Jim Fyvie, Lisa Hall, Tim McKee, Kim Ostin, the greatly missed Jerry Tapper, Jeff Troyer, and Jim Valentine. They also gifted me with the confidence to pursue the mission of 9-1-1 wellness to the greater 9-1-1 family in the U.S.

I am thankful for Rick Jones who listened and first recognized the need for a national standard on 9-1-1 stress management, and who inspired the 2010 launch of the NENA Stress Workgroup. Dee Ann Summersett faithfully co-chaired the workgroup through to completion of the *Standard on Acute/Traumatic and Chronic Stress Management*. Early on, Dr. Bob Cobb and Ty Wooten listened too, and they affirmed the need to put strategic pursuit of 9-1-1 wellness at the top of the industry's agenda.

Jim Lanier co-founded the 911 Wellness Foundation (911WF) and has been my chief collaborator in this cause. Members of the 911WF Board of Directors have lived out the Foundation's mission by enriching our vision, and in their daily service to the industry: Michael Armitage, Natalie Duran, Jay Fitch, Rick Galway, Sara Gilman, Jan Myers, Lora Reed, Dee Ann Summersett, and Jennifer Vanderstelt (deceased). I am grateful to Ron Bloom, Buster Brown, Allyson Burrell, Laurie Flaherty, Lori Forrer, Bill Hinkle, Jim Lake, Ricardo Martinez, Steve Overton, Carlynn Page, and Laurel Simmermeyer. Each of these individuals has uniquely encouraged me.

A big thank you is due to Deborah Gagnon and Ryan Dedmon of the 911 Training Institute for their extraordinary support. I have deep appreciation for my co-editor Tracey Laorenza, a friend and colleague whose writing gifts and 9-1-1 expertise have been invaluable to this book.

Acknowledgments

Finally, I want to thank my wife, Linda Marshall, a faithful life partner and the book's final line-by-line proofreader; and my daughters Ami and Abbi, who know, more than anyone else, that I am still learning to live up to what is written in these pages.

JM

In addition to Jim's thank yous, I would also like to acknowledge some of those for whom this book was written. I have worked alongside some of the finest dispatchers I have had the pleasure of knowing. To the nameless, faceless voices on the other side, thank you for being who you are and for providing such an invaluable service. Not only to the citizens you serve, but to the men and women of your police, fire, ambulance, and public safety departments with whom you work. Without you, there would be chaos. I tip my headset to all of you.

And, like Jim, I have also learned why life-partners are given thanks. In a way they are much like a dispatcher—in the background, handling the distress, angst, and, at times, the lack of faith that everything will work out. So, to the one who helped me find my voice, and encouraged me at every turn, John Trask, I thank you for being my best friend and biggest cheerleader.

Without the help and support of those we have recognized here, this book would not have been possible.

TL

APPENDICES

CHAPTER 17 APPENDIX
Assuring Best Practice in 9-1-1 Employee Assistance Programs

Prepared by Jim Marshall, 911 Training Institute

Scope of Document

This document is intended for use by 9-1-1 directors, their governing bodies and Employee Assistance Program (EAP) with whom they are currently in (or are considering entering into) a contractual relationship. While it offers important information to promote best practice in delivery of EAP services to 9-1-1 centers, it should be considered introductory. Readers are encouraged to read the full chapter for more extensive guidance.

The Purpose of an EAP

The EAP's purpose in contractual relationship with a 9-1-1 center is to provide initial mental health and counseling services at no charge to the employee for a limited number of sessions to incentivize the employee to take initiative for self-care. The goal of such participation (which is confirmed generally by research findings on EAP value) is to prevent development and persistence of psychological problems negatively impacting work performance and retention. As a fundamental expectation of a typical EAP service contract, the EAP provider organization agrees to serve as the first point of contact for employees in distress, though often not for those in crisis. So, once the leaders of a 9-1-1 center (or their governing agency) establish a contractual relationship with an EAP provider, all employees should be informed initially (and periodically reminded) of the available services, the terms by which those are delivered, and how the EAP can be contacted when needed.

A Standard for Best Practice in Selecting EAP Providers

Most 9-1-1 centers (except some dispatch authorities with their own governing boards and private EMS companies) who have EAP benefits receive those services from the EAP provider contracted by their city, county or state governments. Therefore, directors of 9-1-1 centers are typically not involved in original selection of the EAP provider. They may face real limitations in how much they can influence this selection or decisions about EAP contract renewal. The hope is that the information in this document will empower directors to make their *best effort* to educate and influence their organization's EAP decision makers.

Clinician Qualifications to Provide EAP Services to 9-1-1 Professionals

9-1-1 centers and their governing bodies should make every effort to identify and contract with an EAP provider adequately staffed by clinicians who meet the following criteria:
- Specialize in the assessment and treatment of traumatic stress or can expedite referral to those who are so specialized in your community
- Possess expert knowledge about psychological resilience and related skills training
- Have extensive experience utilizing Evidence-Based Treatment (EBT) for PTSD or be prepared to expedite referral to those who do have this experience.
- Are knowledgeable (or willing, as a condition of their EAP contract, to become fully knowledgeable) about the distinct characteristics of the 9-1-1 profession and its culture, and the greater emergency response culture.
- If, in the event the EAP clinicians cannot fulfill the above criteria, they should be trained to effectively screen 9-1-1 employees for PTSD and other serious mental struggles, and to be aware of and refer to those area clinicians who are qualified as defined above.

Special Considerations for Clinicians and agencies seeking to offer EAPs to 9-1-1

9-1-1 telecommunicators collectively represent what is called a *special treatment population*. Such populations are composed of individuals who share specific characteristics that must be recognized by the clinician if assessment and treatment are to be effective. Other special treatment populations include military personnel, police officers, survivors of mass casualty events, certain indigenous people groups, etc. The value of recognizing such groups is that their members are known to struggle with certain mental health problems at a greater rate and with different underlying issues compared to the general population; and members of a special population may have particular beliefs and views related to mental health services that increase their ambivalence about accepting help. Thus, they are at greater risk of not receiving the services they need because they are less apt to seek them and or because mental health providers are not equipped to treat them effectively.

These considerations about special treatment populations apply to 9-1-1 employees and must serve as the foundation for your agency's decisions in selecting the clinical providers and organizations that will be tasked with caring for these personnel. The 9-1-1 employee's ability to accept and participate in mental health services will require that selected clinicians have an understanding of their distinct culture and be qualified to treat the mental health issues to which they are especially at risk. When a 9-1-1 employee elects to seek such services, we can expect that they are in an emotionally vulnerable state and likely ambivalent about openly acknowledging their psychological struggles.

Leaders will be most likely to succeed in selecting an EAP if they keep this first critical moment of initial contact between their employees and a clinician in mind—and all that may be riding on it for the individual and the agency. The information below is provided to increase awareness of EAP providers about 9-1-1 professionals as a special population and the importance of care that recognizes them as such.

9-1-1 as part of the Law Enforcement Culture

The 9-1-1 profession is a subculture of the nation's Law Enforcement Agencies (LEAS, in which 90% of our 9-1-1 centers are still housed). Law Enforcement Officers (LEO) and 9-1-1 telecommunicators share a skepticism of mental health due to a stigma perpetuated in this culture summed up in the motto: *mental health services are for the weak and are not likely helpful*. Police and 9-1-1 professionals ("9-1-1Pros") both often expect that non-emergency responder personnel from such agencies will not "get what we go through"—a belief that is unfortunately often confirmed when they attempt to seek help from well-meaning clinicians who do not specialize in treatment of first responders and miss the mark in their care responses. The stigma and belief noted here are then perpetuated when such treatment failures occur since these emergency responders, as members of any close-knit group, will talk about their experience (selectively), leading to underutilization of services.

9-1-1 as its Own Culture

In addition to these characteristics shared by LEOs, 9-1-1 is also its own group possessing very distinct characteristics. While 9-1-1 professionals share an increased risk of Post-Traumatic Stress Disorder with LEOs, they appear to have a significantly higher rate of PTSD than LEO and firefighters. This has obvious and major implications for the foci of clinical assessment. It is also a key factor related to another distinction of the 9-1-1 community: telecommunicators have experienced a long history during which their role as the Very First Responder has been largely undervalued despite their extraordinary exposure to traumatic events. As a result, 9-1-1Pros are especially sensitive to how their profession is perceived by those outside their profession, including mental health professionals. So, during an initial session when seeking help for work-related stress issues, the telecommunicator is inclined to quickly dismiss a clinician viewed as ignorant about the 9-1-1 profession and that lacks knowledge or at least a humble curiosity about stressors unique to 9-1-1 telecommunicators. The clinician treating these professionals must be psychologically prepared to tolerate extremely emotionally impacting material common in telecommunicators' work experience.

Summary and Implications

It is an ethical responsibility of the 9-1-1 center leadership, whenever possible, to seek contractual relationships with those clinicians who are qualified to treat 9-1-1 telecommunicators. There are significant ramifications if clinicians unqualified to understand, assess and treat 9-1-1Pros staff the EAP: dispatchers will be discouraged by the care they receive resulting in low participation rates; a higher rate of treatment failure; and thus, a higher risk of ongoing stress-related problems impacting personal health, professional performance and the well-being of the 9-1-1 center culture. The information in this document (and the chapter it accompanies) can help 9-1-1 leaders as advocates for their personnel to define and communicate criteria essential to EAP success.

For a thorough introduction for clinicians to the 9-1-1 culture and delivery of evidence-based treatment to this population, see *Reaching the unseen first responder with EMDR therapy: Treating 9-1-1 trauma in emergency telecommunicators.* Marshall, J., & Gilman Sara G. (2015). In M. Luber (Ed.), **Eye Movement Desensitization and Reprocessing (EMDR) Therapy Scripted Protocols and Summary Sheets: Treating Trauma- and Stressor-Related Conditions** (pp. 185-216). New York, NY: Springer Publishing Co.

See also **https://www.9-1-1training.net/seeking-personal-help** where we define what we see as a Best Practice standard and offer insight for clinicians seeking to serve 9-1-1 with EAPs.

CHAPTER 19 APPENDIX
A PSAP Project Guide: Optimizing Six Key PSAP Workplace Conditions

Introduction

Organizations struggle more with problems of many kinds when major stressors are not identified and addressed in the workplace. The Health Safety Executive (HSE) of The United Kingdom has identified six conditions which "…if not properly managed, are associated with poor health and wellbeing, lower productivity and increased sickness absence" (4). These work conditions, which we'll define soon, are:
- Demand
- Control
- Support
- Relationships
- Role
- Change

In essence, these six work conditions represent stress *risk factors*. We have prepared this guide, based on the HSE model, to assist your PSAP in evaluating and planning related to each of these conditions. This process can help you safeguard your employee's resilience, morale, and performance. We will share HSE's definition of all six conditions and then offer you a set of questions to evaluate each of them as risk factors at your PSAP. These questions will also help your team explore and plan strategies to reduce these risks by improving conditions. (The HSE has created a workbook that offers background, detail, and guidance related to this planning model. You can download the workbook here: **http://www.hse.gov.uk/pubns/wbk01.htm.** . While it may be impractical to follow the full HSE model as set forth in the workbook, we highly encourage you to review this tremendous resource in preparation for launching your project.)

Our premise for this project and guide is for you to gain the most valuable information about your PSAP. In order to do that, your evaluation and planning process must strategically engage your employees at all levels of the organization, since they all help shape, and are affected by, those six work conditions.

We propose that you create a formal Resilience Optimization Team for this purpose. (You may prefer to call it a Morale Team or Committee. The name isn't as important as the function.)

Four Action Steps to Launch Your Team

We encourage you to consider taking the following steps in leading your initiative to optimize PSAP work conditions:

1. *Establish* a *Resilience Optimization Team* at your PSAP. (9-1-1 centers have in recent years established "Wellness Committees" or teams. These groups often are more informal and focus more generally on promoting a healthy employee lifestyle. Such groups are important and may either continue independent of the Resilience Optimization Team or, at the leader's discretion, expand their mission to include the tasks outlined here.) Using this team approach, busy leaders can share the load and expedite progress, and avoid planning errors that arise from isolated decision making.
2. Select members from each level of your organization to assure fully representative input. Think strategically about how your group members will be selected: directly by you, by anonymous recommendation or vote of peers, or by just welcoming volunteers. Ensure that line level staff telecommunicators are adequately represented (do not assume that Supervisors speak for the telecommunicators). Consider one telecommunicator from each shift, or at least one telecommunicator representing day shift and one for night shift.
3. Before convening the first meeting of your team, provide members with a clear statement of the group's purpose (see the conclusion of Chapter 19); and consider sharing copies of Chapter 19 to help them grasp the big picture of what you are seeking to accomplish for the center.
4. Convene an initial meeting of your team to:

a. *Reaffirm your goal and the group's purpose:* to do everything possible to support the well-being of all personnel, and to optimize performance. (Consider explaining how this project matters to you, personally. Include any key insights you might have gathered from Chapter 19 and the rest of the book, that may help your team understand and trust the sincerity of your motive for the project.). If there is currently an environment of mistrust between line staff and leadership/supervision, then the leader should strongly consider meeting first with the line staff representatives only to assure them that they are supported by the leader, and that their input is critical to the success of this team. This can also provide an invaluable opportunity for the leader to receive frank and candid feedback on the perceptions of the line staff as it relates to levels of trust. Without trust there is no true relationship.
b. *Introduce this project* and the importance of their participation, based on Chapter 19, and per the Introduction and Premise above. The goal of this first meeting and discussion is to assure your personnel of your investment in this project and get them actively engaged with you in real discussion about optimizing your PSAP work conditions. (So be sure to invite, and make space for, open discussion about Chapter 19).
c. Define the six work conditions you want to evaluate and optimize at your center (see the next section of this guide)
d. Lead your group in an exploratory exercise with the first work condition, Demand, using the questions in the next section. Explain that your objective for this discussion is not to make official plans or produce a product, though many valuable ideas may result. It is just to help the group practice functioning together cohesively, relating as a team to each other and to the evaluation and planning process they will be using through the coming weeks. Before beginning this exploration, offer the following assurances, which will also apply to all future meetings:

i. As a leader, you have only your perspective of the workplace, so to fully understand PSAP work conditions, you need their perspectives too.
ii. Everyone's opinions matter a great deal. No sincere ideas or thoughts will be judged. All input, as long as it is respectful and fits the topic being discussed, will be welcomed and highly valued, since each person has expertise and perspective no one else has. The leader must not underestimate the "chilling effect" that can (and usually will) naturally impede frank and candid conversation when senior leadership is interacting with line staff. Effective leaders are tuned in to the chilling effect when it occurs; they employ empathy, and then work to guide the conversation appropriately.
iii. There will be no negative repercussions for honest concerns, and that notes recorded are strictly for pursuit of improvements. (Ask someone to serve as secretary for this purpose.) Then just guide the flow of questions and discussion that ensues.

e. The leader should also have an open discussion with the group about the results and expectations of their ideas and suggestions before any brainstorming starts. There will be occasions when the group will have ideas and suggestions that on the surface seem very reasonable, but the leader may have to advise them very early in the process that these cannot (or should not) be pursued at this time. And to compound this, the leader might not be able to tell the group why--other than there are factors and considerations (political, logistical, etc.) that the leader cannot share with the group at this time. The leader needs to explain to the group that if/when this occurs that it is not a criticism of their idea or an attempt to stymie creativity or input. In addition, there will be occasions when the leader will evaluate a proposal and come back with a position to the group of "not yet." But this does not mean "no." It means that the leader (who may or may not be able to divulge the reasons) has determined that for the proposal to be successful, the timing is not right to bring it to the other stakeholders. For example, the proposal may require allocation of unbudgeted funds and the organization is in the middle of the fiscal year. However the leader is already waiting on word from agency executives about monies that are anticipated to be available during the last quarter of the fiscal year; so shelving the proposal until the funds are available gives it a much greater chance for success than proposing it when there are no available funds and budgets are already tight.

f. Discuss your project follow-up plans: e.g., the team will meet regularly, will use the same evaluation and planning process practiced today, subgroups may be formed to implement tasks, channels of communication will be established to assure that all agency personnel are aware and can have input in this process.

g. Close meeting with open invitation for ongoing dialog outside of meetings, and sharing or discovered resources.

Important Project Considerations

The Relationship between the six work conditions

We have provided a set of evaluation and planning questions related to each of the six working conditions. These questions are designed to support a fundamental level of discussion of the risk related to each condition. Keep in mind, however, that several of these conditions may be at play at the same time in the workplace, either reducing or increasing stress risks for employees. So, your discussion may necessarily evolve to addressing more than one condition at a time. Here's an example:

Employees at your PSAP may feel excessive *demand* when a *change* occurs: launching a new CAD system. Both these conditions—demand and change--should be explored as part of the discussion of this CAD launch. Why? They can both potentially be managed to decrease stress so that the goal is achieved without exceeding employees' resources. Yet, in this example, a third condition will also be at play: the director's *support* of staff may be needed to hear employee concerns and modify the CAD roll-out plans. So, from the perspective of the Stress-Risk Manager (SRM, Chapter 21), this third condition (support) also needs to be discussed since the SRM's goal is always greater than just achieving technical success; it is also to protect and foster optimal employee resilience, morale and performance.

Chapter 19 Appendix

The Importance of Practicing Mutual Respect

Leaders willing to enter the evaluation and planning process proposed here are taking an emotional risk, because the Q&A process calls for transparent exploration of how they manage the six work conditions. They choose this vulnerable process because they recognize the importance of gaining their employees' perspectives, expertise, trust and collaboration to improve these work conditions and achieve legitimate success as a PSAP team. Yet, employees participating on the Resilience Optimization (or Morale) are also taking a serious risk: they may fear negative consequences of expressing concerns about bosses or peers in an open group in which both are present. Accordingly, leaders and employees must share responsibility for assuring mutually respectful conditions are upheld in all team discussions.

When either party has a concern related to a specific individual's actions, every effort should be made to communicate constructively, without conveying blame and judgement. Consider this approach, using the CAD launch as an example: an employee speaks up to the director who had sent out the email announcing the launch date:

"When you sent the email telling us our 'go-live' was next week, I was upset, because it didn't feel like we had enough time to prepare. I just want to figure out together how we can make the best of this"

In summary, your response defines:
- The *situation*
- How you *felt*, and *why*
- *An offer to help resolve it.*

After acknowledging the employee's concern, the director can reply with the same three elements.

"You feel like you needed more time. This did come about very quickly. I'm frustrated too, because I did tell everyone in June this was coming. But, let's talk this through and see what we can do…"

Leaders and employees on your team can grow in cohesion and become highly productive by practicing mutually respectful communication like this, and by using the question sets below to guide discussion.

Exploring the Six Conditions[1]: Questions to Guide Evaluation & Planning

Risk Factor 1: *Demand*
"Includes issues such as workload, work patterns and the work environment" (HSE 4).

- Make a list of the demands our employees face at our center.
- Which of these demands represent *stressors* (demands that singly or in combination outstrip employee resources of energy, time, and capability)?
- As you review your list, identify:
  o Which demands are stressing your employees the *most*?
  o What steps, if any, have been taken to lessen or modify these demands?
- Define: what new (and/or existing) steps should we follow to reduce them?

Risk Factor 2: *Control*
"How much say do the people have over the way they work?" (HSE 4).

What challenges and factors at our center impact our employees' sense of control? (Include an explanation of how you identified this.)
- How have we sought to increase their sense of control related to these challenges? (Examples: chances to participate in defining the problem, venting about it, defining ways to improve or manage it, such as defining policies related to acceptance/refusal of O.T., bidding for shifts)?
- How do our leaders (at each level) communicate with staff about our efforts to address these challenges?
- What difference do such efforts make in employees' morale and investment in the PSAP? (How did you identify these benefits: employee survey, informal feedback, staff meetings dedicated to inviting such feedback, etc.?)

- What additional or revised efforts by our leaders (at each level) do we need to make to communicate with staff about these challenges?

Risk Factor 3: *Support*
"Includes encouragement, sponsorship and resources provided by the organisation, line management and colleagues" (HSE 4).

- What kinds of support do we provide our people to help them endure, manage, or improve the demands they face? (Describe efforts you've made personally, and through your administrative and supervisory staff, including programs, events, and messages.)
- What difference do such efforts make in morale and your employees' investment in the PSAP?
- What additional initiatives do we need to pursue to increase this support?
- What Support do *you*, the center leader(s) and other members of your team need to help you deal with PSAP challenges?

Risk Factor 4: Managing *Relationships*
"Includes promoting positive working to avoid conflict and dealing with unacceptable behaviour." (HSE 4).

Certainly, the healthier and more supportive the relationships among your employees within and between all levels, the more resources they will have to face adversity. For example, this includes how willing they are to help each other fill the schedule and staff their shifts amidst staffing challenges.

- How do our center's major challenges contribute to relationship struggles in our PSAP?
- Conversely, how do relationship struggles in our center contribute to our major challenges?
- Specifically, how do you attempt to foster positive and truly supportive relationships between your administrative staff, supervisors, and frontliners?
- How could optimal relationships improve your management of the challenges?

- What steps do you need to take to improve relationships within the center? (Explore this between groups and levels of employees.)

Risk Factor 5: *Roles*
"Do people understand their role within the organisation, and does the organisation ensure roles are not conflicting" (HSE 4)?

The Health Safety Executive (HSE) model recognizes that the stress level and success of an organization depends a lot on the way leaders design, communicate about, and manage the *Roles* in which employees serve. So, consider the following questions:
- How clearly defined are the roles in which your employees serve? (Include all levels: managers, supervisors, frontline employees)
- How feasible are these roles (fit skills, ability, allotted time, etc.)?
- What role do your employees have in defining their roles?
- Who is responsible for overseeing performance of employees expected to fill these roles?
- What are the stress impacts of how these roles are managed?
- How have you needed to modify their roles to align expectations with resources and employee fit/abilities, etc.?

Risk Factor 6: *Change*
"How is organisational change (large and small) managed and communicated" (HSE 4)?

- What major changes have been implemented in your PSAP that were initiated by your leaders?
- Reflect on how one or more of these major changes was made: were employees invited to participate in plans to explore and decide on the change? How was the change (and required work to implement it) communicated to staff?
- How have those changes affected employee stress levels?
- What changes in your Change process do you need to implement to make it less stressful? For example: how should we involve our people as stakeholders in the change process to boost buy-in for implementation, help launching it and living well with the change?

- What difference do such efforts make in attitude and morale?

NOTE: As these Resilient Optimization Plans addressing each of the six conditions (risk factors) are implemented, the team should assure that an ongoing process also begins, to assure follow-up efforts are sustained through the year, and that *effectiveness is measured* and documented.

In addition to these six conditions, the Australian federal government identified two other work conditions (related to the six but deserving special attention). These are: low levels of recognition and reward, and organisational injustice. See *Tip Sheet Two: A risk management approach to work-related stress.* Catalogue No. WC01074 WorkCover Publications. Workplace Health & Safety QLD, Department of Justice and Attorney General worksafe.qld.gov.au. No. WC01074 WorkCover Publications. Workplace Health & Safety QLD, Department of Justice and Attorney General worksafc.qld.gov.au.

Work Cited

"Tackling work-related stress using the Management Standards approach: A step-by-step workbook." *Health Safety Executive,* 16 March 2017, www.hse.gov.uk/pubns/wbk01.htm

Made in the USA
Middletown, DE
09 December 2023